AF442667

Gastrointestinal Inflammation and Disturbed Gut Function: The Challenge of New Concepts

FALK SYMPOSIUM 130

Gastrointestinal Inflammation and Disturbed Gut Function: The Challenge of New Concepts

Edited by

G. Holtmann
Gastroenterologie/Hepatologie
Universitätsklinikum Essen
D-45147 Essen
Germany

N.J. Talley
The Nepean Hospital
University of Sydney
Penrith NS 2751
Australia

Proceedings of Falk Symposium 130 (Part I of the Gastroenterology Week Freiburg 2002) held in Freiburg, Germany, October 4–6, 2002

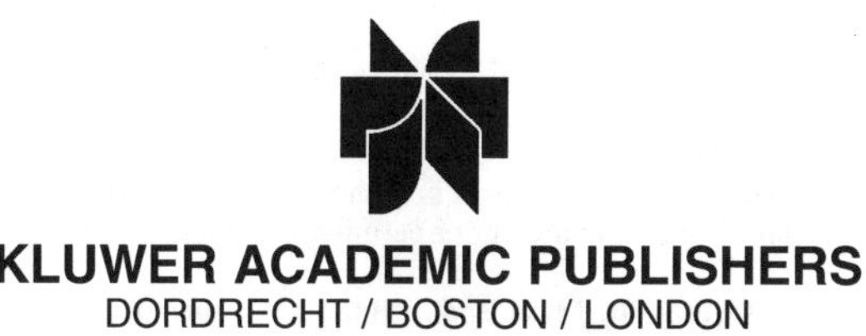

KLUWER ACADEMIC PUBLISHERS
DORDRECHT / BOSTON / LONDON

Library of Congress Cataloging-in-Publication Data is available.

ISBN 0–7923–8783–X

Published by Kluwer Academic Publishers, BV
P.O. Box 17, 3300 AA Dordrecht, The Netherlands.

Sold and distributed in North, Central and South America
by Kluwer Academic Publishers,
101 Philip Drive, Norwell, MA 02061, USA.

In all other countries, sold and distributed
by Kluwer Academic Publishers, Distribution Center,
P.O. Box 322, 3300 AH Dordrecht, The Netherlands.

Printed on acid-free paper

Printed and bound in Great Britain by MPG Books, Bodmin, Cornwall.

Contents

CONTENTS

CONTENTS

CONTENTS

Section VIII: ROLE OF ACUTE BACTERIAL INFECTIONS IN IRRITABLE BOWEL SYNDROME

Section IX: GENETICS AND MOLECULAR MECHANISMS

Section X: THE BRAIN, THE GUT AND THE GENES

List of principal contributors

B Adam
Universitätsklinikum Essen
Gastroenterologie/Hepatologie
Hufelandstr. 55
D-45122 Essen
Germany

K Bielefeldt
University of Iowa
Division of Gastroenterology
4614 JCP
200 Hawkins Drive
Iowa City, IA 52242
USA

J Bienenstock
Departments of Medicine, and
  Pathology and Molecular
  Medicine
McMaster University
Health Science Centre
1200 Main Street West
Hamilton, ON L8N 3Z5
Canada

LA Blackshaw
Nerve-Gut Research Laboratory
Hanson Institute
Frome Road
Adelaide, SA 5000
Australia

L Chang
CNS: Center for Neurovisceral
  Sciences and Women's Health
VAGLAHS, Bldg. 115/CURE
11301 Wilshire Blvd
Los Angeles, CA 90073
USA

SM Collins
McMaster University
Health Science Centre
Rm 4W8
1200 Main Street West
Hamilton, ON L8N 3Z5
Canada

SV Coutinho
Enterology Research Team
Johnson & Johnson Pharmaceutical
  Research and Development
Welsh and McKean Roads
Spring House, PA 19477-0776
USA

R Duchmann
Innere Medizin I
Universitätsklinikum Benjamin Franklin
der Freien Universität Berlin
Hindenburgdamm 30
D-12203 Berlin
Germany

GF Gebhart
College of Medicine
Department of Pharmacology
2-471 Bowen Science Building
Roy J. and Lucille A. Carver
  College of Medicine
University of Iowa
Iowa City, IA 52242-1109
USA

J Hammer
Universitätskliniken Wien
Klinik für Innere Medizin IV
Gastroenterologie/Hepatologie
Währinger Gürtel 18-20
A-1090 Wien
Austria

H Harder
Department of Medicine II
University Hospital of Mannheim
D-68167 Mannheim
Germany

A von Herbay
Pathologisches Institut
Universität Heidelberg
Im Neuenheimer Feld 220/221
D-69120 Heidelberg
Germany

G Holtmann
Abteilung für Gastroenterologie und
    Hepatologie
Universitätsklinikum Essen
Hufelandstr. 55
D-45147 Essen
Germany

P Holzer
Department of Experimental and
    Clinical Pharmacology
University of Graz
Universitätsplatz 4
A-8010 Graz
Austria

W Jänig
Physiologisches Institut
Christian-Albrechts-Universität zu Kiel
Olshausenstr. 40
D-24098 Kiel
Germany

J Kruse
Abteilung für Psychosomatische
    Medizin
Universitätsklinikum Düsseldorf
Bergische Landstr. 2
D-40629 Düsseldorf
Germany

GR Locke
Division of Gastroenterology
Mayo Clinic
200 First Street SW
Rochester, MN 55905
USA

A Madisch
Medical Department I
Univ.-Klinikum C. Gustav Carus der
    Technischen Univ. Dresden
Fetscherstr. 74
D-01307 Dresden
Germany

EA Mayer
Center for Neurovisceral Sciences
    and Women's Health
Departments of Medicine, Physiology,
    Psychiatry and Biobehavioral
    Sciences
Geffen School of Medicine at UCLA
Los Angeles, CA 90073
USA

S Müller-Lissner
Abteilung Innere Medizin
Park-Klinik Weißensee
Schönstr. 80
D-13086 Berlin
Germany

CA O'Morain
Head of Internal Medicine Department
Trinity College Dublin, Adelaide and
    Meath, incorporating National
    Children's Hospital
Tallaght
Dublin 24
Ireland

MA Pezzone
Department of Medicine
Division of Gastroenterology,
    Hepatology and Nutrition
University of Pittsburgh Medical Center
200 Lothrop Street
Pittsburgh, PA 15213
USA

EMM Quigley
Cork University Hospital
Department of Medicine
Clinical Sciences Building
Wilton Road
Cork
Ireland

W Siffert
Institut für Pharmakologie
Universitätsklinikum Essen
Hufelandstr. 55
D-45147 Essen
Germany

RC Spiller
University Hospital
Queen's Medical Centre
Division of Gastroenterology
C Floor, South Block
Nottingham
NG7 2UH
UK

V Stanghellini
Università di Bologna
Policlinico S. Orsola
Department of Internal Medicine and
  Gastroenterology
Via Massarenti 9
I-40138 Bologna
Italy

J Tack
Department of Internal Medicine
Division of Gastroenterology
University Hospital Gasthuisberg
Herestraat 49
B-3000 Leuven
Belgium

NJ Talley
The Nepean Hospital
University of Sydney
Clinical Science Building
PO Box 163
Penrith, NS 2751
Australia

NB Vakil
University of Wisconsin Medical
  School
Aurora Sinai Samaritan Medical
  Center
945 North 12th Street, Rm 4040
Milwaukee, WI 53233-1305
USA

T Wedel
Institut für Anatomie
Universität Lübeck
Ratzeburger Allee 160
D-23538 Lübeck
Germany

PJ Whorwell
Education and Research Centre
Wythenshawe Hospital
Manchester M23 9LT
UK

Preface

In gastrointestinal (GI) practice, a large proportion of patients presents with what are currently classified as functional GI complaints. For decades, psychological causes have been implicated in the initiation and maintenance of symptoms. In recent years, disturbances of GI function including sensory motor abnormalities have been catalogued and are now believed to play a key role in the development of symptoms. While there is now mounting knowledge regarding the epidemiology and pathophysiology of these disorders, there is also sufficient evidence to assume a genetic predisposition that may play a crucial role for the manifestation of these disorders. Furthermore, evidence has accumulated that GI inflammation can trigger and maintain functional disturbances. In particular, acute GI infections appear to play a crucial role in at least a subgroup of patients. These observations and new insights into molecular mechanisms appear to have profound implications for the field, and suggest the functional GI disorders are indeed organic diseases. Based upon the current insights we have to acknowledge an "organification" of the so-called functional GI disorders. In the long term, these new disease concepts will completely change our approach to these patients and may ultimately result in better targetted treatments that hold the promise of cure or at least better control of symptoms.

This book summarizes lectures that were given at the Falk Symposium "Gastrointestinal Inflammation and Disturbed Gut Function: The Challenge of New Concepts" which took place in Freiburg/Breisgau in October 2002. The organizers were glad that some of the world's most recognized researchers from a number of fields could be attracted to contribute to the program. Thus the organizers are grateful to all contributors. Most noteably, this scientific endeavour was made possible by the generous support of Dr. H. Falk and the Falk Foundation. We would like to express our deep appreciation for this financial and logistic support, without which we would not have been able to accomplish this work.

Gerald Holtmann
Nicholas Talley

Section I
Setting the scene: epidemiology

1
Epidemiology of functional bowel disease and inflammatory bowel disease: a common link?

G. R. LOCKE

Historically, functional bowel disease (FBD) and inflammatory bowel disease (IBD) have been considered separate entities. In fact, a diagnosis of FBD has been predicated on the absence of IBD. Recent advances in the understanding of FBD has raised the question as to whether inflammation plays a role in the development of FBD and thus whether these two disease groups should be considered related. Can we break from tradition and find a common link? At present the epidemiology literature has not examined the potential link between FBD and IBD. Many epidemiology studies use one group as a control for the other. The number of differences is significant. Nonetheless, it is reasonable for epidemiological studies of the future to examine the possibility of a connection between these two. The observations from the bench are intriguing. We need to learn whether these observations can be validated in the community.

FUNCTIONAL GASTROINTESTINAL DISORDERS

The functional gastrointestinal disorders have been defined as variable combinations of chronic or recurrent gastrointestinal symptoms not explained by structural or biochemical abnormalities[1]. Through the Rome consensus process, 19 separate functional gastrointestinal disorders have been identified, of which perhaps the most common or the most well known is irritable bowel syndrome. The goal of this approach was to create specific symptom criteria that could then be used to identify patients for research studies. This has proven useful in creating homogeneous populations for clinical trials.

Although this approach has been useful in research, it may not be as useful in clinical practice. In a motility practice one will see patients with classic motility disorders such as achalasia and intestinal pseudo-obstruction and Hirschsprung's disease. However, these disorders are very unusual. Most of the time spent in the motility practice is in seeing patients with gastrointestinal (GI) symptoms for whom standard GI tests such as endoscopy and laboratory studies have been

3

unremarkable. The question that is raised is to what degree there is a motility problem versus a functional disorder. Sometimes it is hard to draw the line. People with functional dyspepsia often have delayed gastric emptying. How does one distinguish that group from patients with gastroparesis? Transit studies can be slightly abnormal in patients with symptoms of irritable bowel syndrome. They may have exaggerated gastrocolic reflexes and high-amplitude contractions of the colon. They may have subtle changes on gastroduodenal manometry. Should these people be considered to have subtle intestinal motility disorders or should they still be considered under the umbrella of irritable bowel syndrome? This issue becomes important because the way physicians view patients with motility disorders is slightly different from the way we view those with functional disorders.

In addition, there is considerable overlap among the functional disorders. Patients will present with symptoms consistent with multiple functional disorders so, for example, 45% of patients with symptoms of irritable bowel syndrome will report symptoms of dyspepsia. Forty-two per cent of patients with irritable bowel syndrome will have symptoms of reflux. Looking at it the other way, 55% of patients with dyspepsia will also have heartburn and 38% of these patients will have symptoms of irritable bowel syndrome. Even though these disorders are common, this overlap is greater than would be expected by chance[2].

In addition, when followed over time, patients will have symptoms of one functional GI disorder at one point in time only to have symptoms of another disorder in the future. This is nicely described in the study of Agreus et al.[3]; they did surveys 1 year apart and found that only 50% of the people with symptoms of irritable bowel syndrome on their first survey continued to have such symptoms on the second survey. Among this group, 22% had dyspepsia, 18% had unspecified symptoms, and only 5% of the group were asymptomatic. This was true for the other functional GI disorders studied.

This leads one to wonder whether the functional GI disorders are one disease or many. They are all technically diagnoses of exclusion. There is significant overlap among symptoms and transition between symptoms over time. The pathophysiology of these conditions is thought similar. There are motor abnormalities, visceral hypersensitivity, and psychological and environmental issues that come into play. Finally, there is significant treatment overlap. Low-dose tricyclic antidepressants are used for multiple functional disorders.

Thus, the question arises whether using symptoms is the best way to categorize these patients. Certainly, more physiological approaches might be more accurate. There may well be subgroups of functional disorders that overlap with other disorders that may share a common pathophysiology. Thus, it seems appropriate to keep an open mind as to how one might view the functional GI disorders. There may come a time when we have very specific tests that describe very specific conditions that will in turn respond to specific therapies. Clinically, this would be ideal for the future.

INFLAMMATION IN FUNCTIONAL DISORDERS: A NEW PARADIGM

Given that there certainly is opportunity for novel thinking regarding functional GI disorders, it is certainly reasonable to consider the role of inflammation.

Patients have been well described who develop functional GI disorders after enteric infections[4]. We will also see patients with inflammatory bowel disease who have symptoms despite minimal disease activity. These symptoms may be very similar to those of irritable bowel syndrome. We will see patients with reflux who will continue to have symptoms of chest pain despite resolution of the reflux oesophagitis. We will see patients with dyspepsia who will have gastric inflammation, and the question has been raised as to whether or not that gastric inflammation gives rise to their symptoms. The goal of this chapter is to look at the relationship between functional GI disorders and inflammatory bowel disease. The issue is whether inflammation plays a role in each of these disease conditions and whether there is some commonality in their pathogenesis. The questions to be addressed are: (1) whether functional bowel disease leads to inflammatory bowel disease or (2) whether inflammatory bowel disease leads to functional bowel disease, and (3) whether there is a common pathophysiological basis for these conditions. The emphasis of this chapter is on epidemiology; thus I will turn to the epidemiology of functional GI disorders (FGID) with special emphasis on irritable bowel syndrome and the epidemiology of inflammatory bowel disease (IBD) (Crohn's disease and ulcerative colitis) to discover if there is an indication of a common pathophysiological basis.

EPIDEMIOLOGY OF FGID AND IBD

The FGIDs are certainly very common. Since patients with these problems do not always seek care, clinic-based data capture only a portion of the disease burden. A number of investigators have done surveys of random samples of the population to ascertain how common these GI symptoms are in unselected members of the community[5]. Symptoms of irritable bowel syndrome have been reported by 10% of the general population. Many other GI symptoms are also common, with dyspepsia affecting perhaps 25%, heartburn perhaps 20%, and constipation and diarrhoea 15% apiece. Thus, functional GI symptoms are quite common. On the other hand, IBD is somewhat unusual. The prevalence of IBD is 229 per 100 000 for ulcerative colitis and 144 per 100 000 for Crohn's disease[6]. It is important to note the denominator. For the FGIDs we are speaking of percentages of the population or numbers per 100, whereas for IBD we are talking about numbers per 100 000; thus there is a 50–100-fold difference in the prevalence of these conditions. This does not support commonality. One may say perhaps we should look at a subgroup of patients with irritable bowel syndrome (IBS). It is important to note that even diarrhoea-predominant IBS is common; in one study it was estimated to be 5.5% of the population[7]. The prevalence of IBS is higher in younger people and decreases slightly over time. Studies have varied in the degree of gender difference; in some studies this is closer to 1 : 1. However, most studies of the community suggest that IBS is twice as common in women as it is in men.

There is similarity with the incidence curve for IBD. Both Crohn's disease and ulcerative colitis tend to have a higher incidence in people in their 20s, and this gradually decreases with age. The gender distribution for each is fairly close to 1 : 1. Data regarding the incidence of IBS are more difficult to determine.

Symptoms of IBS come and go over time, as mentioned earlier. When surveys have been done 1 year apart, 10% of the population will report new symptoms of IBS[8]; however, we cannot really be certain that these symptoms are new; it may be that they just were inactive at the time of the first survey. Thus, the term 'onset' rather than 'incidence' is typically used. There have been studies that try to identify incidence rates. It is important to note that these studies rely on physician diagnoses and thus rely on health-care seeking. Only half the general population with symptoms of IBS will report having seen a physician; thus the incident figures for IBS are an under-representation of the true incidence of the condition. Nonetheless, the figures in the literature are fairly consistent. In one study the figure was 196 per 100 000[9] and in another study 260 per 100 000[10]. Again, it is important to note the order of magnitude difference between IBD and IBS. In IBD the incident rates are 8 or 9 per 100 000 as compared to 200 per 100 000; again a 20-fold increase in number[6].

In summary, if one looks at simple incidence and prevalence, these disorders both affect young people and share the organ system of involvement. However, there is a dramatic difference in numbers, which makes it harder to see the common link.

RISK FACTORS

A number of risk factors have been proposed for IBS. It probably represents a mix of problems, of which perhaps one or several may be present in order to give rise to the condition. Much of the attention in IBS has been focused towards psychiatric diagnoses and psychological distress. It is important to recognize that this is confounded by health-care seeking. Community-based studies have found psychological profiles of IBS sufferers to be similar to those without IBS; however, when patients are seen in health-care systems, especially in academic medical centres, the rates of psychiatric diagnoses and psychological distress in IBS are greatly increased. Still, there is some difference at the level of the population; population-based surveys have shown that histories of physical and sexual abuse are more common in people with IBS in the community as opposed to controls[8,11].

In terms of other risk factors attention is certainly being paid to the role of genetics in IBS. IBS has been found to aggregate in families[2]. There is just slightly double the risk of having IBS if you report having family members with the condition. Twin studies have been done, and they report a higher concordance in monozygotic than dizygotic twins, suggesting a genetic component[12]; however, other studies have shown a role of early adult learning[13]. Children of people with IBS are brought to health care more often for GI symptoms. A hypothesis is that we are taught to be an IBS sufferer. Thus, there remains quite a bit to be learned about nature versus nurture in IBS.

The other major risk factor under consideration for IBS is inflammation and infection. This has been well described even in the early work of Chaudhary and Truelove[14], showing that people will have developed IBS after enteric infections. This rate is roughly 30%. Some have argued that recall bias raises questions regarding the validity of these figures; however, prospective studies have confirmed this.

One specific study deserves mention: Gwee *et al.*, in 1996[4], reported results of a prospective study. Seventy-five patients with acute gastroenteritis admitted to the hospital were identified. Patients with a prior history of IBS symptoms were excluded. The investigators then followed up these patients over time and found that 30% had IBS symptoms at 6 months. They then looked at risk factors for the development of IBS. Women and those with longer duration of illness were more likely to have subsequent IBS. In addition, people with higher levels of anxiety, depression, neuroticism, and somatization at the time of their acute infection were more likely to develop IBS in the future. This demonstrates the interplay between psychological distress and environmental challenges such as infection in producing the condition. Certainly, other chapters in this book will cover the physiological basis of this post-infectious IBS.

If we now look at risk factors for IBD, they have some similarities but also some important differences from IBS. Significant attention has been paid to geographical and ethnic issues in IBD that are not seen in IBS. IBD is much more common in developed countries. Countries which become more developed have increasing rates of IBD. There is perhaps a north–south gradient where, at least in the northern hemisphere, more northerly countries or more northerly aspects of individual countries will have higher rates of IBD than the southern areas. There are significant ethnic differences, with the prevalence of Caucasians being higher than other ethnic groups, at least in the United States[15]. There is also a strong association with Jewish ancestry that has been well described.

IBD also seems to have a genetic component. Patients with IBD will frequently report having relatives with IBD; the reporting ranges from 5% to 17%. Of note, this is much higher than the prevalence of the condition at large. A number of studies have studied familial IBD[16]; certainly these disorders aggregate in families. Studies suggested that specific types of Crohn's disease aggregate in families[17]. Twin studies suggest a genetic component with higher rates in monozygotic twins[18]. Recently, a specific gene has been identified which seems to be associated with specific types of Crohn's disease[19,20].

There may well, however, be environmental influences: married couples have been reported to have developed Crohn's disease, suggesting a common infectious agent. Certainly, many have argued that there could be some role of infection in IBD. Diversion seems to make the bowel disease better; however, despite all the attention paid to infections in IBD, no specific infection has been identified.

IBS AND IBD: IS THERE A LINK?

Having reviewed the epidemiology of IBS and IBD, we see some similarities in terms of types of people affected and types of risk factors under consideration. However, this really does not tell us that there is any link. Thus, we must ask if IBS leads to IBD. Certainly, the symptoms of IBS and IBD are similar, with urgency and diarrhoea. When a patient who has had a prior diagnosis of IBS develops IBD, many have argued that the original IBS diagnosis was probably a misdiagnosis. Thus, prospective follow-up is critical.

One recent study deserves mention. Garcia Rodriguez *et al.*, in 2000, reported the results of a population-based cohort study using an administrative database in England and Wales[10]. They identified general practitioner diagnoses of IBS in 2956 patients; they also identified 9900 with functional dyspepsia and selected 20 000 controls at random. They then followed this group for a subsequent diagnosis of IBD. One would certainly expect to have a high rate of diagnosis in the first year if this is an issue of misdiagnosis. The authors also looked at colorectal cancer and found that to be the case. There was an increase in colorectal cancer the first year, which stabilized in the future. However, the curve for IBD was different. Patients with IBS continued to have higher rates of developing IBD than the patients with functional dyspepsia and the controls. This suggests either a very long lag period of their IBD, or that patients with IBS are more likely to develop IBD. The numbers in this study are in keeping with other studies. The incidence of IBS from which they selected their patients was 260 per 100 000. The incidence of IBD in their control group was 13 per 100 000, which is keeping with other reported rates. The incidence of IBD among the IBS sufferers was 178 per 100 000; thus the relative risk of contracting IBD after IBS was 16.3 (95% CI 6.6–40.7). The risk was more marked in Crohn's disease than in ulcerative colitis, but there was insufficient statistical power in the study to do subgroup analyses. Overall, this is the one study that is highly suggestive of an overlap between IBS and IBD.

The alternative question is to ask if IBD leads to IBS; certainly it can only lead to a portion of IBS given that IBS is so much more common than IBD. Yet the discussion under consideration is the role of inflammation in provoking IBS; thus IBD as an inflammatory condition could well give rise to IBS in the future.

Finally, we can ask if there is a common pathophysiological basis between IBS and IBD. Unfortunately the past literature has tended to use one group as the control for the other. Rates in IBS are compared to rates in IBD, and multiple differences have been identified. Studies really have not focused on the similarities between these two conditions and compared the two relative to some third independent control group. We have seen that they affect young people; we have seen that there are infectious and genetic issues involved in both, but overall the epidemiological literature really has not focused on this topic in order to provide us with further information. A reasonable working hypotheses would be that patients have specific genetic make-up and are often exposed to enteric infections; in some the response is recovery, in some it is IBS and in a few it is IBD. This idea has some validity and appears reasonable to pursue.

SUMMARY

This chapter has looked at the way we think about functional gastrointestinal disorders. The possibility was entertained that these disorders could have a component of inflammation, at least in a subset. The chapter looked at the interaction between IBS and IBD to see if there is a common link. At present I believe this hypothesis is certainly intriguing, but there certainly is not much data to provide support. Our hope is that future studies can address this question more directly and provide us with the answer to the question of functional bowel disease and IBD: is there a common link?

Acknowledgement

The author thanks Karen Kruger and Susan Leachman for their assistance in the preparation of this chapter.

References

1. Drossman DA, Li Z, Andruzzi E *et al.* U.S. householder survey of functional gastrointestinal disorders. Prevalence, sociodemography, and health impact. Dig Dis Sci. 1993;38:1569–80.
2. Locke GR, Zinsmeister AR, Talley N, Fett SL, Melton LJ 3rd. Familial association in adults with functional gastrointestinal disorders. Mayo Clin Proc. 2000;75:907–12.
3. Agreus L, Svardsudd K, Nyren O, Tibblin G. Irritable bowel syndrome and dyspepsia in the general population: overlap and lack of stability over time. Gastroenterology. 1995;109:671–80.
4. Gwee KA, Graham JC, McKendrick MW *et al.* Psychometric scores and persistence of irritable bowel after infectious diarrhoea [comment]. Lancet. 1996;347:150–3.
5. Locke GR. The epidemiology of functional gastrointestinal disorders in North America. Gastroenterol Clin N Am. 1996;25:1–19.
6. Loftus EJ, Sandborn WJ. Epidemiology of inflammatory bowel disease. Gastroenterol Clin N Am. 2002;31:1–20.
7. Talley N, Zinsmeister AR, Melton LJ 3rd. Irritable bowel syndrome in a community: symptom subgroups, risk factors and health care utilization. Am J Epidemiol. 1995;142:76.
8. Talley NJ, Weaver AL, Zinsmeister AR, Melton LJ 3rd. Onset and disappearance of gastrointestinal symptoms and functional gastrointestinal disorders. Am J Epidemiol. 1992;136:165–77.
9. Locke GR, Yawn BP, Wollan PC, Lydick E. The incidence of clinically diagnosed irritable bowel syndrome in the community. Gastroenterology. 1999;116:A76.
10. Rodriguez LG, Ruigomez A, Wallander M-A, Johansson S, Olbe L. Detection of colorectal tumor and inflammatory bowel disease during follow-up of patients with initial diagnosis of irritable bowel syndrome. Scand J Gastroenterol. 2000;35:306–11.
11. Talley NJ, Fett SL, Zinsmeister AR, Melton LJ 3rd. Gastrointestinal tract symptoms and self-reported abuse: a population-based study. Gastroenterology. 1994;107:1040–9.
12. Morris-Yates A, Talley NJ, Boyce P, Nandurkar S, Andrews G. Evidence of a genetic contribution to functional bowel disorder. Am J Gastroenterol. 1998;93:1311–17.
13. Levy R, Whitehead WE, Von Korff M, Feld A. Intergenerational transmission of gastrointestinal illness behavior. Am J Gastroenterol. 2000;95:451–6.
14. Chaudhary N, Truelove S. The irritable colon syndrome. A study of the clinical features, predisposing causes, and prognosis in 130 cases. Q J Med. 1962;31:307–22.
15. Kurata J, Kantor-Fish S, Frankl H, Godby P, Vadheim C. Crohn's disease among ethnic groups in a large health maintenance organization. Gastroenterology. 1992;102:1940–8.
16. Kirsner J, Spencer J. Familial occurrences of ulcerative colitis, regional enteritis and ileocolitis. Ann Intern Med. 1963;59:133–44.
17. Colombel J-F, Grandbastien B, Gower-Rousseau C *et al.* Clinical characteristics of Crohn's disease in 72 families. Gastroenterology. 1996;111:604–7.
18. Tysk C, Lindberg E, Jarnerot G, Floderus-Myrhead B. Ulcerative colitis and Crohn's disease in an unselected population of monozygotic and dizygotic twins: a study of heritability and the influence of smoking. Gut. 1988;29:990–6.
19. Ogura Y, Bonen D, Inohara N *et al.* A frameshift mutation in NOD2 associated with susceptibility to Crohn's disease [comment]. Nature. 2001:411:603–6.
20. Hugot J-P, Chamaillard M, Zouali H *et al.* Association of NOD2 leucine-rich repeat variants with susceptibility to Crohn's disease. Nature. 2001;411:599–603.

2
Extraintestinal manifestations and psychiatric illness in irritable bowel syndrome: is there a link?

L. CHANG

INTRODUCTION

While irritable bowel syndrome (IBS) is characterized by chronic or recurrent abdominal pain or discomfort and altered bowel habits, many IBS patients also report extraintestinal symptoms such as fatigue, muscle pain, sleep disturbances, and sexual dysfunction. The underlying mechanisms of gastrointestinal and extraintestinal manifestations of IBS are not completely understood. The greater reporting of extraintestinal symptoms has been thought to be due to psychiatric illness. While some of these extraintestinal symptoms are often seen in patients with psychiatric disorders, such as fatigue, weight loss and sleep disturbances, some are less often associated with these disorders, such as urinary frequency and urgency, and musculoskeletal pain. This chapter will examine the prevalence of extraintestinal and psychological symptoms in IBS, the co-morbid conditions which overlap with IBS, the evidence supporting and disputing a causative mechanism of psychiatric illness on extraintestinal symptoms in IBS, and a conceptual model based on stress-related central dysregulation resulting in behavioural and physiological alterations which may be responsible for the clinical symptoms seen in IBS.

PREVALENCE OF EXTRAINTESTINAL MANIFESTATIONS IN IBS

In a population of secondary-care IBS patients, up to two-thirds reported extraintestinal symptoms compared to less than 15% of healthy controls[1]. These symptoms ranged from non-specific symptoms such as headaches, back pain, and tiredness to organ-specific symptoms such as urinary frequency and urgency (Table 1). Sleep[2] and sexual disturbances[3] have also been reported by a greater number of patients with functional bowel disorders, including IBS, compared to healthy individuals. Furthermore, studies show that extraintestinal symptoms are

Table 1 Common extraintestinal symptoms reported in IBS

Fatigue
Musculoskeletal pain
Headaches
Sleep disturbances
Sexual dysfunction
Urinary symptoms

more common in IBS patients compared to patients with organic gastrointestinal diseases. When compared to 295 other gastrointestinal outpatients with organic diseases, e.g. inflammatory bowel disease, peptic ulcer disease, gallstones, and reflux oesophagitis, 107 IBS patients had a greater prevalence for extraintestinal symptoms, e.g. lethargy, headaches, back pain and urinary frequency[4]. Furthermore, the presence of these symptoms in conjunction with gastrointestinal symptoms suggestive of IBS increased the relative risk of the patient having the diagnosis of IBS compared to the organic gastrointestinal conditions. One study found that sexual dysfunction was higher in women with IBS compared to women with inflammatory bowel disease and duodenal ulceration[5]. In these studies the higher prevalence of extraintestinal symptoms in patients with functional bowel disorders could not be accounted for by the presence of psychological symptoms. Additional studies have demonstrated that the presence of extraintestinal symptoms has a significant health impact. Extraintestinal symptoms are frequently reported as the worst symptom by IBS patients[6]. Furthermore, IBS patients have a greater number of physician visits for non-gastrointestinal symptoms than do healthy individuals[7].

ROLE OF GENDER AND BOWEL HABIT IN THE PRESENCE OF EXTRAINTESTINAL SYMPTOMS

While gender[8] and bowel habit predominance[9,10] appear to have an impact on the differences in clinical symptoms and physiological responses in IBS, these factors also appear to affect the presence of extraintestinal symptoms. Lee *et al.* surveyed 714 male and female patients with IBS regarding symptoms and bowel patterns[11], and found that women were more likely to report extracolonic viscero- and somatosensory symptoms (urinary urgency, alterations in taste, muscle stiffness, aching) compared to men. After controlling for gender differences in the general population the authors also found that the only health-related quality-of-life domain which was worse in women with IBS than men with IBS was bodily pain. There were no differences in the report of abdominal pain severity between men and women with IBS.

Bowel habit has also been shown to have an effect on the presence of extraintestinal symptoms. Schmulson *et al.* reported that, in a mixed sample of 140 constipation-predominant IBS patients and 216 diarrhoea-predominant IBS patients, the constipation-predominant IBS patients complained more of musculoskeletal symptoms, sleep impairment, decreased appetite, and sexual dysfunction than patients with diarrhoea-predominant IBS[9]. Psychological symptom scores did not differ between the two groups.

OVERLAP OF IBS AND CO-MORBID SYNDROMES

IBS patients are twice as likely as comparison groups to be diagnosed with a non-gastrointestinal chronic pain disorder[12]. Co-morbid conditions which are commonly diagnosed in IBS patients include fibromyalgia (FM), chronic fatigue syndrome, interstitial cystitis, sicca syndrome and chronic pelvic pain (Table 2). An excellent review of these overlapping conditions with IBS has recently been published and should be referred to for details[12].

One of the more well-studied co-morbid conditions seen in IBS patients is FM. IBS and FM are both syndromes characterized by chronic visceral and chronic somatic pain and discomfort, respectively. Patients affected by both disorders are commonly seen in tertiary referral centres and frequently pose a considerable therapeutic challenge. Epidemiological studies have confirmed the clinical impression that these two functional disorders frequently overlap in the same patient, suggesting shared pathophysiological mechanisms[12]. A study of 80 patients demonstrated that 70% of FM patients also had symptoms of IBS, and 65% of IBS patients suffered from FM symptoms[13]. Using the diagnostic criteria for both FM[14] and IBS[15], Sperber *et al.* found that 31.6% of IBS patients met criteria for FM and 32% of FM patients met criteria for IBS[16]. While unequivocal demonstration of peripheral tissue changes underlying the pain is lacking in both syndromes, somatic hypersensitivity is considered the hallmark physical finding of FM[14,17–22], while visceral hypersensitivity is a characteristic finding of IBS[23–26]. These two syndromes have many similar clinical characteristics[27]: (1) female predominance, (2) majority of patients associate stressful life events with initiation or exacerbation of symptoms, (3) increased prevalence of sexual abuse, (4) majority of patients complain of disturbed sleep and fatigue, (5) psychotherapy and behavioural therapies are efficacious in treating symptoms, and (6) low-dose tricyclic antidepressants can improve symptoms. These similarities suggest that these two syndromes may share a common centrally regulated aetiology. Recent brain-imaging studies have shown a greater activation of a subregion of the anterior cingulate cortex in response to a noxious somatic stimulus in FM patients[28,29] and to a colorectal distension stimulus in IBS patients[29,30]. This subregion of the anterior cingulate cortex is thought to

Table 2 Co-morbid conditions which commonly overlap with IBS

• Fibromyalgia
Chronic fatigue syndrome
Interstitial cystitis
Sicca syndrome
Post-traumatic stress disorder (PTSD)
Headaches
Temporomandibular joint disorder
Chronic pelvic pain

---

have cognitive functions such as attentional demand and response selection. The enhanced activation of this region in both IBS and FM patients to visceral and somatic stimuli, respectively, suggests an alteration of normal attentional attribution to specific afferent information from different body regions[29].

PREVALENCE OF PSYCHOLOGICAL SYMPTOMS AND ADVERSE LIFE EVENTS

IBS patients also have a high prevalence of psychological symptoms such as anxiety and depression, particularly in those with severe symptoms and health-care-seeking behaviour[31,32]. In tertiary care centres, the prevalence of psychiatric disorders in IBS patients ranges from 40% to 90%[33,34]. Somatization, anxiety and depressive disorders are also more commonly seen in IBS patients than in healthy controls. Psychosocial factors have been recognized to modify the illness experience and influence health-care utilization and treatment outcome. Factors that adversely affect health status and clinical outcome include a history of emotional, sexual or physical abuse; stressful life events; chronic social stress; anxiety disorders or maladaptive coping styles. Psychosocial trauma and early adverse life events (e.g. parental separation or physical/verbal/sexual abuse history) may profoundly affect symptom severity, daily function, and health outcome[35,36]. Although these adverse events, such as abuse, may be quite prevalent in IBS patients, a significant number have not discussed this with anyone and a smaller number will actually inform their physicians[37]. While psychological symptoms and adverse life events, as well as extraintestinal symptoms, are commonly seen in IBS patients, there is no convincing evidence to suggest that extraintestinal symptoms are commonly reported due to the presence of co-morbid psychological or psychiatric conditions. It is conceivable that the mechanisms underlying the presence of extraintestinal symptoms are similar to those underlying the presence of psychological and psychiatric symptoms.

STRESS-RELATED BIOLOGICAL MECHANISMS UNDERLYING EXTRAINTESTINAL AND PSYCHOLOGICAL SYMPTOMS

Stress is widely believed to play a major role in the pathophysiology and clinical presentation of IBS[38]. It has been postulated that, in the predisposed individual, sustained stress can result in permanent increased stress responsiveness of central stress circuits and vulnerability to develop functional and affective disorders. Stress may be central (e.g. psychological distress) or peripheral (e.g. infection, surgery) in origin. Numerous studies indicate that IBS patients report more lifetime and daily stressful events, including abuse, compared to medical comparison groups or healthy controls[37,39,40]. In IBS patients, stress is strongly associated with symptom onset, exacerbation and severity. Even though the effects of stress on gut function are universal, patients with IBS appear to have greater reactivity to stress compared to healthy individuals.

A current conceptual model of the role of psychosocial factors in IBS suggests that early adverse life experiences influence later physiological functioning, stress responsiveness and susceptibility to developing a functional disorder[38]. A stressor may produce symptoms through changes in gastrointestinal function, central amplification of normal gut signals or a combination of both. The combined effect of altered physiology and psychosocial status via interactions between the central nervous system and periphery will modulate symptom experience, illness behaviours and ultimately clinical outcome.

As individuals are challenged by stressors, alterations in neuroendocrine responses result in increased arousal state which in normal physiological circumstances result in increased performance in an attempt to adapt and to re-establish homeostasis. The inability or failure of this homeostatic mechanism in effectively dealing with the stressful challenge results in failure of the individual to cope, and has been referred to as vital exhaustion. Vital exhaustion is referred to as the mental state at which individuals arrive when their resources for adapting to chronic stress are broken down[41]; it clinically manifests as undue fatigue, irritability, and feelings of demoralization[42]. As the individual moves from a stressful challenge to control and then to actual loss of control, the pattern of effective hormonal and behavioural responses changes[43]. These changes in maintaining control over the environment have been associated with changes in arousal and in the sympathetic nervous system and hypothalamic–pituitary adrenal axis, which are the two main components of the central stress response system[44]. Alterations in the central stress response have also been demonstrated in IBS and other functional syndromes such as FM, chronic fatigue syndrome, and post-traumatic stress disorder[45]. The psychophysiological state associated with non-adaptive responses to sustained stress may explain, at least in part, the significant gastrointestinal, extraintestinal, psychological and health-related quality-of-life impairment experienced by IBS patients. Further characterization of the biological mechanisms responsible for the observed alterations in the stress response systems is needed to fully understand chronic stress-related disorders such as IBS and the other functional pain syndromes that typically overlap with IBS.

SUMMARY

Extraintestinal symptoms and psychological symptoms are highly prevalent in IBS patients. The presence of extraintestinal symptoms may be due to co-morbidity of other chronic functional disorders, such as fibromyalgia, chronic fatigue syndrome, pelvic pain or interstitial cystitis. Similar clinical characteristics between IBS and these other syndromes have raised the possibility of a common underlying mechanism. While it is possible that the presence of extraintestinal symptoms such as fatigue, loss of appetite, sleep and sexual disturbances are symptoms of co-morbid psychiatric illness, studies evaluating the prevalence of extraintestinal symptoms have not found an association of these symptoms with the presence of psychiatric illness. A more likely mechanism may be a conceptual model characterized by stress-related, centrally regulated alterations in behavioural and physiological responses due to the inability or failure of homeostatic mechanisms to effectively deal with the stressful challenge resulting in symptoms of vital exhaustion and psychological distress. While some of the clinical symptoms may be related to breakdown in central response systems (anxiety, depression, pain), some may also be related to peripheral alterations (pelvic pain, bowel habit alterations, and urinary symptoms).

References

1. Whorwell PJ, McCallum M, Creed FH, Roberts CT. Non-colonic features of irritable bowel syndrome. Gut. 1986;27:37–40.
2. Fass R, Fullerton S, Tung S, Mayer EA. Sleep disturbances in clinic patients with functional bowel disorders. Am J Gastroenterol. 2000;95:1195–2000.
3. Fass R, Fullerton S, Naliboff B, Hirsh T, Mayer EA. Sexual dysfunction in patients with irritable bowel syndrome and non-ulcer dyspepsia. Digestion. 1998;59:79–85.
4. Maxton DG, Morris J, Whorwell PJ. More accurate diagnosis of irritable bowel syndrome by the use of 'non-colonic' symptomatology. Gut. 1991;32:784–6.
5. Guthrie E, Creed FH, Whorwell PJ. Severe sexual dysfunction in women with the irritable bowel syndrome: comparison with inflammatory bowel disease and duodenal ulceration. Br Med J. (Clinical Research Edition) 1987;295:577–8.
6. Maxton DG, Morris JA, Whorwell PJ. Ranking of symptoms by patients with the irritable bowel syndrome. Br Med J. 1989;299:1138.
7. Drossman DA, Li Z, Andruzzi E et al. U.S. householder survey of functional gastrointestinal disorders. Prevalence, sociodemography and health impact. Dig Dis Sci. 1993;38:1569–80.
8. Chang L, Heitkemper MM. Gender differences in irritable bowel syndrome. Gastroenterology. 2002;123:1686–701.
9. Schmulson M, Lee OY, Chang L, Naliboff B, Mayer EA. Symptom differences in moderate to severe IBS patients based on predominant bowel habit. Am J Gastroenterol. 1999;94:2929–35.
10. Schmulson M, Chang L, Naliboff B, Lee OY, Mayer EA. Correlation of symptom criteria with perception thresholds during rectosigmoid distension in irritable bowel syndrome patients. Am J Gastroenterol. 2000;95:152–6.
11. Lee OY, Mayer EA, Schmulson M, Chang L, Naliboff B. Gender-related differences in IBS symptoms. Am J Gastroenterol. 2001;96:2184–93.
12. Whitehead WE, Palsson O, Jones KR. Systemic review of the comorbidity of irritable bowel syndrome with other disorders: what are the causes and implications? Gastroenterology. 2002; 122:1140–56.
13. Veale D, Kavanagh G, Fielding JF, Fitzgerald O. Primary fibromyalgia and the irritable bowel syndrome: different expressions of a common pathogenetic process. Br J Rheumatol. 1991; 30:220–2.
14. Wolfe F, Smythe HA, Yunus MB et al. The American College of Rheumatology 1990 criteria for the classification of fibromyalgia, a report of the Multicenter Criteria Committee. Arthritis Rheum. 1990;33:160–72.
15. Thompson WG, Dotevall G, Drossman DA, Heaton KW, Kruis W. Irritable bowel syndrome: guidelines for the diagnosis. Gastroenterol Int. 1989;2:92–5.
16. Sperber AD, Atzmon Y, Neumann L et al. Fibromyalgia in the irritable bowel syndrome: studies of prevalence and clinical implications. Am J Gastroenterol. 1999;94:3541–6.
17. Scudds RA, Rollman GB, Harth M, McCain GA. Pain perception and personality measures as discriminators in the classification of fibrositis. J Rheumatol. 1987;14:563–9.
18. Tunks E, Crook J, Norman G, Kalaher S. Tender points in fibromyalgia. Pain. 1988;34:11–19.
19. Granges G, Littlejohn G. Pressure pain threshold in pain-free subjects, in patients with chronic regional pain syndromes, and in patients with fibromyalgia syndrome. Arthritis Rheum. 1993; 36:642–6.
20. Gibson SJ, Littlejohn GO, German MM, Helme RD, Granges G. Altered heat pain thresholds and cerebral event-related potentials following painful CO_2 laser stimulation in subjects with fibromyalgia syndrome. Pain. 1994;58:185–93.
21. Lautenbacher S, Rollman GB, McCain GA. Multi-method assessment of experimental and clinical pain in patients with fibromyalgia. Pain. 1994;59:45–53.
22. McDermid AJ, Rollman GB, McCain GA. Generalized hypervigilance in fibromyalgia: evidence of perceptual amplification. Pain. 1996;66:133–44.
23. Mertz H, Naliboff B, Munakata J, Niazi N, Mayer EA. Altered rectal perception is a biological marker of patients with irritable bowel syndrome. Gastroenterology. 1995;109:40–52.

24. Munakata J, Naliboff B, Harraf F *et al*. Repetitive sigmoid stimulation induces rectal hyperalgesia in patients with irritable bowel syndrome. Gastroenterology. 1997;112:55–63.
25. Naliboff BD, Munakata J, Fullerton S *et al*. Evidence for two distinct perceptual alterations in irritable bowel syndrome. Gut. 1997;41:505–12.
26. Bouin M, Plourde V, Boivin M *et al*. Rectal distension testing in patients with irritable bowel syndrome: sensitivity, specificity, and predictive values of pain sensory thresholds. Gastroenterology. 2002;122:1771–7.
27. Chang L. The association of functional gastrointestinal disorders and fibromyalgia. Eur J Surg Suppl. 1998;583:32–6.
28. Gracely RH, Petzke F, Wolf JM, Clauw DJ. Functional magnetic resonance imaging evidence of augmented pain processing in fibromyalgia. Arthritis Rheum. 2002;46:1333–43.
29. Chang L, Berman S, Mayer EA *et al*. Brain responses to visceral and somatic stimuli in patients with irritable bowel syndrome with and without fibromyalgia. Am J Gastroenterol. 2003;98:1354–61.
30. Naliboff BD, Derbyshire SWG, Munakata J *et al*. Cerebral activation in irritable bowel syndrome patients and control subjects during rectosigmoid stimulation. Psychosom Med. 2001;63:365–75.
31. Drossman DA, McKee DC, Sandier RS *et al*. Psychosocial factors in the irritable bowel syndrome. A multivariate study of patients and nonpatients with irritable bowel syndrome. Gastroenterology. 1988;95:701–8.
32. Whitehead WE, Bosmajian L, Zonderman AB, Costa Jr PT, Schuster MM. Symptoms of psychological distress associated with irritable bowel syndrome. Gastroenterology. 1988;95:709–14.
33. Irwin C, Falsetti SA, Lydiard RB, Ballenger JC, Brock CD, Brener W. Comorbidity of posttraumatic stress disorder and irritable bowel syndrome. J Clin Psychiatry. 1996;57:576–8.
34. Walker EA, Gelfand AN, Gelfand MD, Katon WJ. Psychiatric diagnoses, sexual and physical victimization, and disability in patients with irritable bowel syndrome or inflammatory bowel disease. Psychol Med. 1995;25:1259–67.
35. Drossman DA, Leserman J, Hu JB. Gastrointestinal diagnosis, abuse history, and effects on health status. Gastroenterology. 1996;111:1159–61.
36. Drossman DA, Creed FH, Olden KW, Svedlund J, Toner BB, Whitehead WE. Psychosocial aspects of the functional gastrointestinal disorders. Gut. 1999;45:II25–II30.
37. Drossman DA, Leserman J, Nachman G *et al*. Sexual and physical abuse in women with functional or organic gastrointestinal disorders. Ann Intern Med. 1990;113:828–33.
38. Mayer EA, Naliboff BD, Chang L, Coutinho SV. Stress and the gastrointestinal tract: V. Stress and irritable bowel syndrome. Am J Physiol Gastrointest Liver Physiol. 2001;280:G519–24.
39. Mayer EA. The neurobiology of stress and gastrointestinal disease. Gut. 2000;47:861–9.
40. Mayer EA, Craske MG, Naliboff BD. Depression, anxiety and the gastrointestinal system. J Clin Psychiatry. 2001;62:28–36.
41. McEwen B. Protective and damaging effects of stress mediators. N Engl J Med. 1998:338:171–9.
42. Appels A. Mental precursors of mycardial infarction. Br J Psychiatry. 1990;156:465–71.
43. Henry JP. Psychological and physiological responses to stress: the right hemisphere and the hypothalamo–pituitary–adrenal axis, an inquiry into problems of human bonding. Acta Physiol Scand Suppl. 1997;640:10–25.
44. Elenkov IJ, Wilder RL, Chrousos GP, Vizi ES. The sympathetic nerve – an integrative interface between two supersystems: the brain and the immune system. Pharmacol Rev. 2000;52:585–638.
45. Clauw DJ, Chrousos GP. Chronic pain and fatigue syndromes: overlapping clinical and neuroendocrine features and potential pathogenic mechanisms. Neuroimmunomodulation. 1997;4:134–53.

3
Evidence of bidirectional cross-sensitization of the distal colon and lower urinary tract: a possible aetiology of concurrent irritable bowel syndrome and interstitial cystitis

M. A. PEZZONE, W. C. de GROAT and M. O. FRASER

INTRODUCTION

Chronic pelvic pain is a poorly understood but sufficiently debilitating clinical condition primarily affecting women. Few diagnostic and treatment options are available for this understudied patient population which is estimated at 9.2 million in the United States[1]. The causes of chronic pelvic pain are numerous but may include primary gynaecological, urological, gastrointestinal, musculoskeletal, neuronal, or psychological origins, as well as combinations thereof. Chronic pelvic pain encompasses pain syndromes of the pelvic cavity (irritable bowel syndrome and interstitial cystitis) and the pelvic floor (vulvodynia, orchialgia, urethral syndrome, and prostadodynia)[2]. The colorectum and urinary bladder are two of the larger pelvic organs thought to be affected primarily in these disorders; thus it is not surprising that irritable bowel syndrome (IBS) and interstitial cystitis (IC), analogous disorders of pelvic visceral pain and urgency, are two of the commonest causes of reported chronic pelvic pain.

IBS is an intestinal disorder characterized by chronic or recurrent lower abdominal pain or discomfort associated with altered stool consistency and frequency[3]. It is the most common gastrointestinal cause of chronic pelvic pain, affecting 50% of such women presenting to gynaecological clinics[4–7]. Up to 20% of the US population report symptoms consistent with this disorder which is not explained by structural or biochemical abnormalities[8]. IBS sufferers, 70% of whom are female, incur 74% more direct health-care costs than non-IBS sufferers and have more physician visits for both gastrointestinal and non-gastrointestinal complaints[9]. IBS alone results in an estimated US$8 billion in direct medical costs annually[10].

Afflicting women almost exclusively, IC is a chronic pelvic disorder that affects the urinary bladder and is characterized by unpleasant urinary symptoms such as urinary frequency, urgency, discomfort, pain (suprapubic, pelvic, and perineal), and dyspareunia[11,12], all in the absence of organic disease. Over 700 000 women in the USA suffer with IC[13], and associated yearly direct and indirect costs exceed US$430 million (1982 figures[14]). Health-care costs aside, IC, IBS, and other causes of chronic pelvic pain impact dramatically upon one's quality of life, and their predilection for women also adds to the burden of this understudied population and raises further questions regarding possible aetiologies and the role of female sex hormones.

Although the aetiologies of both IBS and IC have been studied extensively (albeit mutually exclusively), few have considered a common underlying mechanism responsible for the development of these and other causes of chronic pelvic pain. Interestingly, as many as 40–60% of patients with IBS also exhibit symptoms consistent with IC[5,15,16], while 38% of patients with IC also have symptoms consistent with IBS (30% with known IBS diagnoses). The high concurrence rate of IBS and IC and other causes of chronic pelvic pain suggest a common predisposition or a shared aetiological factor. Because the symptoms associated with both IBS and IC have been attributed primarily to the development of altered visceral perceptions or visceral afferent sensitization, dysregulation or sensitization of pelvic afferent nerves could lead to visceral hyperalgesia, which could manifest itself in numerous ways affecting various aspects of gastrointestinal, urogenital, and/or pelvic floor function. Infectious, idiopathic, inflammatory, metabolic, or other neuropathic mechanisms could lead to sensitization of the nerves that sense and regulate normal physiological functioning producing pain and aberrant smooth muscle activity in response to normally non-noxious or physiological stimuli. Previously, no-one has adequately investigated the hypothesis that afferent sensitization of one pelvic organ may adversely influence and sensitize the other via direct neuronal connections or reflexes or via changes in central processing. We hypothesize that shared afferent innervation and/or convergence of afferent pathways of the pelvic organs could lead to 'co-sensitization' and account for an overlap of pelvic floor pain disorders and, in a sense, lead to 'referred' pelvic pain.

MATERIALS AND METHODS

Animals

Female Sprague–Dawley rats, 200–250 g in weight, were purchased from Hilltop Lab Animals, Inc. (Scottsdale, PA) and were housed in standard polypropylene cages with *ad libitum* access to food and water in the University of Pittsburgh's Central Animal Facility. All studies were approved by the University of Pittsburgh's Institutional Animal Care & Use Committee and found to meet the standards for humane animal care and use as set by the Animal Welfare Act and the NIH Guide for the Care and Use of Laboratory Animals.

Colon-to-bladder cross-sensitization

Trinitrobenzenesulphonic acid (TNBS) colitis

Under 4% isoflurane anaesthesia, 2,4,6-TNBS (5% aqueous solution; Sigma) was instilled intrarectally as previously described by Morris *et al.*[17] and modified by Appleyard and Wallace[18] to induce colitis. Briefly, TNBS (50 mg/ml) dissolved in 50% ethanol (v/v) was administered via a trans-anal approach (total volume 0.5 ml) using a PE-90 catheter with the tip placed approximately 8 cm proximal to the anal verge. Control animals received 0.5 ml of normal saline.

Micturition patterns

30–90 days following intrarectal TNBS treatment, rats were placed in metabolism cages (Nalgene metabolic cage, Nalgene Co., Rochester, NY) that measure voided urine. Urine was collected for a 24 h period into a specially designed cup mounted on a force transducer (Force displacement transducer FT03, Grass Instruments Co., Quincy, MA). A Transbridge transducer amplifier (World Precision Instruments, Sarasota, FL) was used to amplify the signal from the force transducer which was later processed using a Windaq data-acquisition system (Windaq, DATAQ Instruments Inc., Akron, OH) hooked up to a computer. Micturition parameters evaluated were: (1) total urine output per 24 h; (2) number of micturitions per 24 h; (3) voided volume/micturition.

Tissue processing/histology

Urinary bladders and distal colonic segments (2 cm sections with their centres 8 cm from the anal verge – the site of TNBS administration) were harvested after pentobarbital overdose (100 mg/kg) and placed in 4% buffered paraformaldehyde for 4 h and cryoprotected in 30% sucrose in PBS overnight. Tissues were cut into 8 μm sections and mounted on polylysine-coated slides. Mast cells were stained with Giemsa and quantified.

Bladder-to-colon cross-sensitization

Experimental set-up

Rats were anaesthetized with urethane (Sigma, St Louis, MO) 1.2 g/kg subcutaneously and subjected to a midline laparotomy. A transvesical flared-tip PE-50 catheter (Fisher Scientific, Hanover Park, IL) for urinary bladder filling and pressure recording was inserted through the bladder dome via a small cystotomy and ligated in place, effectively anchoring the catheter and sealing the cystotomy. The catheter tubing was externalized via the proximal aspect of the ventral abdominal incision. The intravesical catheter was connected to a blood pressure transducer (World Precision Instruments, Sarasota, FL) and a syringe pump (Harvard Apparatus, Holliston, MA) via three-way stopcocks. Normal saline was infused into the bladder at a rate of 0.1 ml/min for continuous cystometry. A Transbridge transducer amplifier (World Precision Instruments, Sarasota, FL) was used to amplify the signal from the pressure transducer which was later processed using a PowerLab 8s unit data-acquisition system (ADInstruments,

Mountain View, CA) connected to a Macintosh G3 computer. Intravesical catheters were calibrated using a pressure gauge.

Intracolonic balloons were fashioned from condom reservoir tips and PE-50 tubing. The balloon tip, which approximated the dimensions of a rat stool pellet, was inserted through the anus with its proximal tip positioned 4 cm from the anal verge and fastened in place to the tail with tape. Via three-way stopcocks the intracolonic balloon was connected to a blood pressure transducer for measurement of intracolonic pressure and a 1 ml syringe filled with saline for balloon distension. Intracolonic pressure signals were amplified and acquired as above. Balloons were calibrated and zeroed outside the animal. Balloon compliance was calculated as previously described[19].

Fine-wire electrodes were fashioned from stainless-steel polyurethane-coated wire (0.05 μm in diameter; M. T. Giken Co Ltd, Tokyo, Japan) and were percutaneously inserted into the external urethral sphincter (EUS) and the lower abdominal wall musculature for electromyography (EMG) recording. The EMG signals were amplified using an IsoDAM8A biological amplifier (World Precision Instruments, Sarasota, FL) and acquired by the Power Lab unit. The EMG signals were filtered (high frequency 3 kHz, low frequency 10 Hz) and acquired at a rate of 1000 samples/s. EMG frequencies were measured from the raw EMG signals using the Power Lab unit and expressed as spikes per second.

The initial recording period consisted of a 45–60 min interval of baseline activity with continuous bladder filling (normal saline) at a rate of 0.1 ml/min to allow the animal to recover from the experimental manipulations. Control recordings were then obtained for a 30 min interval. Urinary bladder contraction frequency, EUS EMG activity and frequency, abdominal EMG activity and frequency, and colonic pressure and contraction parameters were measured during this saline infusion control period.

Colorectal distension

With the continuous infusion of saline into the bladder (saline cystometry), graded colorectal distensions were performed. The intracolonic balloon was distended by graded infusions of 0.1 ml at 5 min intervals for a total of five infusions (0.5 ml). Five minutes after the last infusion the intracolonic balloon was returned to its predistension volume; 15–20 min later the control distensions were repeated once more in some animals in order to verify that the control distensions did not induce colonic afferent sensitization. Urinary bladder contraction frequency, EUS EMG activity and frequency, abdominal EMG activity and frequency, and colonic contractions were measured as above.

Acute cystitis

Acute urinary bladder irritation was performed using intravesical infusions of protamine sulphate and potassium chloride as previously described[20]. Briefly, following control (saline) cystometry, the saline infusion was replaced with 10 mg/ml protamine sulphate. Protamine sulphate infusions were maintained for 30 min and were subsequently followed by 300 mM KCl infusion at the same infusion rate. Graded colorectal distensions and cystometric recordings were then made 30–40 min after initiating KCl infusion, when bladder irritation was both maximal and stable.

Statistical analysis

All data are expressed as mean ± SE. Student's *t*-test was used for comparison of 24 h voiding pattern and CMG parameters. ANOVA for repeated measures was utilized to determine differences in colorectal distension effects before and after bladder irritation. A *p*-value less than 0.05 was considered significant.

RESULTS

Colon-to-bladder cross-sensitization

In awake rats previously pretreated with intracolonic TNBS (30–90 days prior), a 30% reduction in bladder voiding volume (0.92 vs 0.65 ml per void) ($p < 0.05$) was observed (Fig. 1A). In addition, a 50% increase in bladder voiding frequency (1.43 vs 2.25 voids per hour) ($p < 0.05$) was recorded when compared to saline-treated controls (Fig. 1B). These observed urinary voiding patterns in animals previously treated with intracolonic TNBS are consistent with the development of chronic cystitis.

Figure 2 illustrates colonic mast cell densities at the site of initial colonic irritation 30–90 days following the administration of intracolonic TNBS. Colonic mast cell counts were dramatically increased following intracolonic TNBS and are quantified in Fig. 3 ($p < 0.0001$). In correlation with the physiological effects of chronic TNBS colitis upon lower urinary tract function, urinary bladders from animals previously treated with intracolonic TNBS demonstrated increased numbers of mast cells as in the directly treated colonic tissue (Fig. 4). Preliminary assessment of these slides revealed as many as 30 mast cells per high-power field in a rat previously treated with intracolonic TNBS but only a maxium (average) of two per high-power field in intracolonic saline-treated controls.

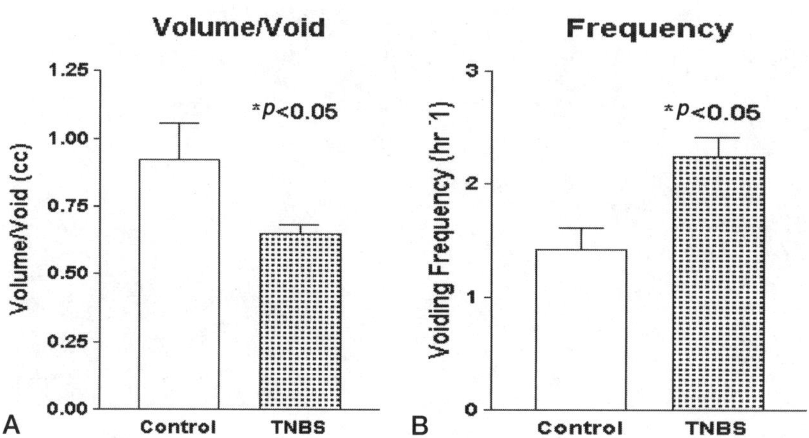

Fig. 1 Voiding volume and frequency in awake rats 30–90 days following the induction of TNBS colitis

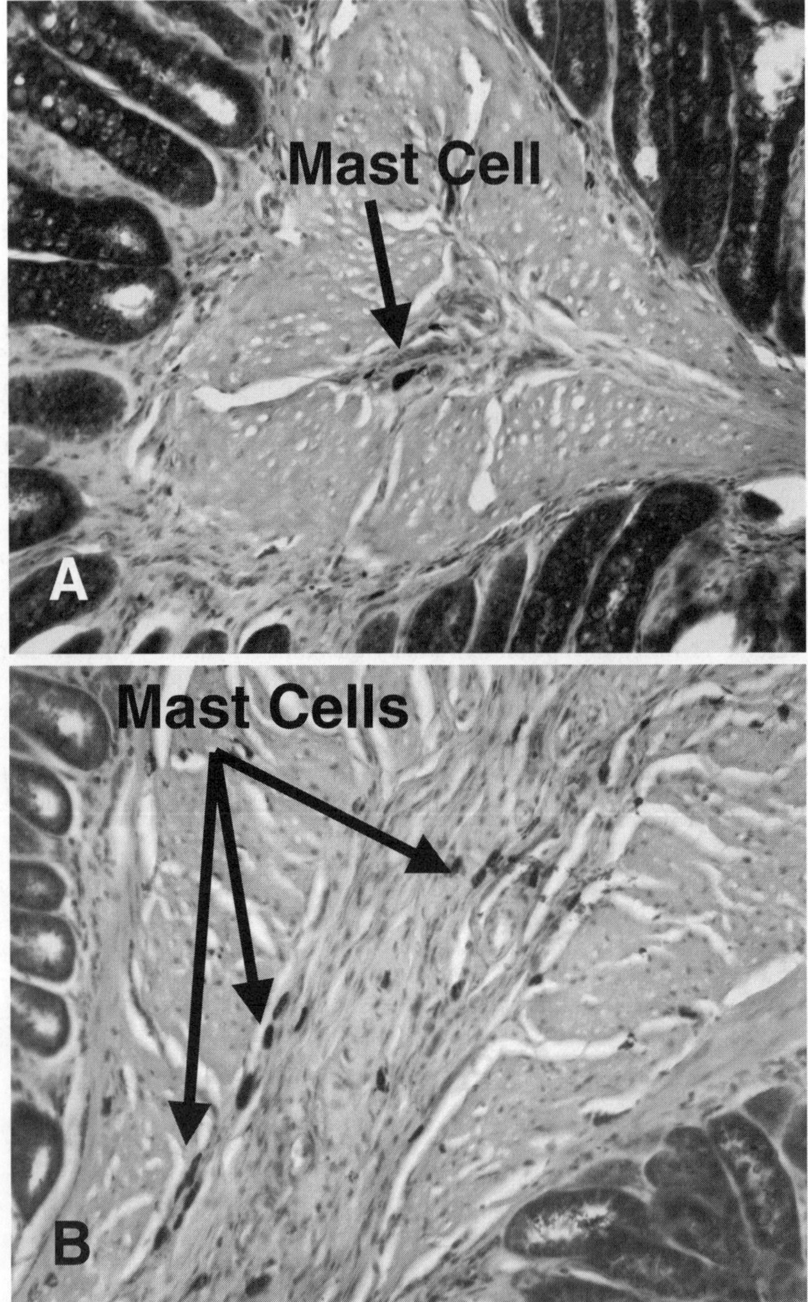

Fig. 2 Giemsa stain of the distal colon illustrating increased colonic mast cell density 30–90 days following the induction of TNBS colitis

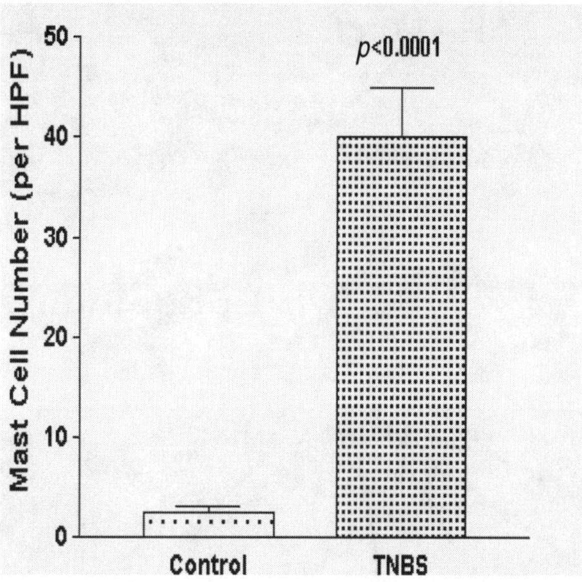

Fig. 3 Colonic mast cell counts quantified in rats treated 30–90 days prior with intracolonic saline or TNBS

The mast cells, as shown in Fig. 4, were predominantly located near the bladder epithelium and lamina propria where C-fibre afferent innervation which governs bladder activity is most prominent.

Bladder-to-colon cross-sensitization

In the second set of experiments, abdominal EMG activity was utilized as a bioassay for colorectal sensitivity in order to determine the effects of acute cystitis on distal colonic sensory thresholds to colorectal distension.

In Fig. 5 abdominal EMG activity, intravesical and intracolonic pressures are recorded in an animal before and after the induction of acute cystitis. Bladder contractions occurred at a rate of 0.26 contractions per minute at a fill rate of 0.1 ml/min, while graded colorectal distensions (CRDs) to $60\,cmH_2O$ produced no notable changes in abdominal wall EMG activity prior to the induction of acute cystitis (Fig. 5A).

Note the expected increase in bladder contraction frequency following intravesical irritation with protamine sulphate and KCl (Fig. 5B). A statistically significant ($p < 0.01$) four-fold increase in bladder contraction frequency was measured (one contraction per minute). Following acute cystitis, increases in baseline abdominal wall EMG activity were noted at colorectal distension pressures much lower than $60\,cmH_2O$, indicating bowel hypersensitivity (or cross-sensitization in this model). In Fig. 6 normalized abdominal wall baseline EMG recordings are represented for each colonic distension volume both before and after bladder irritation.

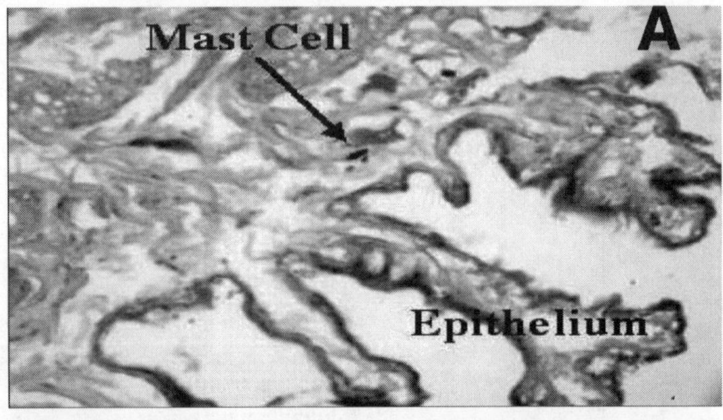

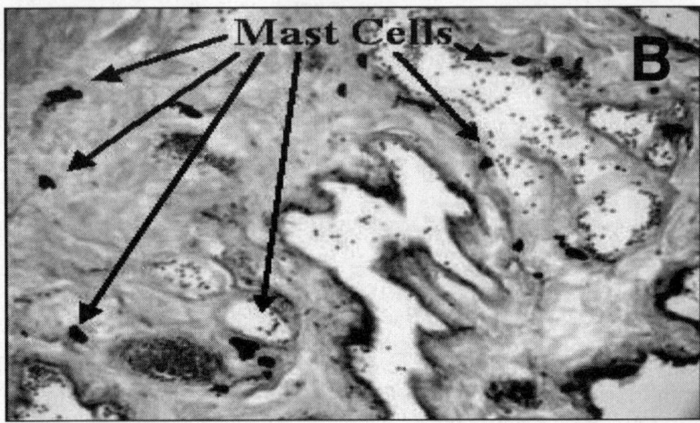

Fig. 4 Giemsa stain of the urinary bladder illustrating mast cells in rats treated 30–90 days prior with intracolonic saline or TNBS

Statistically significant differences were noted at the 0.4 and 0.5 ml CRD distension levels ($p < 0.05$).

DISCUSSION

We report compelling evidence of bidirectional cross-sensitization in both chronic (distal colon-to-bladder) and acute (bladder-to-distal colon) visceral pain models. In chronic TNBS colitis urinary bladder voiding patterns were found to be consistent with chronic cystitis and may be indicative of cross-sensitization. Bladder mast cell counts were increased similar to that seen in the colon, and appeared to be concentrated in areas of the bladder rich in afferent C-fibre innervation, perhaps a consequence of neurogenic inflammation.

Neural influences on the gut, urinary bladder, and pelvic organs are extensive; therefore, so is the potential for their dysregulation. The convergence of afferent innervation of the distal colon and lower urinary tract may account for the high concurrence rate of such chronic pelvic pain disorders as IBS and IC. The colon

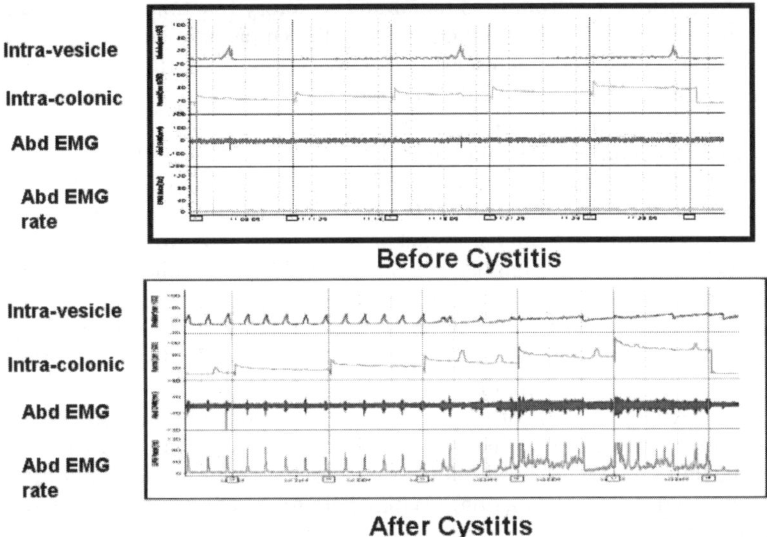

Fig. 5 Evidence of colorectal sensitivity as evidenced by increased abdominal EMG activity following acute cystitis

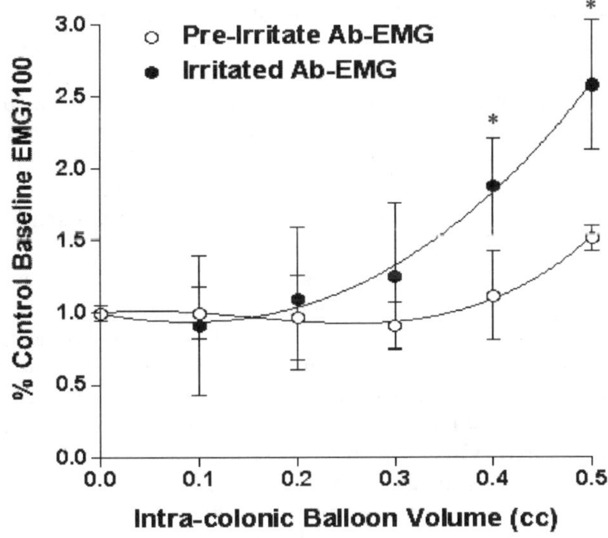

Fig. 6 Basal EMG activity following CRD and acute cystitis ($*p < 0.05$)

and rectum, the predominant sites of dysfunction in IBS, function primarily in water resorption and the storage and elimination of faeces when appropriate (continence). Likewise, the urinary bladder, the pelvic organ primarily affected in IC, is involved in the storage and the periodic elimination of urine. Besides

25

providing extrinsic control of the motor and secretory functions of the colon and lower urinary tract, the autonomic nerves, both sympathetic and parasympathetic, are also the route by which sensory (afferent) fibres reach these organs. These afferents detect and relay information about noxious stimuli and thereby trigger painful sensations in the central nervous system (CNS).

Afferent innervation of the colon and bladder consists of: (1) mucosal afferents supplying the anal canal and passing through pelvic and pudendal nerves to sacral parasympathetic segments; (2) distal colonic afferents passing through pelvic, hypogastric and lumbar splanchnic nerves; (3) more proximal colonic afferents passing through lumbar colonic and lumbar splanchnic nerves as well as through the vagus nerve, urinary bladder lumbar afferents projecting exclusively into the hypogastric nerve, and urinary bladder sacral afferents passing through the pelvic nerve to the spinal cord[21,22]. Functionally, these afferents: (1) detect physical and chemical stimuli providing feedback for subsequent reflexes or responses; (2) form synapses with noradrenergic neurons in sympathetic prevertebral ganglia, likewise mediating reflexes or responses; (3) may independently modulate local blood flow, secretory processes, motility, and intrinsic nervous system function; (4) may help maintain visceral tissues such as colonic or bladder mucosa via release of trophic factors; and (5) influence second-order neurons in the spinal cord via release of transmitters or retrograde transport of neurotrophic substances[21]. Afferent signals mediating pain from the pelvic organs are thought to primarily originate from the pelvic nerves rather than their lumbar counterparts (lumbar splanchnic nerves)[23].

Disorders such as IBS and IC may coexist, in part, due to altered or aberrant neuronal reflexes from the initially sensitized organ which progressively affects the interactions with the previously unaffected organ. Other possibilities include sphincteric interactions with indirect cross-over effects such as bladder irritation resulting in anal sphincter activation[24] leading indirectly to distal colonic over-distension and subsequent afferent stimulation and sensitization. Left unchecked, symptoms in both systems may eventually emerge. The unique model described here markedly enhances the level of sophistication of models required to study such bladder–bowel–sphincteric interactions.

Experimental evidence supporting the development of cross-sensitization or afferent plasticity of one pelvic organ induced by the irritation of another is limited to non-existent. It has been previously hypothesized by Wesselmann *et al.*[25] that a painful pelvic (possibly inflammatory) condition could develop in the referred zone of another inflamed pelvic organ via altered central mechanisms. For example, vulvar vestibulitis or prostatitis could develop in patients with IC. Historically, 'referred' visceral pain, as described originally by Head in 1893, represented hyperalgesia in the somatic (referred) region of a given visceral structure[26]. Possible mechanisms of referred pain could include an antidromic axon reflex via a single primary afferent supplying two (dichotomizing) structures (one visceral and one somatic), viscerosomatic convergence in the spinal cord, or a sympathetic reflex[27]. Perhaps through these same pathways, cross-sensitization of two pelvic viscera may occur, accounting for the substantial overlap of chronic pelvic pain disorders.

Consistent with the physiological effects upon lower urinary tract function, urinary bladders from animals previously treated with intracolonic TNBS demonstrated increased numbers of mast cells as in the directly treated colonic tissue. A preliminary assessment of these bladder specimens remarkably revealed as many as 30 mast cells per high-power field in a rat previously treated with intracolonic TNBS, but only two per high-power field in a saline-treated control. The mast cells were predominantly located near the bladder epithelium and lamina propria where C-fibre afferent innervation is most prominent. As one may expect, these findings are quite astonishing and unprecedented. The TNBS-treated animals showed no signs of a systemic inflammatory response as they gained weight appropriately after the resolution of the acute phases of the colitis and exhibited behaviours no different from those of controls. Moreover, during retrieval of bladder and colonic tissue there were no apparent adhesions noted between the two organs; nor was there any evidence at all of any locally spread inflammatory mass (i.e. non-neurogenic). The combination of both the histological and physiological findings provides strong support for cross-sensitization (bowel-to-bladder) in this model. The chronicity of the model and the associated findings probably indicate that significant central and/or peripheral sensitization has occurred in this setting. It is our impression that the mast cells are a marker of a neurogenic process; furthermore, the role of neurogenic mastocytosis as a marker and/or causal factor in the development of cross-sensitization of pelvic visceral organs needs to be studied in greater detail.

In conclusion, these data support the notion that co-morbidity of pelvic pain/urgency syndromes is not coincidental, but rather causal in nature. Clearly, further research is warranted to expand on the current findings.

Acknowledgement

This study was supported by NIH grant K08 DK02488 to M.A.P.

References

1. Mathias SD, Kuppermann M, Liberman RF, Lipschutz RC, Steege JF. Chronic pelvic pain: prevalence, health-related quality of life, and economic correlates. Obstet Gynecol. 1996;87:321–7.
2. Wesselmann U. Neurogenic inflammation and chronic pelvic pain. World J Urol. 2001;19:180–5.
3. Thompson WG, Longstreth GF, Drossman DA, Heaton KW, Irvine EJ, Muller-Lissner SA. Functional bowel disorders and functional abdominal pain. In: Drossman DA, Corazziari, E, Talley N, Thompson WG, Whithead WE, editors. The Functional Gastrointestinal Disorders, 2nd edn. McLean, VA: Degnon Associates, 2000:351–75.
4. Hogston P. Irritable bowel syndrome as a cause of chronic pain in women attending a gynaecology clinic. Br Med J. 1987;294:934–5.
5. Prior A, Wilson K, Whorwell PJ, Faragher EB. Irritable bowel syndrome in the gynecological clinic. Survey of 798 new referrals. Dig Dis Sci. 1989;34:1820–4.
6. Walker EA, Katon WJ, Jemelka R. The prevalence of chronic pelvic pain and irritable bowel in two university clinics. J Psychosom Obstet Gynaecol. 1991;12s:65–70.
7. Walker EA, Gelfand AN, Gelfand MD, Green C, Katon WJ. Chronic pelvic pain and gynecological symptoms in women with irritable bowel syndrome. J Psychosom Obstet Gynaecol. 1996;17:39–46.
8. Drossman DA. Review article: an integrated approach to the irritable bowel syndrome. Aliment Pharmacol Ther. 1999;13:3–14.
9. Drossman DA, Li Z, Andruzzi E *et al.* U.S. householder survey of functional gastrointestinal disorders. Prevalence, sociodemography, and health impact. Dig Dis Sci. 1993;38:1569–80.

10. Talley NJ, Gabriel SE, Harmsen WS, Zinsmeister AR, Evans RW. Medical costs in community subjects with irritable bowel syndrome. Gastroenterology. 1995;109:1736–41.
11. Ratner J. Women's Health. 1992;1:63–8.
12. Koziol JA. Epidemiology of interstitial cystitis. Urol Clin N Am. 1994;21:7–20.
13. ICA Website (www.ichelp.org).
14. Doggweiler R, Blankenship J, MacDiarmid SA. Review on chronic pelvic pain from a urological point of view. World J Urol. 2001;19:160–5.
15. Alagiri M, Chottiner S, Ratner V, Slade D, Hanno PM. Interstitial cystitis: unexplained associations with other chronic disease and pain syndromes. Urology. 1997;49s:52–7.
16. Whorwell PJ, McCallum M, Creed FH, Roberts CT. Non-colonic features of irritable bowel syndrome. Gut. 1986;27:37–40.
17. Morris GP, Beck MS, Herridge MS, Depew WT, Szewczuk MR, Wallace JL. Hapten-induced model of chronic inflammation and ulceration in the rat colon. Gastroenterology. 1989;96:795–803.
18. Appleyard CB, Wallace JL. Reactivation of hapten-induced colitis and its prevention by anti-inflammatory drugs. J Am Physiol Soc. 1995;269:G119–25.
19. Turler A, Moore BA, Pezzone MA, Overhaus M, Kalff JC, Bauer AJ. Colonic postoperative inflammatory ileus in the rat. Ann Surg. 2002;236:56–66.
20. Fraser MO, Chuang YC, Lavelle JP et al. A reliable, nondestructive animal model for interstitial cystitis: intravesical low-dose protamine sulfate combined with physiological concentrations of potassium chloride. Urology. 2001;57:112.
21. Janig W, Haupt-Schade P, Kohler W. Afferent innervation of the colon: the neurophysiological basis for visceral sensation and pain. In: Mayer EA, Raybould HE, editors. Basic and Clinical Aspects of Chronic Abdominal Pain. Amsterdam: Elsevier, 1993:71–86.
22. Sengupta JN, Gebhart GF. Gastrointestinal afferent fibers and sensation. In: Johnson LR, editor. Physiology of the Gastrointestinal Tract, 3rd edn. New York: Raven Press, 1994:483–519.
23. Janig W, Koltzenburg M. On the function of spinal primary afferent fibres supplying colon and urinary bladder. J Auton Nerv Syst. 1990;30:S89–96.
24. Thor KB, Muhlhauser MA. Vesicoanal, urethroanal, and urethrovesical reflexes initiated by lower urinary tract irritation in the rat. J Am Physiol Soc. 1999;46:R1002–12.
25. Wesselmann U, Burnett AL, Heinberg LJ. The urogenital and rectal pain syndromes. Pain. 1997;73:269–94.
26. Head H. On disturbances of sensation with special reference to the pain of visceral disease. Brain. 1893;16:1–113.
27. Wesselmann U. Neurogenic inflammation and chronic pelvic pain. World J Urol. 2001;19:180–5.

4
Are dissociative mental disturbances responsible for visceral hyperalgesia in patients with functional abdominal pain?

J. KRUSE, N. SCHMITZ, B. CLAR, W. WÖLLER, P. ENCK

During the last few years there has been an increasing interest in investigating the association between history of sexual abuse and gastrointestinal disorders. Studies in the clinical setting showed an even higher frequency of abuse history in patients with functional gastrointestinal disorders. On the other hand, adult females with a history of abuse described gastrointestinal symptoms as their most common somatic complaints.

Patients with a history of childhood abuse are prone to develop a variety of psychiatric disorders. These features are commonly seen among patients with GI disorders. Walker[1] found that patients with functional GI disorders who had been severely abused were more likely to suffer from anxiety disorders, major depression and alcohol abuse. Psychological complaints can up-regulate and enhance the patients' symptom perception (i.e. sensation intensity). They are associated with health-related quality of life and health care behavior. For example, Creed[2] reported that psychological distress was an independent and significant predictor of health-related quality of life in addition to abdominal symptoms in patients with severe irritable bowel syndrome (IBS).

The association between mental disorders and health care behaviour (e.g. number of doctor visits) was demonstrated in several studies[3]. Patients with IBS who had not consulted a doctor for this symptom were significantly less psychologically disturbed than their clinical counterparts.

Traumatic life experiences like childhood abuse are predominantly associated with dissociation and PTSD. However, the impact of dissociation and PTSD on patients with functional gastrointestinal disorders has rarely been investigated to date.

Dissociation is a central neurophysiological process resulting in disturbed self-perception and self-consciousness and may serve as a coping mechanism for individuals facing the trauma of abuse. It is a process and resulting condition at the same time. It is manifested by problems with the integration of mental functions such as identity and memory or consciousness. Amnesia and derealization are aspects of dissociation but peripheral sensory and motor functions can also be affected. For instance, pseudoneurological symptoms, such as psychogenic impaired vision, hearing defects, paralyses and ataxia, are dissociative phenomena. Dissociative phenomena have an impact on the ability of an individual to select which of his or her recollections and sensations are to be chosen for immediate attention. A close association between dissociation and traumatic life experiences has been suggested[4]. Here, dissociation is considered to be a strategy for coping with traumatic life experiences; it shows a reduced capacity to integrate traumatic life experiences into one's life.

At the beginning of the 20th century Janet[5] suggested that memories of traumatic experiences may be stored outside of conscious awareness and expressed in somatic symptoms. In recent years, studies have suggested new evidence for a relationship between somatization and dissociation. Therefore the question has been raised whether dissociation is also connected with functional abdominal pain.

The goal of the present study was to evaluate whether dissociation is associated with symptom perception and health care behaviour in patients with functional abdominal pain.

We investigated 160 female patients with functional lower abdominal pain recruited in a primary care setting. All patients had abdominal pain for at least six months that was poorly related to gut function and was associated with some loss of daily activities. It was not possible for the patients to disregard the symptoms. More than 50% of the patients reported to have been woken up by the pains in the night. The patients had no other gastrointestinal disorder that would explain the abdominal pain. The patients fulfilled the diagnostic criteria of functional abdominal pain syndroms or unspecified functional abdominal pain according to the Rome II criteria.

Dissociation was assessed using the FDS, the German adaptation of the Dissociative Experiences Scale (DES). The FDS includes all DES items and has been extended by the scale conversion[6]. This is a 44-item, self-report questionnaire designed to assess dissociative experiences, including disturbances in memory, identity, awareness, cognition and conversion not occurring under the influence of alcohol or drugs. The possible response options increase in increments of 10% and range from 0% (this never happens) to 100% (this always happens). The participant was asked to circle the corresponding percentage of time she had had the particular experience described in each item. We computed a DES total score. Fig. 1 shows the distribution of the DES total scores.

The subjects in our sample showed a high medical service utilization in the previous year (Fig. 2). During the last year more than 40% of the patients visited their physicians more than 4 times because of abdominal pain. 50% of the patients had had an X-ray examination or a gastroscopy/coloscopy. 29% of the patients had been hospitalized during the last 12 months. 29% of the patients reported at least one day out of work because of their abdominal complaints.

When comparing the patient sample with a reference sample of healthy subjects, we found a similar pattern of the DES sumscores, indicating that subjects with FAP did not have an increased level of dissociative experiences. In accordance with Drossmann[7] and Talley[8] we found that a high number (more than

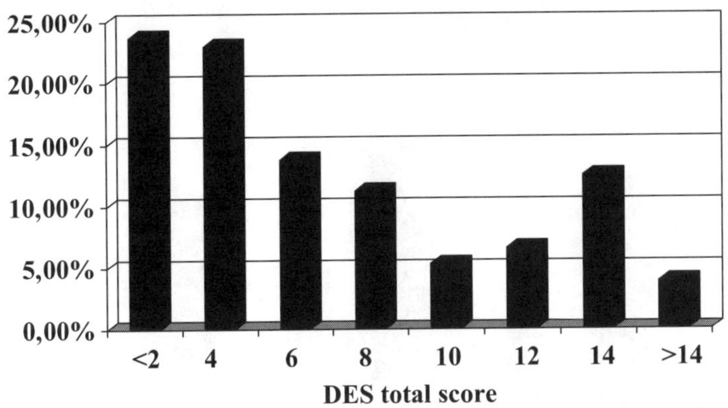

Fig. 1 Distribution of the DES total score

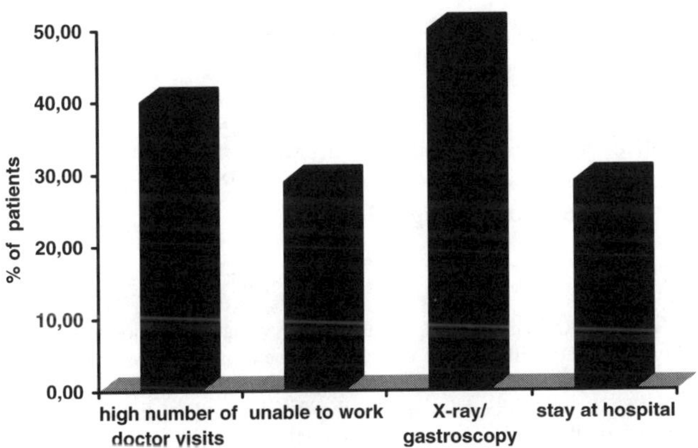

Fig. 2 Medical care utilization

50%) of our patients reported either violence or sexual attacks in their childhood. As expected, patients reporting a history of childhood violence and sexual abuse had higher scores of dissociation on the DES global scale. Our findings for the nonabused group fell well within this normal range. Supporting the specific link between abuse and dissociation, the means for our abused group indicated significantly more pathology.

Dissociation (DES) was more frequent in patients who consulted physicians more frequently, had a greater number of days off work and in those who reported more pain (Fig. 3).

SUMMARY

Dissociation of self-perception was found in a subgroup of patients with LAP, and especially in those with experienced sexual trauma. Dissociation seems to be

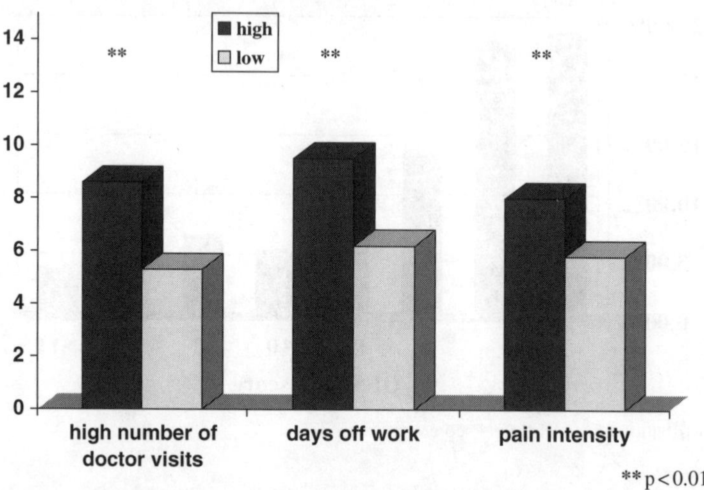

Fig. 3 Health care behavior and dissociation (DES mean values)

associated with excessive health-care utilization, but it still needs to be determined whether altered visceral perception in LAP is a consequence of such a dissociative central neurophysiological process.

References

1. Walker EA, Gelfand AN, Gelfand MD, Katon WJ. Psychiatric diagnoses, sexual victimization, and disability in patients with irritable bowel syndrome or inflammatory bowel disease. Psychol Med. 1995; 25:1259–67
2. Creed F, Ratcliffe J, Fernandez L *et al*. Health related quality of life and health care costs in severe, refactory irritable bowel syndrome. Ann Intern Med. 2001; 134:860–8.
3. Talley NJ, Boyce PM, Jones M. Predictors of health care seeking for irritable bowel syndrome: a population based study. Gut. 1997;41:394–8
4. Putnam FW. Dissociation as an extreme response to trauma. In: Kulft RP, ed., Childhood antecedents of multiple personality. Washington DC: American Psychiatry. 1985.
5. Janet P. The major symptoms of hysteria. New York: Macmillian. 1907.
6. Bernstein EM, Putnam FW. Development, reliability, and validity of a dissociation scale. J Nerv Ment Dis. 1986; 174:727–35.
7. Drossman DA, Leserman J, Nachman G *et al*. Sexual and physical abuse in women with functional or organic gastrointestinal disorders. Ann Intern Med. 1990;113:828–33.
8. Talley NJ, Fett SL, Zinsmeister AR, Melton III JL. Gastrointestinal tract symptoms and self-reported abuse: a population-based study. Gastroenterology. 1994;107:1040–49.
9. Talley NJ, Fett SL, Zinsmeister AR. Self-reported abuse and gastrointestinal disease in outpatients: Association with irritable bowel-type symptoms. Am J Gastroenterol. 1995;90:366–71.

Section II
Basic mechanisms of gastrointestinal inflammation

5
Current knowledge regarding the initiation and regulation of gastrointestinal inflammation in inflammatory bowel disease

R. DUCHMANN

NORMAL INTESTINAL IMMUNE RESPONSES

Immune responses to luminal antigens generally result in two major pathways, one leading to protective immunity or inflammatory immune responses, the other to tolerance or down-regulation of inflammatory immune responses (Fig. 1). Although many of the mechanisms that direct these responses are still not well understood, it is quite clear that regulation occurs in a broader context in which the antigen is perceived by the organism as dangerous or harmless. T cells are critically involved in the regulatory process and, within the specific context, differentiate into a variety of subpopulations which each regulate immune responses by a well-defined spectrum of effector functions.

In the context of a bacterial infection it is well established that bacterial products induce the production of interleukin (IL)-12 by macrophages. IL-12 then leads to differentiation into Th1 cells, which are characterized by their cytokine secretion profile (IL-2, interferon (IFN)-γ) and are important regulators of the antibacterial immune response. Allergic reactions or worm infections in contrast induce Th2 cells, which develop under the influence of IL-4 and are characterized by secretion of cytokines IL-4, IL-5 and IL-10[1]. Complementary T cell subpopulations characterized by cytokine secretion profile or phenotype regulate immune tolerance or suppress inflammatory immune responses. These include transforming growth factor beta (TGF-β) secreting Th3 cells in oral tolerance, and Tr1 cells which down-regulate inflammation in animal models by production of IL-10[2–4]. Surface expression of CD4CD25$^+$ characterizes yet another T cell population which has strong suppressor activity and is important for the control of autoimmune diseases. Thus, animals lacking CD4CD25$^+$ T cells develop a variety of autoimmune diseases whereas transfer of CD4CD25$^+$ T cells is therapeutic[5].

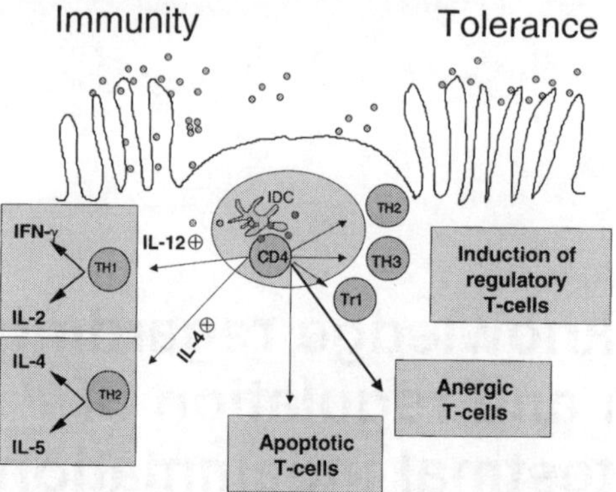

Fig. 1 Immunity vs. tolerance. Intestinal immune responses in the intestine are tightly regulated by T cells. Antigens that are seen by the organism in the context of danger will favour T cell differentiation to inflammatory subtypes Th1 or Th2. Immune responses towards antigens that are seen by the organism in a context signalling no harm, in contrast, do not elicit an inflammatory response and are down-regulated by mechanisms of peripheral tolerance including T cell anergy, T cell apoptosis or effects of regulatory suppressor T cells

INFLAMMATORY BOWEL DISEASES

The inflammatory bowel diseases (IBD), Crohn's disease (CD) and ulcerative colitis (UC), are immune-mediated, chronic inflammatory diseases of the intestine and often associated with extraintestinal manifestations. The large clinical overlap between IBD and rheumatic diseases suggests that both forms of chronic inflammatory diseases share at least some pathogenetic pathways. Although the aetiology of IBD is still unknown, extensive knowledge regarding disease pathogenesis and mechanisms of disease is available. In essence, numerous studies indicate that, in genetically susceptible individuals, the normal intestinal flora acts as an endogenous stimulus that is required to generate IBD through a variety of immune abnormalities[6,7] (Fig. 2).

From epidemiological and twin studies it has long been established that IBD have a genetic component. Using modern techniques, decisive progress was recently made in studies associating CD with mutations at the single gene level[8,9]. It is now clear that 25–33% of CD patients carry a mutation in the NOD2/CARD15 gene, that carriers of one or several NOD2/CARD15 gene mutations have a 3–40-fold increased risk for CD and that NOD2/CARD15 mutations are associated with involvement of the terminal ileum[10]. Altogether, these studies identified mutations in the NOD2/CARD15 gene, which also occur in about 15% of the normal population, as the single highest known risk factor for the development of CD. In addition to a genetic susceptibility it is clear that the immune system is essential in mediating the inflammatory process and may contribute to the disease by one or a larger number of primary abnormalities. In this review the central role of T cells for the dysregulated immune response and the essential role of the intestinal flora to provide the endogenous stimulus required to drive the immune system along the dysregulated pathways will be addressed in more detail.

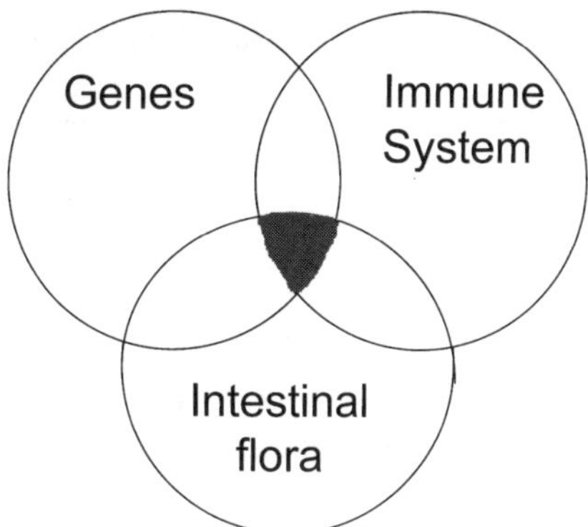

Fig. 2   Major factors in IBD pathogenesis. Current data suggest that IBD is driven by the intestinal flora, involves a dysregulated T cell response and develops in the genetically susceptible host

INTESTINAL FLORA

Most of our knowledge regarding the composition of the resident intestinal flora is still based on very laborious microbiological and phenotypic analyses of faecal samples or luminal aspirates. These data suggest that the normal intestinal flora is a very complex ecosystem consisting of an astonishingly large number and variety of bacteria. Estimates indicate that the intestinal flora comprises 10 times more bacteria than the body contains cells, and that the intestinal flora harbours more than 400 different bacterial species. The normal flora colonizes the intestinal tract shortly after birth and in adults characteristic population levels are maintained in defined regions along the alimentary canal. The highest number and complexity of bacteria and bacterial species is found in the terminal ileum and colon[11,12]. There is evidence for immune tolerance to the intestinal flora. How the immune system normally regulates its responses to the huge amount of stimulatory molecules within the normal flora to prevent chronic inflammation, however, is still incompletely understood[11,13–15].

ANIMAL MODELS

Within the past 10–20 years animal models have decisively shaped our understanding of IBD pathogenesis[6]. Results from a large variety of models, including different knockout or transgenic models, T cell transfer models, spontaneous and chemically induced models, have been very stringent in demonstrating that chronic intestinal inflammation is dependent on the presence of luminal bacteria (Fig. 3). Thus, it is a common observation in most models that intestinal inflammation develops in normally housed but not in germ-free animals and that CD4 T cells are crucially involved in disease pathogenesis. In the following, a selection of data relevant to the role of T cells and luminal bacteria in animal models of IBD pathogenesis will be discussed.

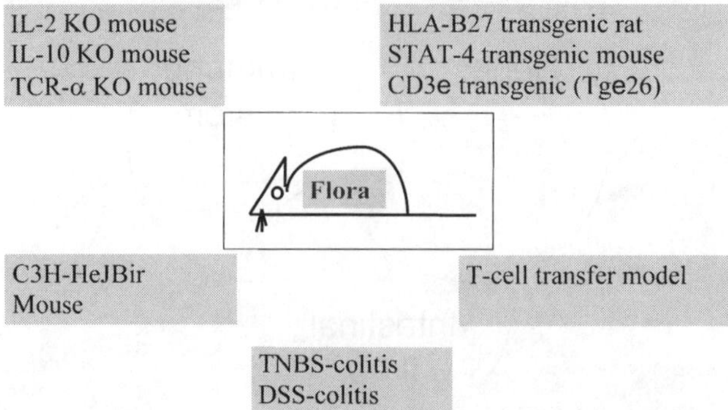

Fig. 3 Animal models of IBD. Chronic intestinal inflammation develops as a consequence of a large variety of immune abnormalities. A dysregulated T cell response to normal intestinal flora is the basic mechanism in the majority of animal models

TRINITROBENZENESULPHONIC ACID (TNBS) INDUCED COLITIS

Colitis induced by rectal administration of the hapten TNBS is a granulomatous colitis that is driven by Th1 cells and shares many histological and immunological features with CD[16]. Mice with TNBS-induced colitis show the same abrogation of tolerance to their flora as was observed in human IBD, indicating that the intestinal flora constitutes the essential T cell stimulus in that model[13,14]. The finding that antibodies to IL-12 restore tolerance to self-intestinal flora in this model indicates that antibacterial T cell responses in TNBS colitis are mediated by IL-12. Thus, IL-12 is not only an important counterregulator of TGF-β-mediated oral tolerance but also counterregulates tolerance to normal intestinal flora.

C3H-HeJBir MICE

C3H-HeJBir mice spontaneously develop a Th1-driven colitis early in life and show a highly restricted humoral response to bacterial antigens but not to food or epithelial antigens. CD4$^+$ T cells from colitic C3H-HeJBir mice are strongly reactive towards antigens from the enteric bacterial flora but not to epithelial or food antigens, and show a much higher precursor frequency of bacteria-reactive CD4$^+$ cells compared to non-colitic control mice. T cells from C3H-HeJBir mice stimulated with enteric bacterial antigens and transferred into SCID mice induce colitis[17,18].

STAT-4 TRANSGENIC MICE

Constitutive expression of STAT-4, an intracellular signalling molecule essential for the induction of IL-12, leads to a chronic colitis mediated by Th1 cells. Similar to the C3H-HeJBir model, transfer of STAT-4 transgenic T cells stimulated by bacterial antigens induces disease in immunodeficient hosts[19].

T CELL TRANSFER MODEL

In the T cell transfer model, intestinal inflammation develops after adoptive transfer of CD4[+] T cells into immunodeficient hosts. Highlighting the role of different immunoregulatory T cell subpopulations in inducing or controlling disease, it was shown that CD45RB[high] CD4[+] T cells induce colitis when injected into immunodeficient (SCID or RAG) mice, whereas co-transfer of CD4[+] T cell subsets expressing the cell surface markers CD45RB[low] or CD4CD25 prevents disease[5,20]. Similar to the above-mentioned (and in fact most) animal models of IBD, T cell transfer colitis is mediated by Th1 cells, depends on the presence of a normal flora[21] and shows signs of antigen-driven activation and oligoclonal expansion of T cells[22] (and own observation). In addition to these T cell populations it was shown that T regulatory (Tr1) cells which produce IL-10 as a consequence of repeated administration of antigen in the presence of IL-10 also prevent colitis in this model[23].

EVIDENCE FOR A ROLE OF THE INTESTINAL FLORA IN IBD

Since the possibilities for experimental interventions in humans are more limited than in experimental animal models, evidence for a role of intestinal bacteria in IBD pathogenesis is circumstantial (Fig. 4). However, the induction of an inflammatory response by infusion of faeces into excluded ileum[24], the association of sites of disease predilection with those showing highest bacterial load, increased T and B cell responses to flora antigen[11,12], and the effectiveness of antibiotic therapy in active and in fistulizing CD and of probiotic therapy for remission maintenance in ulcerative colitis[25,26] and pouchitis[27], provide good and independent evidence. There is congruent evidence from different laboratories that cellular and humoral immune responses to bacteria from the normal intestinal flora are increased in IBD. Data from our own laboratory indicate that tolerance to the intestinal flora observed in controls is abrogated in active IBD[13].

REGULATORY ABNORMALITIES IN IBD

Studies determining the cytokine secretion profile of CD4[+] T cells from IBD patients demonstrated that lamina propria CD4[+] T cells isolated from CD

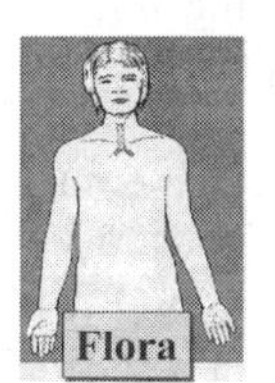

Colon and terminal ileum show highest bacterial concentrations and are the most affected sites in IBD

Cellular and humoral immune responses to bacteria from the normal intestinal flora are increased in IBD

Diversion of fecal stream proximally to the ileocolonic anastomosis protects against disease recurrence

Infusion of autologous ileal effluent triggers recurrence of CD in the terminal ileum within days

Antibiotic therapy is beneficial in fistulizing and in active CD

Probiotic therapy is effective for remission maintenance in ulcerative colitis and pouchitis

Fig. 4 Observations suggesting an involvement of the intestinal flora in IBD

patients produce more IFN-γ but less IL-4 or IL-5 than control T cells, indicative of a Th1 response. In contrast, lamina propria T cells from UC patients produced more IL-5 and did not show increased production of IFN-γ[28], indicative of a Th2-type response. Integrating the data from animal models and IBD patients, data therefore suggest that CD results from a dysregulated immune response to antigens from the normal flora and increased generation of Th1 cells. In UC, in contrast, the normal flora apparently drives the immune response towards pathways that are characterized by an increased generation of Th2-type cells[7].

The reasons for the apparent immunological and clinical differences between CD and UC remain incompletely understood. In CD it is suggested that abnormalities including the increased production of the soluble mediator IL-12[29], IL-6 *trans*-signalling[30] and cell–cell interactions mediated by CD44 variants[31,32] drive the differentiation of T cells towards Th1 regulators of inflammation. During these processes, IL-12 increases the action of IL-18, which is also increased in CD[33], through up-regulation of its receptor on T cells, counterregulates tolerance to normal intestinal flora[14] and induces lamina propria T cells to produce IFN-γ, which in turn activates macrophages to produce proinflammatory cytokines. In addition to this regulatory abnormality, data indicate that activation-induced cell death by apoptosis, an important mechanism to take inflammatory cells out of the system, is defective in CD[34,35]. In UC, in contrast, low levels of IL-12 seem to favour the differentiation of Th2-type cells more prone to B cell help and the production of autoantibodies. Whether the balance is further tipped to inflammation through decreased generation of regulatory (suppressor) cells is not well established. At least for CD4CD25 T cells as yet unpublished data from our laboratory for the first time suggest that this might be the case.

SUMMARY

In a comprehensive model of the initiation and dysregulation of immune responses in IBD pathogenesis (Fig. 5), it is suggested that IBD is a consequence of a dysregulated immune response of CD4$^+$ T cells to luminal, most likely bacterial, antigens. Although this may be due to a single abnormality with different phenotypic expression, current data seem to favour the concept that more than one abnormality can lead to chronic intestinal inflammation (e.g. indicated by the large number of different abnormalities leading to chronic intestinal inflammation in animal models). In IBD these abnormalities may eventually combine to individual or subgroup-specific patterns and overrule the normally counter-inflammatory tone of the mucosal immune system, mediated by regulatory T cells, T cell anergy and apoptosis.

The important role of T cells becomes evident from various animal models of IBD, in which gut inflammation can be induced and transferred by T cells. In addition increased numbers of activated T cells are present in the intestinal mucosa and peripheral blood of IBD patients. The exact mechanisms resulting in T cell activation in IBD are still unclear; however, most of the available information provides evidence that colitic T cells are driven by antigens from the normal intestinal flora. Thus in most animal models of IBD inflammation develops in the presence of an intestinal flora but not in germ-free mice, indicating that it acts as

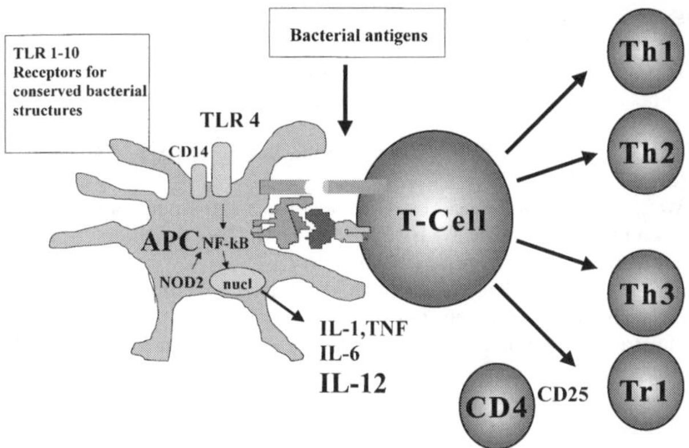

Fig. 5 Comprehensive model of immune dysregulation in IBD. Receptors of the innate immune system recognize conserved bacterial products and are expressed on antigen-presenting cells. Signals received by the antigen-presenting cell through any of these receptors affect the differentiation of the antigen-presenting cell. Soluble mediators secreted by the antigen-presenting cell or molecules expressed on its cell surface profoundly influence the quality of antigen-specific T cell responses. Once T cells have been instructed to differentiate into a certain type of regulatory cell that is distinguishable by its cytokine secretion profile (e.g. Th1, Th2, Th3, Tr1) and sometimes phenotype (e.g. CD4$^+$ CD25$^+$ T cells), they become pivotal players to induce or suppress intestinal inflammation. In IBD it is suggested that one or more abnormalities along these pathways leads to an increased generation of inflammatory T cell populations (Th1/Th2). The role of bacteria in this model may be dual and may include both an abnormal activation of the antigen-presenting cell through receptors of the innate immune system and an abnormal activation of T cells via its antigen-specific T cell receptor

an endogenous stimulus required to generate disease. Why the intestinal flora elicits a 'physiological inflammation' in healthy individuals, but leads to chronic inflammation in IBD, remains incompletely understood. Recent data, however, strongly suggest that receptors of the innate immune system, which bridge the gap between the innate immune system and adaptive T cell responses, are critically involved. These receptors have evolved to recognize conserved bacterial products and may be involved in IBD pathogenesis by shifting immune responses to pathological pathways. For example, recognition of microbial products by Toll-like receptors expressed on dendritic cells has been shown to trigger dendritic cell differentiation and profoundly influences the quality of antigen-specific T cell responses. In addition, mutations within the NOD2/CARD15 gene have been identified as the most important single risk factor for CD. The NOD2/CARD15 gene in turn codes for an intracellular protein that is involved in recognition of bacterial products and participates in signalling pathways mediating activation of NF-κB or apoptosis. Once T cells have been instructed to differentiate into a certain type of regulatory cell that is distinguishable by its cytokine secretion profile (e.g. Th1, Th2, Th3, Tr1) and sometimes phenotype (e.g. CD4$^+$CD25$^+$ T cells), they become pivotal players to induce or suppress intestinal inflammation. The molecular mechanisms that contribute to the establishment and maintenance of cytokine memory in regulatory T cell subpopulations is not yet clear, but there is increasing evidence that Th1 cells associated with CD are controlled by transcription factors T-bet and Stat-4, whereas Th2 cells associated with ulcerative colitis are controlled by GATA-3.

References

1. Mosman T. Cytokines and immune regulation. In: Rich, Fleischer, Schwartz, Shearer, Strobes, editors. Clinical Immunology, Principles and Practice. St. Louis: Mosby, 1995: 217–30.
2. Roncarolo MG, Bacchetta R, Bordignon C, Narula S, Levings MK. Type 1 T regulatory cells. Immunol Rev. 2001;182:68–79.
3. Mowat A, Weiner H. Oral tolerance: physiological basis and clinical applications. In: Orgra PL, Mestecky J, Lamm ME, Strober W, Bienenstock J, McGhee J, editors. Mucosal Immunology, 2nd edn. New York: Academic Press, 1999:587–618.
4. Weiner HL. The mucosal milieu creates tolerogenic dendritic cells and T(R) 1 and T(H) 3 regulatory cells. Nat Immunol. 2001;2:671–2.
5. Read S, Malmstrom V, Powrie F. Cytotoxic T lymphocyte-associated antigen 4 plays an essential role in the function of CD25(+) CD4(+) regulatory cells that control intestinal inflammation. J Exp Med. 2000;192:295–302.
6. Blumberg RS, Saubermann LJ, Strober W. Animal models of mucosal inflammation and their relation to human inflammatory bowel disease. Curr Opin Immunol. 1999;11:648–56.
7. Blumberg RS, Strober W. Prospects for research in inflammatory bowel disease. J Am Med Assoc. 2001;285:643–7.
8. Hugot JP, Chamaillard M, Zouali H et al. Association of NOD2 leucine-rich repeat variants with susceptibility to Crohn's disease. Nature. 2001;411:599–603.
9. Ogura Y, Bonen DK, Inohara N et al. A frameshift mutation in NOD2 associated with susceptibility to Crohn's disease. Nature. 2001;411:603–6.
10. Sachar D. Genomics and phenomics in Crohn's disease. Gastroenterology. 2002;122:1161–2.
11. Duchmann R. The role of resident intestinal bacteria. In: Holoman J, Glasa J, editors. Chronic Inflammatory Bowel Diseases. Progress and Controversies. Progress in Hepato-Pharmacology, Vol. 5, 2000:17–31.
12. Duchmann R. Gut flora: future implications. In: Rogler G, Kullmann F, Rutgeerts P, Sartor RB, Schölmerich J, editors. IBD at the End of its First Century. Lancaster: Kluwer, 2000:42–50.
13. Duchmann R, Kaiser I, Hermann E, Mayet W, Ewe K, Meyer zum Buschenfelde KH. Tolerance exists towards resident intestinal flora but is broken in active inflammatory bowel disease (IBD). Clin Exp Immunol. 1995;102:448–55.
14. Duchmann R, Schmitt E, Knolle P, Meyer zum Buschenfelde KH, Neurath M. Tolerance towards resident intestinal flora in mice is abrogated in experimental colitis and restored by treatment with interleukin-10 or antibodies to interleukin-12. Eur J Immunol. 1996;26:934–8.
15. Duchmann R, Neurath MF, Meyer zum Buschenfelde KH. Response to self and non-self intestinal microflora in health and inflammatory bowel disease. Res Immunol. 1997;148:589–94.
16. Neurath MF, Fuss I, Kelsall BL, Stuber E, Strober W. Antibodies to interleukin 12 abrogate established experimental colitis in mice. J Exp Med. 1995;182:1281–90.
17. Cong Y, Brandwein SL, McCabe RP et al. CD4+ T cells reactive to enteric bacterial antigens in spontaneously colitic C3H/HeJBir mice: increased T helper cell type 1 response and ability to transfer disease. J Exp Med. 1998;187:855–64.
18. Cong Y, Weaver CT, Lazenby A, Elson CO. Colitis induced by enteric bacterial antigen-specific CD4+ T cells requires CD40-CD40 ligand interactions for a sustained increase in mucosal IL-12. J Immunol. 2000;165:2173–82.
19. Wirtz S, Finotto S, Kanzler S et al. Cutting edge: chronic intestinal inflammation in STAT-4 transgenic mice: characterization of disease and adoptive transfer by TNF- plus IFN-gamma-producing CD4+ T cells that respond to bacterial antigens. J Immunol. 1999;162:1884–8.
20. Powrie F, Mauze S, Coffman RL. CD4+ T-cells in the regulation of inflammatory responses in the intestine. Res Immunol. 1997;148:576–81.
21. Aranda R, Sydora BC, McAllister PL et al. Analysis of intestinal lymphocytes in mouse colitis mediated by transfer of CD4+, CD45RBhigh T cells to SCID recipients. J Immunol. 1997; 158:3464–73.
22. Matsuda JL, Gapin L, Sydora BC et al. Systemic activation and antigen-driven oligoclonal expansion of T cells in a mouse model of colitis. J Immunol. 2000;164:2797–806.
23. Groux H, O'Garra A, Bigler M et al. A CD4+ T-cell subset inhibits antigen-specific T-cell responses and prevents colitis. Nature. 1997;389:737–42.

24. D'Haens GR, Geboes K, Peeters M, Baert F, Penninckx F, Rutgeerts P. Early lesions of recurrent Crohn's disease caused by infusion of intestinal contents in excluded ileum. Gastroenterology. 1998;114:262–7.
25. Kruis W, Schutz E, Fric P, Fixa B, Judmaier G, Stolte M. Double-blind comparison of an oral *Escherichia coli* preparation and mesalazine in maintaining remission of ulcerative colitis. Aliment Pharmacol Ther. 1997;11:853–8.
26. Rembacken BJ, Snelling AM, Hawkey PM, Chalmers DM, Axon AT. Non-pathogenic *Escherichia coli* versus mesalazine for the treatment of ulcerative colitis: a randomised trial. Lancet. 1999;354:635–9.
27. Gionchetti P, Rizzello F, Venturi A *et al.* Oral bacteriotherapy as maintenance treatment in patients with chronic pouchitis: a double-blind, placebo-controlled trial. Gastroenterology. 2000;119:305–9.
28. Fuss IJ, Neurath M, Boirivant M *et al.* Disparate CD4+ lamina propria (LP) lymphokine secretion profiles in inflammatory bowel disease. Crohn's disease LP cells manifest increased secretion of IFN-gamma, whereas ulcerative colitis LP cells manifest increased secretion of IL-5. J Immunol. 1996;157:1261–70.
29. Neurath MF, Duchmann R, Meyer zum Buschenfelde KH. [Cytokines in chronic inflammatory intestinal diseases]. Dtsch Med Wochenschr. 1996;121:735–41.
30. Atreya R, Mudter J, Finotto S *et al.* Blockade of interleukin 6 *trans* signaling suppresses T-cell resistance against apoptosis in chronic intestinal inflammation: evidence in Crohn disease and experimental colitis *in vivo*. Nat Med. 2000;6:583–8.
31. Wittig B, Seiter S, Schmidt DS, Zuber M, Neurath M, Zoller M. CD44 variant isoforms on blood leukocytes in chronic inflammatory bowel disease and other systemic autoimmune diseases. Lab Invest. 1999;79:747–59.
32. Wittig BM, Johansson B, Zoller M, Schwarzler C, Gunthert U. Abrogation of experimental colitis correlates with increased apoptosis in mice deficient for CD44 variant exon 7 (CD44v7). J Exp Med. 2000;191:2053–64.
33. Monteleone G, Trapasso F, Parrello T *et al.* Bioactive IL-18 expression is up-regulated in Crohn's disease. J Immunol. 1999;163:143–7.
34. Boirivant M, Marini M, Di Felice G *et al.* Lamina propria T cells in Crohn's disease and other gastrointestinal inflammation show defective CD2 pathway-induced apoptosis. Gastroenterology. 1999;116:557–65.
35. Itoh J, de la Motte C, Strong S, Levine A, Fiocchi C. Decreased bax expression by mucosal T cells favours resistance to apoptosis in Crohn's disease. Gut. 2001;49:35–41.

6
Is the normal gut inflamed?
And does it matter?

A. von HERBAY

INTRODUCTION

The question asked in the title appears to be unconventional. According to the principles of general pathology an organ is either normal or inflamed. However, among the various functions that serve the gut (i.e. transport, digestion and absorption, endocrine secretion, epithelial barrier, immunological barrier), this question continues to be a real matter of debate[1]. To find a contemporary answer it should be recognized that there is a further, more basic question behind this one: how to define what is normal in the gut and what is abnormal?

A definition one can possibly agree with may be: 'A normal gut is characterized by features which are commonly present in healthy persons among a distinct population.'

THE SPECTRUM OF NORMAL GUT MUCOSAL MORPHOLOGY

Following that definition the mucosa of the small intestine has a remarkebly variable morphology, as becomes evident by light microscopy.

The normal gut mucosa – in newborns, babies, and young children

Structural development of the intestinal tract starts *in utero*, but has not finished at birth[2]. This ongoing process is reflected by the continued development of mucosal morphology after birth.

1. In a newborn child the mucosal villi are fairly slim and tall. Just a few leucocytes are present within the lamina propria. No mucosa-associated lymphoid tissue (MALT) has yet organized (Fig. 1a).
2. In babies of few months age the villi become finger-shaped, there are some more leucocytes in the lamina propria, and development of MALT has started (Fig. 1b).

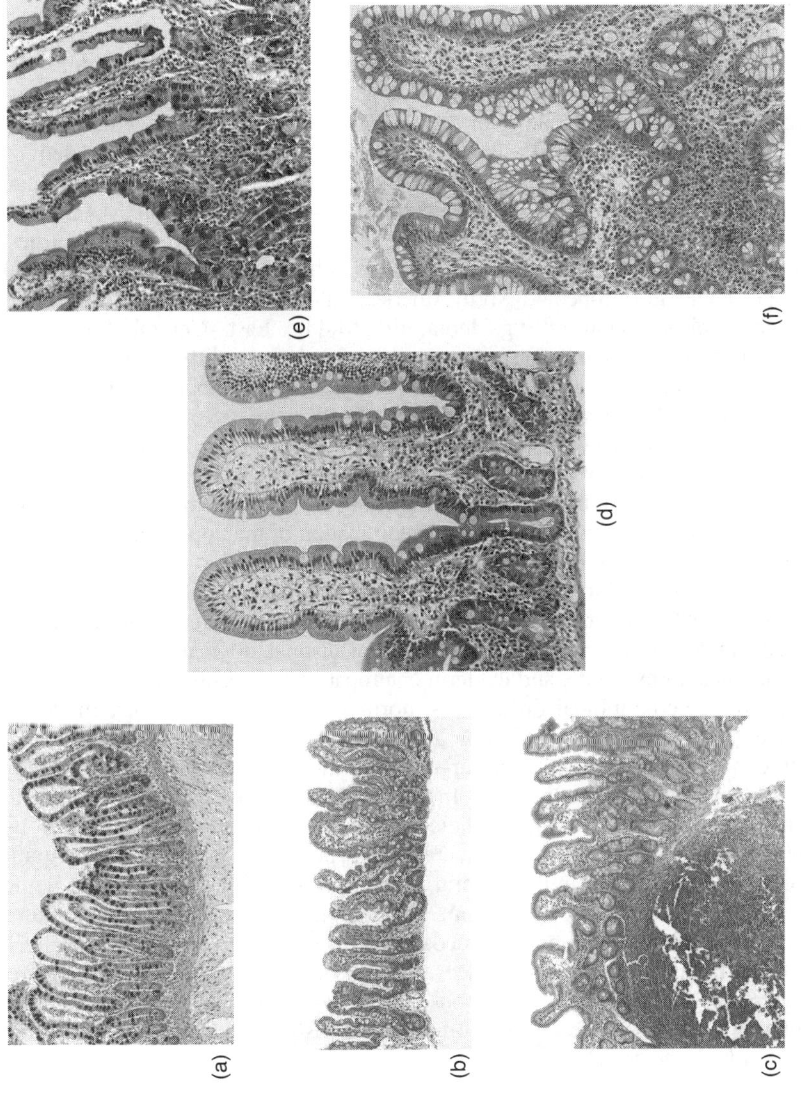

Fig. 1 The spectrum of normal gut mucosal morphology: (a) mucosa in a healthy newborn (1 day old); (b) mucosa in a healthy baby (3 months); (c) mucosa in a healthy toddler (21 months); (d) mucosa in a healthy adult from Germany (52 years); (e) mucosa in a healthy adult after travelling to Central America (31 years); (f) ileal pouch mucosa in an asymptomatic adult after restorative proctocolectomy.

3. In toddlers the villi are finger-shaped, and there is a moderate but considerable number of diverse leucocytes in the lamina propria. In addition, MALT is well developed, and lymphoid follicles with enlarged germinal centres may be present (Fig. 1c).

The normal gut mucosa – in adults

Textbooks commonly illustrate the mucosa from adults[2]. In healthy adults the mucosal villi are finger-shaped, and crypt depth is moderate. The ratio of villous height to crypt depth varies along the small bowel. In the distal duodenum, where biopsies are usually obtained[3], the ratio is approximately 2–3 : 1. The lamina propria contains a moderate number of leucocytes, and some lymphocytes are commonly present within the villous epithelium (Fig. 1d). In addition, MALT with follicles is well developed, albeit this is more occasionally met in mucosal biopsies.

Of note, these histological features (Fig. 1d) characterize the small intestinal mucosa of adults in Europe and North America, but not all over the world. Persons living in tropical countries, e.g. India, the Middle East, Central Africa, the Carribbean, and Central and South America, frequently have different mucosal features[4–7]. When analysed, asymptomatic adults, e.g. from Zambia (Central Africa), commonly have shorter villi, increased crypt depth, increased number of mitoses per crypt, and also an increased number of leucocytes in the lamina propria, as compared with black or white persons from South Africa, or from Great Britain[7,8]. Current theories concerning the aetiopathogenesis of this phenomenon focus on the role of infection or continuing bacterial contamination of the upper small intestine[7]. As the 'tropical mucosa' (Fig. 1e) is different from that of European persons, it is traditionally considered to reflect tropical enteropathy, and a relationship with tropical sprue has been suggested[4,5]. However, considering the common occurrence of 'tropical mucosa' in asymptomatic people from distinct tropical populations, this apparently is a normal state, and the term enteropathy is a misnomer[8].

Apart from geographical differences, normal mucosal morphology may also reflect that physiological conditions are different in a distinct population. An example is given by patients after surgery, e.g. after restorative proctocolectomy with ileo-anal pouch anastomosis. In a pelvic faecal neo-reservoir (i.e. ileal pouch), the mucosa of asymptomatic adults is commonly characterized by moderately reduced villous height, increased crypt depth, and an increased number of leucocytes in the lamina propria, as compared with a non-operated ileum (Fig. 1f). Despite its difference from prevalvular ileal mucosa, these features characterize a normal ileal pouch mucosa[9].

In brief, the normal intestinal mucosa cannot be illustrated by a single figure, albeit this may be suggested by textbooks. There is a spectrum of normal mucosal morphology among different persons, which also includes variable normal numbers of leucocytes (Fig. 1a–f).

THE NORMAL GUT IS AN ECOSYSTEM

The spectrum of normal gut mucosa (Fig. 1a–f) can be understood better when it is appreciated that the gut is an ecological system[10]. There are four major factors which contribute to this: (1) intestinal microbial flora (or microflora), (2) intestinal immune system, (3) intestinal epithelial cells, and (4) intestinal motility.

The intestinal microflora

The human gut contains a complex mix of bacteria. Previous studies by means of conventional culture and typing techniques revealed that there are more than 400 bacterial species along the large and small intestine[11]. Together they contribute to intraluminal metabolism[12,13], and refer to colonization resistance[14].

Recent studies, by means of polymerase chain reaction (PCR) amplification of bacterial DNA, have extended the traditional view, as they permit detection of bacteria without cultivation. By monitoring the diversity of 16S ribosomal DNA in faecal samples of healthy babies for more than 10 months, and by analysing the DNA sequences, 19 of 34 (56%) cloned ribosomal DNA sequences did not correspond to known bacterial sequences[15]. This indicates there are still many more as yet uncultured and unidentified bacteria, which also participate in neonatal gut colonization[15].

The enteric bacterial flora has effects on mucosal morphology. Until birth the gut lumen is filled with meconium which is sterile (cf. Fig. 1a). Just after birth the bacteria enter the intestinal tract by a peroral route, and they start to colonize the gut[16–18]. As early as after 1 month, an individual microbial flora has developed (cf. Fig. 1b). Previously it was assumed that the individual microflora remains rather stable thereafter, but this view has been challenged by recent DNA studies[15].

The effect of the developing intestinal microflora on mucosal morphology in humans (cf. Fig. 1a–c) is paralled by germ-free (gnotobiotic) animals, as compared with conventionally reared animals[13]. Further, variability among the human enteric microflora may also explain, at least in part, the spectrum of normal mucosal morphology in healthy adults (Fig. 1d–f).

The intestinal immune system

The intestinal immune system is acquired after birth, and its postnatal development is driven by the microbial colonization[19]. The structural basis of the mucosa-associated lymphoid tissue (MALT) is well known: it comprises solitary or aggregated lymphoid follicles with B and T cells; furthermore various leucocytes in the lamina propria (plasma cells, lymphocytes, macrophages and others), and intraepithelial lymphocytes[20]. Despite the presence of so many immunocompetent cells the immunological tone of the intestinal tract is apparently highly regulated[20].

Several studies have revealed that, in allegedly healthy persons, mucosal leucocytes (i.e. immune cells) are in a state of activation[1]. One example was given by an experiment with lamina propria leucocytes (LPL) and intraepithelial lymphocytes (IEL), which were isolated from the duodenal mucosa of healthy European adults[21]. It was shown that a subset of LPL (approximately 2% of LPL), as well as subset of IEL (approximately 4% of IEL), is capable to spontaneously secrete interferon-gamma, or interleukin-4 (approximately 1% of LPL and IEL, respectively), which contrasts to peripheral blood mononuclear cells and also to LPL and IEL from colon mucosa. It was concluded that these cytokines are probably involved in the normal homeostasis of the human intestinal mucosa[21].

Another example is given by a recent study of mucosal T cells in healthy adults from Central Africa (Zambians; with a 'tropical mucosa', cf. above), in comparison with black adults and white adults from South Africa (without a 'tropical mucosa', cf. above)[8]. In black Zambians there was a moderate but significant increase of mucosal T cells expressing MHC class II molecules (HLA-DR; approximately 85% vs. 70%), and CD69/activation inducer molecule (approximately 75% vs. 60%). These data indicate a different state of T cell activity in a tropical vs. non-tropical population, while persons are asymptomatic[8].

Considering the presence of immunocompetent cells, and the evidence for their activity, it is tempting to assume that this already reflects inflammation, and indeed this situation is frequently described as a physiological or controlled inflammation[1,20]. However, considering that all these phenomena commonly take place in healthy persons, this should perhaps be regarded as reflecting a normal state.

The intestinal epithelium

Beside its role as a barrier, and in the processing and uptake of nutrients and antigens, the intestinal epithelial cells may also actively participate in immunological processes. Under certain conditions epithelial cells are capable of secreting various interleukins (IL-1, IL-6, IL-7, IL-8, IL-l0, IL-12, IL-15), cytokines (e.g. tumour necrosis factor-alpha, transforming growth factor-beta), and defensins; they may also express receptors for cytokines[22-25].

Further, intestinal epithelial cells (IEC) may express distinct surface molecules and restriction elements, such as the class Ib molecule CD1d and a novel CD8 ligand, gp180, which allow IEC to present antigens to T cells in the lamina propria. These molecules come together to activate a subpopulation of CD8$^+$ regulatory T cells whose function is to suppress immune responses in an antigen non-specific fashion[22].

Interactions in the intestinal ecosystem

Complex interactions between the major constituents of the intestinal ecosystem are difficult to study *in vivo*. Recently an elegant *in-vitro* experiment was performed which provides interesting information. Intestinal epithelial cells (CaCo-2 cells) were cultured either alone, or together with human leucocytes (peripheral blood mononuclear cells). Then cultures were incubated with strains of non-pathogenic bacteria (*Lactobacillus sakei*, *L. johnsonii*, mutants of *Escherichia coli*), and enteropathogenic *E. coli* (EPEC). As a result, epithelial cells only produced chemokine mRNA (TNF-alpha, MCP-1, IL-1beta, IL-8) when they were co-cultured with the leucocytes[26]. Apparently, the differential recognition of non-pathogenic bacteria by intestinal epithelial cells required the presence of leucocytes. These results support the hypothesis that bacterial signalling at the mucosal surface is dependent on a network of cellular interactions[27]. As a consequence, the presence of leucocytes within intestinal mucosa is necessary for maintaining health, i.e. the normal state.

SUMMARY AND ANSWERS

In healthy persons there is a spectrum of normal gut mucosal morphology, which includes a variable normal number of mucosal immune cells. In parallel, there are different states of mucosal immunological activity, which should therefore also be regarded as normal.

From this point of view the normal gut is not inflamed, it just adapts to its respective normal environment; and this does matter, since normal mucosal immunological activity protects from disease. What really matters, however, is to recognize the borderline.

References

1. O'Farrelly C. Just how inflamed is the normal gut? Gut. 1998;42:603–4.
2. Keljo DJ, Gariepy CE. Anatomy, histology, embryology, and developmental anomalies of the small and large intestine. In: Feldman M, Friedman LS, Sleisenger MH, editors. Sleisenger & Fordtran's Gastrointestinal and Liver Disease, 7th edn. Philadelphia: Saunders, 2002:1643–63.
3. Segal GH, Petras RE. Histology of the normal small intestine. In. Sternberg SS, editor. Histology for Pathologists, 2nd edn. New York: Raven Press, 1997:495–518.
4. Klipstein FA, Falaiye JM. Tropical sprue in travellers and expatriates from the tropics living in the continental United States. Medicine. 1969;48:475–91.
5. Klipstein FA. Tropical sprue in travellers and expatriates living abroad. Gastroenterology. 1981;80:590–600.
6. Wood GM, Gearty JC, Cooper BT. Small bowel morphology in British Indian and Afro-Caribbean subjects: evidence of tropical enteropathy. Gut. 1991;32:256–9.
7. Farthing MJG. Tropical malabsorption and tropical diarrhea. In: Feldman M, Friedman LS, Sleisenger MH, editors. Sleisenger & Fordtran's Gastrointestinal and Liver Disease, 7th edn. Saunders, 2002:1842–53.
8. Veitch AM, Kelly P, Zulu IS, Segal I, Farthing MJG. Tropical enteropathy: a T-cell mediated crypt hyperplastic enteropathy. Eur J Gastroenterol Hepatol. 2001;13:1175–81.
9. von Herbay A. Histopathologische Diagnostik chronisch-entzündlicher Darmerkankungen. Historischer Rückblick und aktuelle Übersicht. Pathologe. 1999;20:276–87.
10. Gaskins HR, Lien EL. Developmental ecology of the neonatal intestine. Introduction. Am J Clin Nutr. 1999;69(Suppl.):1027S
11. Hanson LA, Yolken RH, editors. Probiotics, other Nutritional Factors, and Intestinal Microflora. Philadelphia: Lippincott-Raven, 1999.
12. Collins MD, Gibson GR. Probiotics, prebiotics, and synbiotics: approaches for modulating the microbial ecology of the gut. Am J Clin Nutr. 1999;69(Suppl.):1052–7S.
13. Gregg CR, Toskes PP. Enteric bacterial flora and small bowel bacterial overgrowth syndrome. In: Feldman M, Friedman LS, Sleisenger MH, editors. Sleisenger & Fordtran's Gastrointestinal and Liver Disease, 7th edn. Philadelphia: Saunders, 2002:1783–93.
14. van der Waaij D, Berghuis de Vries JM, Lekkerkerk van der Wees JEC. Colonization resistance of the digestive tract in conventional and antibiotic-treated mice. J Hyg Camb 1971;69:405–11.
15. Favier CF, Vaughan EE, De Vos WM, Akkermans ADL. Molecular monitoring of succession of bacterial communities in human neonates. Appl Environ Microbiol. 2002;68:219–26.
16. Sanderson IR. The physicochemical environment of the neonatal intestine. Am J Clin Nutr. 1999;69(Suppl.):1028–34S.
17. Mackie RI, Sghir A, Gaskins HR. Developmental microbial ecology of the neonatal gastrointestinal tract. Am J Clin Nutr. 1999;69(Suppl.):1035–45S.
18. Dai D, Walker WA. Protective nutrients and bacterial colonization in the immature human gut. Adv Pediatr. 1999;46:353–82.
19. Cebra JJ. Influences of microbiota on intestinal immune system development. Am J Clin Nutr. 1999;69(Suppl.):1046–51S.
20. Sartor RB. Mucosal immunology and mechanisms of gastrointestinal inflammation. In: Feldman M, Friedman LS, Sleisenger MH, editors. Sleisenger & Fordtran's Gastrointestinal and Liver Disease, 7th edn. Philadelphia: Saunders, 2002:21–51.

21. Carol M, Lambrechts A, van Gossum A, Libin M, Goldman N, Mascart-Lemone F. Spontaneous secretion of interferon-γ and interleukin-4 by human intraepithelial and lamina propria gut lymphocytes. Gut. 1998;42:643–9.
22. Campbell N, Yio XY, So LP, Li Y, Mayer L. The intestinal epithelial cell: processing and presentation of antigen to the mucosal immune system. Immunol Rev. 1999;172:315–24.
23. O'Neil DA, Porter EM, Elewaut D *et al*. Expression and regulation of the human beta-defensins hBD-1 and hBD-2 in intestinal epithelium. J Immunol. 1999;163:6718–24.
24. Ohta N, Hiroi T, Kweon MN *et al*. IL-15-dependent activation-induced cell death-resistant Th1 type CD8 alphabeta+NK1.1+ T cells for the development of small intestinal inflammation. J Immunol. 2002;169:460–8.
25. de Winter H, Elewaut D, Turovskaya O *et al*. Regulation of mucosal immune responses by recombinant interleukin 10 produced by intestinal epithelial cells in mice. Gastroenterology. 2002;122:1829–41.
26. Haller D, Bode C, Hammes WP, Pfeifer AM, Schiffrin EJ, Blum S. Non-pathogenic bacteria elicit a differential cytokine response by intestinal epithelial cell/leucocyte co-cultures. Gut. 2000;47:79–87.

Section III
Disturbed function in inflammatory bowel disease

7
Symptomatic inflammatory bowel disease in remission – it could be irritable bowel syndrome

P. J. WHORWELL

The prevalence of irritable bowel syndrome (IBS) varies considerably according to the population under study and the definition used. However, a figure of 10–15% would seem to be a reasonable estimate[1]. IBS certainly does not appear to prevent the development of other diseases, thus it might be expected that 10–15% of patients with any disease would therefore suffer symptoms consistent with this diagnosis. Therefore, 10–15% of patients with conditions such as angina, arthritis or inflammatory bowel disease will suffer symptoms of IBS, although it is possible that, if the primary disease is sufficiently severe, it might mask the presence of IBS. The fact that any individual, irrespective of what is wrong with him/her, can suffer from IBS confirms that the approach where IBS is considered as a diagnosis of exclusion is entirely illogical.

Although post-dysenteric IBS (PD-IBS) was first described many years ago, this condition has recently been the centre of much attention. It appears to follow any form of dysenteric illness and is more common in females, after prolonged illness or when there is pre-existing psychological comorbidity. The subject has recently been comprehensively reviewed by Spiller[2]. Mucosal biopsies from the colon of patients with IBS are typically normal, but recently it has been shown that subtle inflammatory changes may be present, particularly in those with PD-IBS[3–5]. In addition, there has been a report suggesting that anti-inflammatory cytokines might be somewhat deficient in some IBS patients[6], and all this has led to the concept that inflammation may be important in the pathogenesis of some cases of IBS, especially when it follows gastrointestinal infection[7]. Whether the syndrome following infection is identical to other forms of IBS, or represents an IB(like)S form, of disorder remains to be determined[8].

Patients with inflammatory bowel disease (IBD) not uncommonly continue to complain of abdominal symptoms, despite apparently being in clinical remission. The symptoms are often reminiscent of IBS and pain is sometimes more of a problem than the disorder of bowel habit. Endoscopy is usually normal or shows only minimal change; likewise other markers of activity such as erythrocyte sedimentation rate, C-reactive protein and white cell scanning are also normal or equivocal. Characteristically, these patients do not respond to steroids but these drugs are often continued with the result that patients become Cushingoid without any symptomatic benefit. All these factors raise the possibility that, under certain circumstances, IBD might be able to provoke a syndrome similar to that observed in PD-IBS.

Although the pathophysiology of IBS is incompletely understood, changes in visceral sensitivity[9] and motor activity[10] of the gastrointestinal tract are thought to be important. Thus it would be of interest to know more about these two phenomena in patients with IBD.

There seems little doubt that patients with active colitis have increased rectal sensitivity[11,12] and it was originally thought that patients with quiescent colitis appeared to have normal sensitivity[11,12]. However, there has been a recent report suggesting that patients with mild activity, somewhat surprisingly, have reduced sensitivity[13]. It is also interesting to note that, in animals, changes in visceral sensitivity associated with inflammation have been shown to persist once the inflammatory process has settled down[14]. Lastly, we have shown that experimentally induced diarrhoea can result in changes in rectal sensitivity in healthy female subjects[15], raising the possibility that the diarrhoea associated with IBD might lead to sensitization, irrespective of the inflammatory process. Motor activity has also been assessed in patients with quiescent ulcerative colitis and those with Crohn's disease, and appears to be affected. Furthermore, the changes do not necessarily appear to be confined to the inflamed segment of bowel[16–19]. Work in animals has revealed a similar situation to that observed with visceral sensitivity in that motor changes induced by inflammation appear to persist following its resolution[20,21].

It would therefore seem reasonable to assume that, based on epidemiological evidence, at least 10–15% of patients with IBD will suffer concurrent IBS. Furthermore, one could speculate that additional patients might suffer from a syndrome similar to that seen in PD-IBS. This would lead to the prediction that, if IBS symptoms were sought in an IBD population, one might expect a prevalence even higher than that observed in the general population.

Many years ago we looked at the prevalence of IBS in patients with ulcerative colitis in remission and found it to be 33%[22]. More recently, Simren and colleagues have undertaken a similar evaluation and found an identical figure[23]. In addition, they also looked at the prevalence of IBS symptomatology in Crohn's disease patients in remission and reported a figure of 57%[23]. It would therefore appear that the prediction that excessive numbers of IBD patients might suffer symptoms consistent with a diagnosis of IBS is correct, and this results from the combination of patients with pre-existing IBS and those in whom the problem has been initiated by inflammation, if indeed the two conditions are different.

In conclusion, IBS should be seriously considered as the cause of continuing symptoms in patients with IBD in remission. The recognition of this possibility is critical to management as it can lead to the avoidance of the inappropriate use of steroids, especially as these drugs have been shown to be unhelpful in PD-IBS[24]. We have previously shown that the presence of bloating, lethargy, backache, nausea and urinary symptoms can help to substantiate the diagnosis of IBS[25]. Thus, the presence of these additional symptoms in an IBD patient who is in apparent mucosal remission may make the physician feel more confident in making the diagnosis of IBS.

References

1. Camilleri M, Heading RC, Thompson WG. Consensus report: Clinical perspectives, mechanism, diagnosis and management of irritable bowel syndrome. Aliment Pharmacol Ther. 2002;16:1407–30.
2. Spiller RC. Post-infectious IBS. In: Camilleri M, Spiller RC, editors. Irritable Bowel Syndrome: Diagnosis and Treatment. London: Saunders, 2002:85–94.
3. Gwee KA, Leong YL, Graham C *et al.* The role of psychological and biological factors in post-infective gut dysfunction. Gut. 1999;44:400–6.
4. Spiller RC, Jenkins D, Thornley JP *et al.* Increased rectal mucosal enteroendocrine cells, t-lymphocytes and increased gut permeability following acute *Campylobacter* enteritis and in post-dysenteric irritable bowel syndrome. Gut. 2000;47:804–11.
5. Chadwick VS, Chen W, Shu D *et al.* Activation of the mucosal immune system in irritable bowel syndrome. Gastroenterology. 2002;122:1778–83.
6. Chan J, Gonsalkorale W, Perrey M *et al.* IL-10 and TGF-beta genotypes in irritable bowel syndrome: evidence to support an inflammatory component? Gastroenterology. 2000;118(Suppl. 1): A184.
7. Collins SM, Pich ET, Rampole P. The putative role of inflammation in the irritable bowel syndrome. Gut. 2001;49:743–5.
8. Lea R, Whorwell PJ. Infection and irritability. Gut. 2002;51:305–6.
9. Houghton LA. Evidence of abnormal rectal sensitivity in IBS. In: Camilleri M, Spiller RC, editors. Irritable Bowel Syndrome: Diagnosis and Management. London: Saunders, 2002: 69–76.
10. Wood JD. Neuropathophysiology of irritable bowel syndrome. J Clin Gastroenterol. 2002;35(Suppl.):s11–22.
11. Rao SS, Read NW, Davison PA, Bannister JJ, Holdsworth CD. Ano-rectal sensitivity and responses to rectal distension in patients with ulcerative colitis. Gastroenterology. 1987;93:1270–5.
12. Loening-baucke V, Metcalf AM, Shirazi S. Ano-rectal manometry in active and quiescent ulcerative colitis. Am J Gastroenterol. 1989;84:892–7.
13. Chang L, Munakata J, Meyer EA *et al.* Perceptual responses in patients with inflammatory and functional bowel disease. Gut. 2000;47:497–505.
14. Mao Y, Wang L, Chen Y, Blennerhassett PA, Collins SM, Tougas G. Long term effects of acute *Trichinella spiralis* infection on substance P levels in NIH Swiss mice. Gastroenterology. 2000;118:A149.
15. Houghton LA, Wych J, Whorwell PJ. Acute diarrhoea induces rectal sensitivity in women but not men. Gut. 1995;37:270–3.
16. Manousos ON, Salem SN. Abnormal motility of the small intestine in ulcerative colitis. Gastroenterologia. 1965;104:249–57.
17. Rao SS, Read NW, Brown C, Bruce C, Holdsworth CD. Studies on the mechanism of bowel disturbance in ulcerative colitis. Gastroenterology. 1987;93:934–40.
18. Chrysos E, Athanasakis E, Tsiaoussis J *et al.* Recto-anal motility in Crohn's disease patients. Dis Colon Rectum. 2001;44:1509–13.
19. Annese V, Bassotti G, Napolitano G, Usai P, Andriulli A, Vantrappen G. Gastrointestinal motility disorders in patients with inactive Crohn's disease. Scand J Gastroenterol. 1997;32:1107–17.
20. Barbara G, Vallance BA, Collins SM. Persistent intestinal neuro-muscular dysfunction after acute nematode infection in mice. Gastroenterology. 1997;113:1224–32.
21. Barbara G, De Giorgio R, Deng Y, Vallance B, Blennerhassett P, Collins SM. Role of immunologic factors and cyclo-oxygenase$_2$ in persistent post-infective enteric muscle dysfunction in mice. Gastroenterology. 2001;120:1729–36.
22. Isgar B, Harman M, Kaye MD, Whorwell PJ. Symptoms of irritable bowel syndrome in ulcerative colitis in remission. Gut. 1983;24:190–2.

23. Simren M, Axelsson J, Gillberg R, Abrahansson H, Svedlund J, Bjornsson ES. Quality of life in inflammatory bowel disease in remission: the impact of IBS like symptoms and associated psychological factors. Am J Gastroenterol. 2002;97:389–96.
24. Dunlop S, Jenkins D, Naesdal J, Borgaonker M, Collins S, Spiller R. Randomised double-blind placebo controlled trial of prednisolone in post-infectious irritable bowel syndrome. Gastroenterology. 2002;122:(Suppl.):A60.
25. Maxton DG, Morris J, Whorwell PJ. More accurate diagnosis of irritable bowel syndrome by the use of non-colonic symptomatology. Gut. 1991;32:784–6.

8
The symptomatic IBD patient in remission – a manifestation of IBS? – Cons

S. MÜLLER-LISSNER

BACKGROUND

Persistence of irritable bowel syndrome (IBS) symptoms after infective diarrhoea is well established: 6 months after infectious diarrhoea about one-quarter of patients still have IBS symptoms[1,2]. Patients with post-infectious IBS have more intramucosal enteroendocrine cells and CD8 lymphocytes than controls, and similar numbers as in acute *Campylobacter* enteritis[3]. It could also be shown that the colonic epithelial layer of IBS patients harbours more intraepithelial *Escherichia coli* than do controls[4]. Animal studies revealed that the mucosal content of neurotransmitters may be affected by experimental infection: infection of rats with *Trichinella spiralis* led to suppression of norepinephrine release and an increase of substance P[5,6].

RATIONALE

The rationale for the question asked in this contribution is the following. The prevalence of symptoms compatible with IBS in ulcerative colitis in remission is considerable, namely between 30% and 50%[7–9]. In addition, patients with IBS were reported to be at increased risk of developing ulcerative colitis. In one study the relative risk of developing ulcerative colitis after the diagnosis of IBS in 2956 patients (GP diagnosis) during a follow-up of 3 years was 16.3[10]. However, this could not be confirmed in another study with 112 IBS patients who had been diagnosed between 1961 and 1963, fulfilled the Rome I criteria, and were followed up for a mean of 29 years (1–32 years)[11]. It could hence be speculated that a proportion of apparent IBS patients would in fact suffer from inflammatory bowel disease (IBD), be it infectious or idiopathic, i.e. that mild IBD may hide itself behind the label IBS.

PHYSIOLOGICAL STUDIES IN IBS AND IBD

The rectum behaves abnormally in ulcerative colitis. When saline was infused into the rectum of patients with ulcerative colitis the contractile response was increased when compared to controls[12,13] and anal incontinence occurred earlier[13]. This was more pronounced in active colitis than in inactive colitis. However, no assessment of subjective sensation was performed in these older studies, but increased intestinal sensation has been identified in recent years to be an important feature in most patients with IBS[14].

A different picture emerged when perception thresholds to rectal balloon distension were assessed. One study compared IBD patients with inactive or mild ulcerative colitis and IBS patients with healthy controls[15]. In the other study patients with mostly inactive ileal Crohn's disease without any macroscopic or microscopic colonic involvement were studied in comparison to IBS and controls[16]. Both studies specifically excluded patients with abdominal pain or fulfilling the Rome criteria for IBS. It turned out that the rectal pressures to elicit discomfort increased in the following order: IBS < controls < IBD. This was true for both types of IBD, inactive ulcerative colitis and ileal Crohn's disease (Fig. 1).

In another study the modulation of a somatic nociceptive reflex by rectal balloon distension was studied in IBS, IBD, and controls. It was found that both slow ramp and rapid phasic distension of the rectum dampened the nociceptive reflex in IBD but facilitated it in IBS (Fig. 2). Rectal compliance was similar between all three groups[17].

Hence, rectal sensation of patients with IBS and IBD diverts from normal in the opposite direction. IBS is characterized by lower thresholds and thus increased sensibility, whereas IBD patients are less sensitive to rectal stimulation and exhibit a higher threshold.

How can this be explained? One explanation is descending facilitation or inhibition, respectively, of spinal afferent signal transduction (Fig. 3). Another explanation would be altered central processing of the signal by the hypothalamus. It has been shown that the CNS projection of painful and non-painful distension

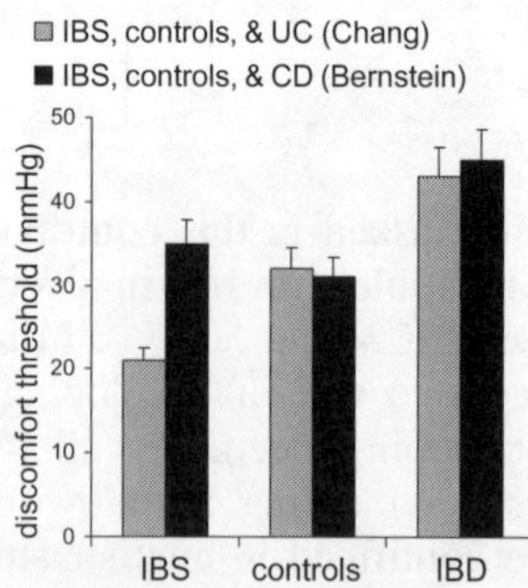

Fig. 1 Perception thresholds to rectal balloon distension in quiescent IBD and IBS. Studies compared 11 patients with inactive ulcerative colitis, 18 IBS patients, and 13 controls (Chang, data from ref. 15), and 12 patients with ileal Crohn's disease (three active), nine diarrhoea-predominant IBS patients, and nine controls (Bernstein, data from ref. 16), respectively. The threshold for discomfort was significantly increased in IBD patients, but normal or even decreased in IBS patients

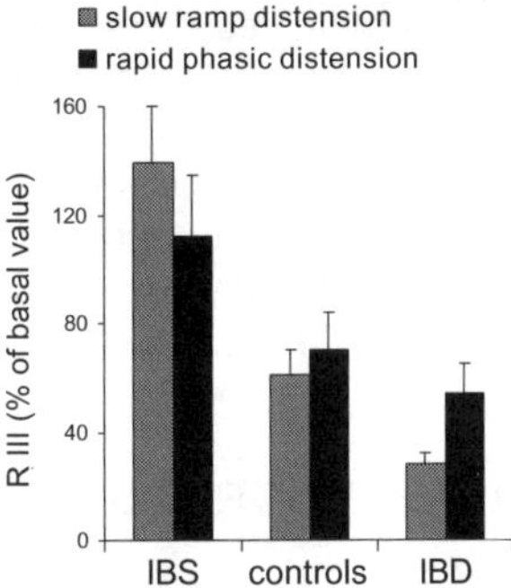

Fig. 2 Modulation of the RIII nociceptive reflex at the lower limb by rectal balloon distension in 14 IBS patients, six patients with inactive IBD (type not specified), and 10 controls. Rectal ballon distension significantly increases the nociceptive reflex in IBS, but lowers it in IBD (data from ref. 17)

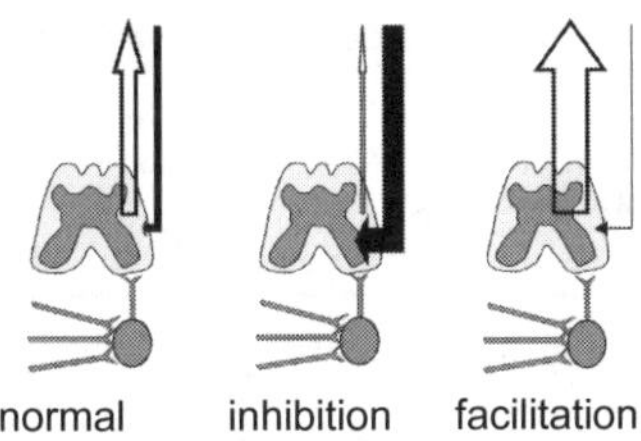

Fig. 3 Schematic drawing of modulation of spinal transduction of peripheral signals by descending inhibition and facilitation ('gating'). This mechanism is amenable to common experience: e.g. an object falling on your feet will hurt more if you see the event coming but will hurt less if you are distracted by another event

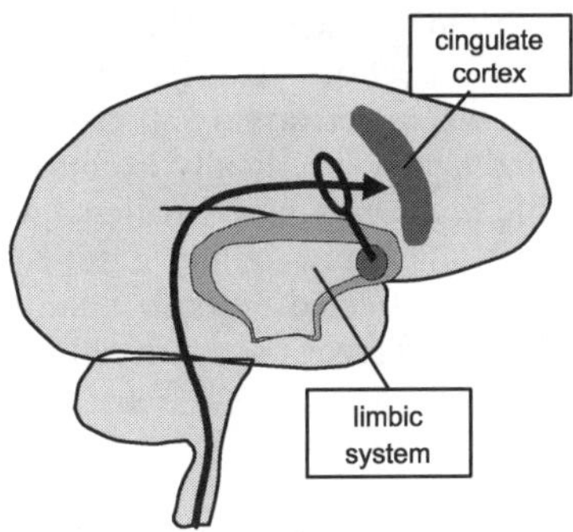

Fig. 4 Painful and non-painful distension of the rectum is projected into the cingulate cortex of the CNS. IBS patients exhibit central hypersensitivity to painful stimuli which is explained by a modulatory function of the limbic system[18]. In IBD patients this modulation could work in the opposite direction than in IBS patients

in IBS to the cingulate cortex is modulated by the limbic system, hence inducing central hypersensitivity to painful stimuli (Fig. 4)[18]. IBD patients have the experience of a chronic or chronic recurrent disease which may severely affect their lives. It is conceivable that these patients behave in a different way than IBS patients, and potentially also than healthy controls, in that they do not pay much attention to sensations from the gut induced by an experimental intervention which they know is not threatening their health.

EVIDENCE FROM THERAPEUTIC TRIALS

An additional argument against a pathophysiological overlap between IBD and IBS can be derived from a therapeutic trial. If residual mucosal inflammation as seen in ulcerative colitis were the basis of IBS, anti-inflammatory treatment such as the one used in ulcerative colitis would be expected to beneficially affect symptoms. Therefore, anti-inflammatory treatment was applied to 31 patients with post-infectious IBS more than 3 months after the acute infection in a randomized double-blind placebo-controlled trial. However, 30 mg of prednisolone for 3 weeks proved no better than placebo on symptoms or cellular infiltrate[19].

Table 1   The symptomatic IBD patient in remission – no manifestation of IBS! The following arguments are against a common pathophysiology

Higher thresholds for rectal discomfort in IBD patients, but not in IBS
Suppression of somatic pain response by rectal painful stimuli in IBD, but not in IBS
No therapeutic effect of anti-inflammatory treatment in post-infectious IBS
'IBS symptoms' are non-specific

CONCLUSIONS

When reviewing the available data it turns out that there is no evidence that the symptomatic IBD patient in remission suffers from a manifestation of IBS. The respective arguments are listed in Table 1. However, some words of caution seem appropriate. First, post-infectious IBS may not be the appropriate model for mild ulcerative colitis when performing a therapeutic trial. Second, the physiological studies quoted above specifically excluded IBD patients with IBS symptoms. It is conceivable that symptomatic patients would behave differently, i.e. similar to IBS patients. If this were the case, however, I would rather conclude that such patients are affected by both conditions, IBD and IBS, and not that they represent different degrees of severity of the same disorder.

References

1. Gwee KA, Graham JC, McKendrick MW *et al*. Psychometric scores and persistence of irritable bowel after infectious diarrhoea. Lancet. 1996;347:150–3.
2. Neal KR, Hebden J, Spiller R. Prevalence of gastrointestinal symptoms six months after bacterial gastroenteritis and risk factors for development of the irritable bowel syndrome: postal survey of patients. Br Med J. 1997;314:779–82.

3. Spiller R, Jenkins D, Thornley JP *et al*. Increased rectal mucosal enteroendocrine cells, T lymphocytes, and increased gut permeability following acute *Campylobacter* enteritis and in post-dysenteric irritable bowel syndrome. Gut. 2000;47:804–11.

4. Swidsinski A, Khilkin M, Kerjaschki D *et al*. Association between intraepithelial *Escherichia coli* and colorectal cancer. Gastroenterology. 1998;115:281–6.

5. Swain MG, Agro A, Blannerhasset P, Stanisz A, Collins SM. Increased level of substance P in the myenteric plexus of *Trichinella*-infected rats. Gastroenterology. 1991;100:675–82.

6. Swain MG, Blannerhasset P, Collins SM. Impaired sympathetic nerve function in the inflamed rat intestine. Gastroenterology. 1991;102:1916–21.

7. Cruz-Santamaria DM, Rey E, Mendoza JL, Paredes JG, Diaz-Rubio M. Irritable bowel syndrome in ulcerative colitis in remission. DDW 2002.

8. Isgar B, Harman M, Kaye MD, Whorwell PJ. Symptoms of irritable bowel syndrome in ulcerative colitis in remission. Gut. 1983;24:190–2.

9. Simren M, Axelsson J, Gillberg R, Abrahamsson H, Svedlund J, Bjornsson ES. Quality of life in inflammatory bowel disease in remission: the impact of IBS-like symptoms and associated psychological factors. Am J Gastroenterol. 2002;97:389–96.

10. Garcia Rodriguez LA, Ruigomez A, Wallander S, Johansson S, Olbe L. Detection of colorectal tumor and inflammatory bowel disease during follow-up of patients with initial diagnosis of irritable bowel syndrome. Scand J Gastroenterol. 2000;35:306–11.

11. Owens DM, Nelson DK, Talley NJ. The irritable bowel syndrome: long-term prognosis and the physician–patient interaction. Ann Intern Med. 1995;122:107–12.

12. Farthing MJ, Lennard-Jones J. Sensibility of the rectum to distension and the anorectal distension reflex in ulcerative colitis. Gut. 1978;19:64–9.

13. Rao SSC, Read NW, Stobart JAH, Haynes WG, Benjamin S, Holdsworth CD. Anorectal contractility under basal conditions and during rectal infusion of saline in ulcerative colitis. Gut. 1988;29:769–77.

14. Thompson WG, Longstreth GF, Drossman DA, Heaton KW, Irvine EJ, Müller-Lissner SA. Functional bowel disorders and functional abdominal pain. Gut. 1999;45(Suppl. II):II43–47.

15. Chang L, Munataka J, Mayer EA *et al*. Perceptual responses in patients with inflammatory and functional bowel disease. Gut. 2000;47:497–505.

16. Bernstein CN, Niazi N, Robert M *et al*. Rectal afferent function in patients with inflammatory and functional intestinal disorders. Pain. 1996;66:151–61.

17. Coffin B, Bouhassira D, Sabate JM, Barbe L, Jian R. Different mechanisms are implicated in the control of pain in patients with inflammatory bowel disease or irritable bowel syndrome. DDW 2002.

18. Mertz H, Morgan V, Tanner G *et al*. Regional cerebral activation in irritable bowel syndrome and control subjects with painful and nonpainful rectal distention. Gastroenterology. 2000;118:842–8.

19. Dunlop S, Jenkins D, Naesdal J, Borgaonker M, Collins S, Spiller R. Randomised double-blind placebo-controlled trial of prednisolone in post-infectious irritable bowel syndrome. DDW 2002.

9
Herbal preparation in functional dyspepsia – *Helicobacter pylori* status is not a predictor for treatment success: results of a double-blind, randomized, placebo-controlled, multicentre trial

A. MADISCH, G. HOLTMANN, G. MAYR, B. VINSON and J. HOTZ[†]

INTRODUCTION

Functional dyspepsia is highly prevalent in western countries and it represents a major reason to seek medical advice[1–4]. The pathophysiology of this disorder remains inadequately understood, even though various mechanisms may play a role in the development of symptoms[3,5]. To date there is no cure for this disorder, and the available treatments are aimed at the relief of symptoms. Even though the efficacy of some currently established treatments (e.g. antisecretory agents or prokinetics) has been proven in placebo-controlled trials, these treatments yield sufficient relief of symptoms only in a proportion of patients[6–9].

Various herbal medications are used in many countries for the treatment of patients with functional dyspepsia, but controlled data supporting the efficacy of these treatments are widely lacking.

For this reason we aimed to investigate, in a placebo-controlled, randomized trial, the efficacy of a herbal preparation that contained six plant extracts (STW-5-II) for the treatment of patients with functional dyspepsia over an 8-week treatment period. Additionally, this clinical trial aimed to assess possible predictive variables for treatment success, especially the *Helicobacter pylori*

[†] Deceased.

status, because several herbal preparations are effective against *H. pylori* and thus metabolic products of *H. pylori* might alter the efficacy of the ingredients.

PATIENTS AND METHODS

Study design and recruitment of patients

The clinical trial was carried out as a randomized, placebo-controlled, double-blind, multicentre study. Outpatients presenting with persistent or recurrent dyspepsia for at least 6 months were recruited by gastroenterologists in private practice or in hospitals. The patients ranged in ages from 21 to 70 years. To be eligible for the trial, patients had to fulfil the Rome I criteria for functional dyspepsia[10]. Patients with symptoms of irritable bowel syndrome or gastro-oesophageal reflux disease (retrosternal pain, burning or regurgitation) dominating the clinical picture were excluded from the study. Structural lesions and other organic diseases were ruled out following a range of clinical evaluations, including upper gastrointestinal endoscopy (during the preceding 6 weeks), abdominal ultrasound, blood counts and serum chemistries. The inclusion and exclusion criteria are summarized in Table 1. At entry, at least three of the dyspeptic symptoms assessed with the gastrointestinal symptom score (GIS) had to be moderate to very severe, based upon the patient's judgement.

Written informed consent was obtained from all patients prior to inclusion in the trial. The study protocol and consent form were approved by an independent ethics committee at each study centre in accordance with the revised Declaration of Helsinki.

Treatment schedule

Prior to randomization the patients had to avoid any medication affecting the gastrointestinal tract for at least 7 days. Each patient was randomly treated

Table 1 Demographic and baseline characteristics of study patients for the various treatment groups

Characteristic	Group A Active (n = 30)	Group B Placebo (n = 30)	p-Value
Female gender (%)	70	70	NS
Age, years, mean ± SD	45.1 ± 13.0	45.2 ± 13.0	NS
Duration of symptoms			
> 6 months– < 12 months	7	11	NS
1– < 2 years	6	7	NS
2– < 5 years	8	7	NS
5 years and more	9	5	NS
H. pylori status (*H. pylori*-positive)	7	6	NS
Median days with dyspepsia in the past 3 months	11.0	11.0	NS
GIS at baseline (mean ± SD)	12.0 ± 4.3	12.5 ± 3.6	NS

NS ($p > 0.15$), no significant difference between the treatment groups at Chi-quadrat test, *F*-Test and Kruskal–Wallis Test; GIS, gastrointestinal symptom score.

during two sequential 4-week treatment periods, either actively with the herbal preparation (active treatment, AT) or with the placebo.

Assessment of dyspeptic symptoms

Primary target variables

At the baseline, and after 4 and 8 weeks, the intensity of dyspeptic symptoms was evaluated by patients' judgement using a Likert scale (absent, 0; mild, 1; moderate, 2; severe, 3; very severe, 4). Symptoms were assessed separately (epigastric pain, sickness, nausea, vomiting, fullness, early satiety, retrosternal discomfort and regurgitation of acid (not dominating the clinical picture), lack of appetite, or bowel cramps (not dominating the clinical picture) and a sum score (GIS) was calculated.

Patients also reported their overall complete relief of symptoms after 4 and 8 weeks. The efficacy of the treatment was also assessed based upon the *H. pylori* status at baseline.

Secondary target variables

The correlation of psychological stress and dyspeptic symptoms, as well as the correlation of dyspeptic symptoms and dyspepsia-related limitations on daily life activities/absenteeism from work, were evaluated based upon data from patients' diary cards.

Randomization, blinding, herbal preparation and placebo

The active medication used in the trial was a herbal preparation (AT) with extracts from bitter candy tuft, matricaria flower, peppermint leaves, caraway, licorice root and lemon balm. A placebo of identical appearance and similar taste was prepared. Treatments were given orally in a double-blind fashion (3 × 20 drops daily). Patients, investigators and study centres maintained strict blinding.

Assessment of *H. pylori* status

Assessment of the *Helicobacter* status was carried out during the endoscopic evaluation utilizing a rapid urease test or histology, using two biopsies from the antrum and one biopsy from the corpus.

Target variables and data analyses

The primary target variables for the assessment of the treatment response were from the global summary score of gastrointestinal symptoms. First, for each individual symptom, a separate analysis of covariance for the differences of symptom intensities during treatment minus symptom intensities at the baseline was performed with medication as the treatment factor and baseline values as the covariate. These analyses yielded adjusted changes in symptom intensities that eliminated the variation in treatment effects that was due to differences in the baseline values. Secondly, these adjusted efficacy variables were standardized and added to O'Brien's global efficacy variable. Logistic regression analyses assess possible predictive variables for treatment success.

Data analyses were done on the basis of intention-to-treat (ITT) analyses. The overall level of significance was controlled using a closed test procedure and *a priori* ordered hypotheses (significance level $p < 0.05$). Statistical analyses were performed utilizing the Statistical Analysis System (SAS version 6.11).

RESULTS

Study population

A total of 60 patients were recruited and randomly assigned to active treatment or placebo. During treatment period II, four patients dropped out from the active treatment group (one due to an adverse event, one due to non-compliance), and two patients dropped out from the placebo group due to insufficient relief of symptoms.

Overall, 75% of the patients were female ($n = 45$). The age ranged from 19 to 71 years with a mean $\pm$ SD of 45.1 ± 13.8 years. The baseline characteristics before treatment are given in Table 2. Patient groups were similar in terms of age, sex, weight, height, medication prescribed in the previous 3 months, smoking, alcohol consumption, GIS at baseline, duration of symptoms, *H. pylori* status and mean days with dyspepsia in the past 3 months.

Follow-up of dyspepsia

GIS scores of the various treatment groups at the baseline and after 4 and 8 weeks of treatment are summarized in Table 3. Patients treated with the active medication improved significantly better compared to patients during placebo treatment ($p < 0.001$) (Table 2).

After 4 weeks, 20.3% ($n = 12$) of those on active treatment and 10.2% ($n = 6$) of those on the placebo reported complete relief of symptoms ($p > 0.05$ vs. placebo); the corresponding rates after 8 weeks were 43.3% ($n = 26$) and 3.3% ($n = 2$) ($p < 0.001$ vs. placebo) (Fig. 1).

Predictors for treatment success

Psychological stress at the baseline and impaired ability to cope with daily life activities within the preceding 3 months of the study were positive predictive variables for a favourable response ($p < 0.001$).

Table 2 Mean ($\pm$ SD) GIS score at baseline and after 4 and 8 weeks of treatment

	Baseline	4 weeks	P-value vs. baseline	8 weeks	P-value vs. 4 weeks
Group A, active ($n = 30$)	12.3 ± 4.7	6.0 ± 4.9	< 0.001	3.9 ± 3.8	< 0.001
Group B, placebo $n = 30$	12.2 ± 3.9	10.1 ± 5.0	NS	9.7 ± 4.9	NS

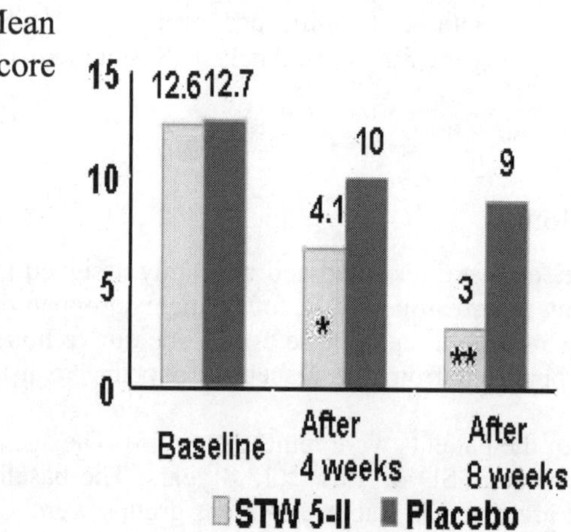

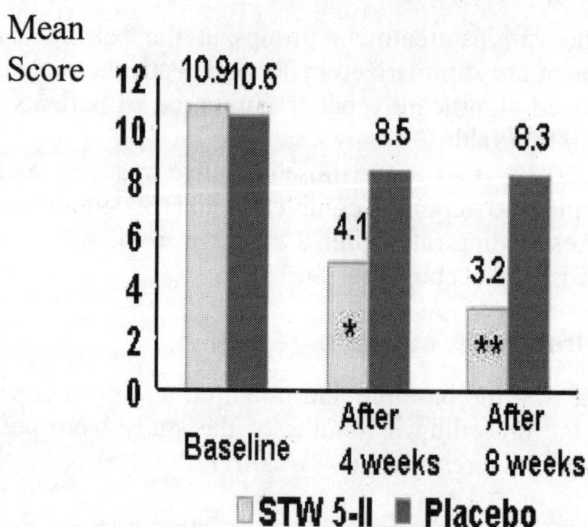

Fig. 1 Efficacy based upon the baseline *H. pylori* (*Hp*) status. No difference between *H. pylori*-positive and negative patients regarding the decrease of GIS after 4 and 8 weeks of treatment ($p = 0.94$ at logistic regression analyses)

No significant association was found between the response to treatment and the predominant type of symptom (i.e. ulcer- or dysmotility-type), the duration of symptoms, a history of functional dyspepsia in relatives, or the *H. pylori* status ($p > 0.05$ for all).

Adverse events and tolerability

No serious side-effects occurred. Four patients in an active treatment period and six patients in a placebo period reported adverse side-effects. In two patients there was a causal link to the treatment, one patient within the placebo treatment (headache, periorbital edema – therapy was interrupted) and one patient within the active treatment (sweating, feeling faint – therapy was continued). Other patients reported incidences of the common cold. Blood chemistry before and after treatment showed no abnormal values.

Tolerability was assessed by the investigators and patients and was found to be very good and good, respectively.

DISCUSSION

The results of this multicentre, randomized, double-blind, placebo-controlled study in patients with functional dyspepsia demonstrate the efficacy of the herbal preparation tested for the relief of dyspepsia. Although several herbal preparations are effective against *H. pylori* and thus metabolic products of *H. pylori* might alter the efficacy of the ingredients, the *H. pylori* status had no influence on the efficacy of the herbal treatment.

Treatments considered efficacious in functional dyspepsia include prokinetics[11] and anticholinergic agents[12], antisecretory drugs[7,8,13,14], sucralfate[15], bismuth and antibiotics[16]. These treatments yield no significant or only a moderate improvement in symptoms. The wide range of therapies prescribed reflects the uncertainty regarding pathogenesis and the lack of satisfactory treatment[6,9,17]. More recently a large, controlled trial on the efficacy of *H. pylori* eradication in functional dyspepsia failed to provide sufficient evidence that *H. pylori* eradication is efficacious[18,19].

Herbal preparations have been used in many countries for the treatment of functional dyspepsia. In spite of this, data to support their use have been widely lacking.

To our knowledge this study is the first randomized trial in functional dyspepsia that tested a herbal preparation for a treatment period of up to 8 weeks. Our findings, however, are in good accordance with two recently published double-blind, placebo-controlled trials that demonstrated a significant improvement of symptoms in patients with irritable bowel syndrome during treatment with a traditional Chinese herbal medicine or a commercially available herbal[20,21]. In addition, May *et al.*, in a double-blind, placebo-controlled trial, demonstrated significant effectiveness of a peppermint oil/caraway oil combination in functional dyspepsia[22]. In a further double-blind equivalence study, Madisch *et al.* showed a comparable efficacy of the same peppermint oil/caraway oil combination to cisapride in patients with functional dyspepsia, but the inadequacy of this study was the missing placebo group[23]. The mechanisms of action remain to be determined. However, it appears that effects on muscle tone or anti-inflammatory effects may play a role. Indeed, experimental studies demonstrated the spasmolytic effects of peppermint oil and a pain-reducing effect in patients with irritable bowel syndrome[20–27]. There is no doubt that further studies are required to identify the mechanisms of action of herbal preparations in patients with functional gastrointestinal disorders. So far, very little is known regarding the mechanism of action of herbals that result in an improvement of symptoms. However, from *in-vitro* studies[28], spasmolytic and anti-inflammatory effects of the ingredients have been observed.

In conclusion, the double-blind, randomized, placebo-controlled trial demonstrated a highly significant and clinically relevant efficacy of the tested herbal preparation in patients with functional dyspepsia after 4 and 8 weeks. Further studies are needed to determine the precise mechanisms of action.

Acknowledgement

This study was sponsored by Steigerwald Arzneimittelwerk GmbH, Darmstadt, Germany. PFK Pharmaforschung Kaufbeuren was responsible for monitoring at the study sites, data collection and source data verification. The authors thank Dr Gunthild Mayr for invaluable help with the study design, organization and all administrative aspects of the trial. The following physicians participated in this study (in alphabetic order): Eiling R, Essen; Feldmann M, Essen; Heydenreich CJ, Essen; Holtmann G, Essen; Krupp P, Bad Zwischenahn; Melderis H, Hamburg; Nemnich H, Hamburg; Rehn L, Essen; Rösch W, Frankfurt.

References

1. Talley NJ, Colin-Jones D, Koch KL, Koch M, Nyrén O, Stanghellini V. Functional dyspepsia: a classification with guidelines for diagnosis and management. Gastroenterol Int. 1991;4:145–60.
2. Barbara L, Camilleri M, Corinaldesi R *et al*. Definition and investigation of dyspepsia. Consensus of an international *ad hoc* working party. Dig Dis Sci. 1989;34:1272–6.
3. Richter JE. Dyspepsia: organic causes and differential characteristics from functional dyspepsia. Scand J Gastroenterol Suppl. 1991;182:11–16.
4. Talley NJ, Holtmann G. Approach to the patient with dyspepsia and related functional gastro-intestinal complaints. In: Yamada T, Alpers DH, Laine L, Owyang C, Powell DW, editors. Textbook of Gastroenterology, 3rd edn. Philadelphia: Lippincott, Williams & Wilkins, 1999: 660–82.
5. Talley NJ, Phillips SF. Nonulcer dyspepsia: potential causes and pathophysiology. Ann Intern Med. 1988;108:865–79.
6. Talley NJ. Drug treatment of functional dyspepsia. Scand J Gastroenterol Suppl. 1991;182: 47–60.
7. Talley NJ, Lauritsen K. The potential role of acid suppression in functional dyspepsia: the BOND, OPERA, PILOT, and ENCORE studies. Gut. 2002;50(Suppl. 4):iv36–41.
8. Bolling-Sternevald E, Lauritsen K, Aalykke C *et al*. Effect of profound acid suppression in functional dyspepsia: a double-blind, randomized, placebo-controlled trial. Scand J Gastroenterol. 2002;37:1395–402.
9. Talley NJ. Review article: Dyspepsia: how to manage and how to treat? Aliment Pharmacol Ther. 2002;16(Suppl. 4):95–104.
10. Drossman DA, Whitehead WE, Corazziari E, Richter JE, Talley NJ, Thompson WG. The functional gastrointestinal disorders and their diagnosis: a coming of age. In: Drossman DA, Richter JE, Talley NJ, Thompson WG, Corazziari E, Whitehead WE, editors. The Functional Gastrointestinal Disorders. Boston: Little, Brown, 1994:1–23.
11. Rösch W. Cisapride in non-ulcer dyspepsia. Results of a placebo-controlled trial. Scand J Gastroenterol. 1987;22:161–4.
12. Stephens CJ, Lever L, Hoare AM. Dicyclomine for idiopathic dyspepsia. Lancet. 1988;1:1004.
13. Talley NJ, McNeil D, Hayden A, Piper DW. Randomized, double-blind, placebo-controlled crossover trial of cimetidine and pirenzepine in nonulcer dyspepsia. Gastroenterology. 1986;91: 149–56.

14. Talley NJ, Meineche-Schmidt V, Pare P *et al.* Efficacy of omeprazole in functional dyspepsia: double-blind randomised placebo-controlled trials. Aliment Pharmacol Ther. 1998;12:1055–65.
15. Otu AA. Perforated peptic ulcer in south-eastern Nigeria 1973–1982. Scand J Gastroenterol Suppl. 1986;124:219–22.
16. Azpiroz F, Malagelada JR. Isobaric intestinal distension in humans: sensorial relay and reflex gastric relaxation. Am J Physiol. 1990;258:G202–7.
17. Holtmann G, Talley NJ. Functional dyspepsia. Current treatment recommendations. Drugs. 1993;45:918–30.
18. Talley NJ, Vakil N, Ballard DE, Fennerty B. Absence of benefit of eradicating *Helicobacter pylori* in patients with non-ulcer dyspepsia. N Engl J Med. 1999;341:1106–11.
19. Blum AL, Talley NJ, O'Morain C *et al.* Lack of effect of treating *Helicobacter pylori* infection in patients with nonulcer dyspepsia. Omeprazole plus clarithromycin and amoxicillin effect one year after treatment (OCAY) Study Group. N Engl J Med 1998;339:1875–81.
20. Bensoussan A, Talley NJ, Hing M, Menzies R, Guo A, Ngu M. Treatment of irritable bowel syndrome with Chinese herbal medicine: a randomized controlled trial. J Am Med Assoc. 1998;280:1585–9.
21. Madisch A, Holtmann G, Plein K, Mayr G, Sassin I, Hotz J. Benefit of a herbal preparation in patients with irritable bowel syndrome: results of a double-blind, randomized, placebo-controlled multicenter trial. Gastroenterology. 2000;118:A4440.
22. May B, Köhler S, Schneider B. Efficacy and tolerability of a fixed peppermint oil and caraway oil in patients suffering from functional dyspepsia. Aliment Pharmacol Ther. 2000;14:1671–7.
23. Madisch A, Heydenreich C-J, Wieland V, Hufnagel R, Hotz J. Equivalence of a fixed peppermint oil and caraway oil combination preparation as compared with cisapride in functional dyspepsia. A multicenter, double-blind, randomized trial. Drug Res. 1999;49:925–32.
24. Veldhuyzen van Zanten SJ, Talley NJ, Bytzer P, Klein KB, Whorwell PJ, Zinsmeister AR. Design of treatment trials for functional gastrointestinal disorders. Gut. 1999;45(Suppl. 2):69–77.
25. Talley NJ, McNeil D, Hayden A, Colreavy C, Piper DW. Prognosis of chronic unexplained dyspepsia. A prospective study of potential predictor variables in patients with endoscopically diagnosed nonulcer dyspepsia. Gastroenterology. 1987;92:1060–6.
26. Duthie HL. The effect of peppermint oil on colonic motility in man. Br J Surg. 1981;68:820–4.
27. Hills JM, Aaronson PI. The mechanism of action of peppermint oil on gastrointestinal smooth muscle. An analysis using patch clamp electrophysiology and isolated tissue pharmacology in rabbit and guinea pig. Gastroenterology. 1991;101:55–65.
28. Okpanyi SN, Mark M, Wahl MA. Gastrointestinal motility modulation with Iberogast®. Acta Hort. 1993;3332:227–35.

10
Intestinal gas dynamics and tolerance are modified by the different components of nutrients

H. HARDER, A. C. HERNANDO-HARDER,
H.-J. KRAMMER and M. V. SINGER

INTRODUCTION

Functional intestinal symptoms, which means symptoms without any demonstrable cause, are common[1,2] and tend to arise postprandially[3,4]. Especially symptoms such as fullness and abdominal bloating are frequently attributed to intestinal gas, but may reflect a broad spectrum of problems[5] (Fig. 1). There is evidence that intestinal gas, besides various other factors, particularly visceral sensitivity, may be involved in generating abdominal complaints[6–9]. Nevertheless, in contrast to patients with irritable bowel syndrome, handling of intestinal gas in healthy persons is generally a dynamic and efficient process, virtually unperceived, and large amounts of gas are accommodated, propulsed and evacuated without any symptom perception[10]. Mechanisms governing intestinal gas dynamics and roles of interacting mechanical and/or chemical stimuli are poorly understood; however, impaired gas handling may lead to gas retention, distension, and symptoms[9,11–16]. Meal-related factors such as the amount and consistency of ingested food, time for eating, eating under stress conditions and composition of the meal (fatty, fibre- or protein-rich diet) are commonly thought responsible for the occurrence of postprandial complaints[3]. We hypothesized that different intraluminal nutrients exert specific effects, both on handling of intestinal gas and visceral symptom perception, mainly influenced by the meal composition. Thus our specific aim was to study the effect of different intraluminal nutrients mimicking physiological postprandial flow rates on: (a) intestinal gas dynamics, (b) basal abdominal and rectal perception and perception thresholds with concomitant intestinal gas load. We assigned (c) types of symptoms and symptom distribution to specific components of nutrients. Furthermore we (d) correlated nutrient-induced gas

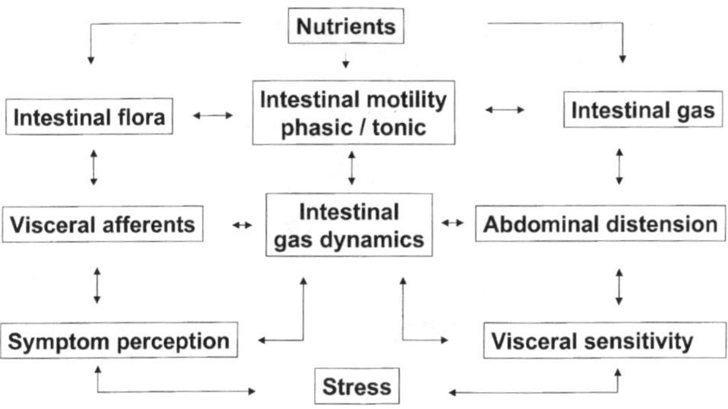

Fig. 1 Intestinal interactions/gas

retention with objective distension and symptom generation. Distending the intestine may, independently from the specific effect of the nutrient ingested, stimulate afferent input[3], heighten visceral sensitivity by so-called 'spatial summation phenomena' and disrupt normal tonic and phasic intestinal motility[17].

MEASUREMENT OF INTESTINAL GAS DYNAMICS

Participants

Thirty-two healthy individuals (20 women and 12 men; age range 22–42 years) participated in the study after giving written informed consent. Subjects completed a pre-entry questionnaire to determine the absence of gastrointestinal symptoms, including constipation, difficult gas evacuation, feeling of excessive abdominal gas or excessive gas evacuation. The protocol for the study had been previously approved by the ethics committee of the University of Mannheim.

Intraluminal tubes

Ileal tube assembly

We used a multilumen polyvinyl tube assembly (3.2 mm OD) that incorporated a gas infusion channel (1.2 mm ID) with multiple side holes at the tip of the tube (120 cm distal to the angle of Treitz), a nutrients infusion channel (1.2 mm ID) opening in duodenum (Fig. 2).

Rectal tube assembly

We used an intrarectal Foley catheter (20 French) which was inserted into the rectum with multiple eccentric located openings for gas recovery.

Measurement of gas transit

Jejunal gas infusion

Gas was infused continuously into the proximal jejunum at 12 ml/min using a modified volumetric pump (B. Braun Melsungen AG). We infused a gas mixture

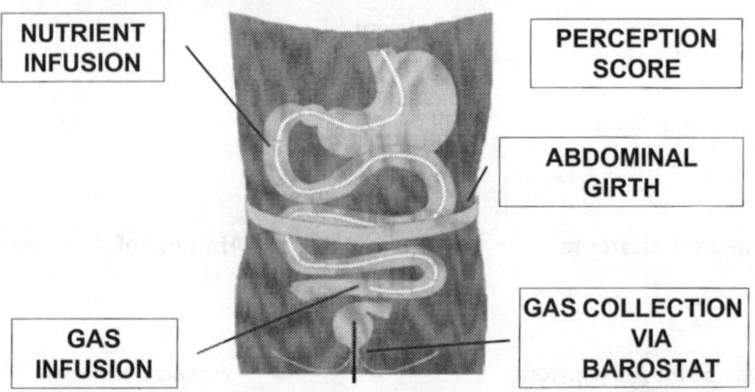

Fig. 2 Measurement of intestinal gas dynamics

containing 88% nitrogen, 6.5% carbon dioxide, and 5.5% oxygen, bubbled into water for saturation, mimicking the partial pressures of venous blood gases to minimize diffusion across the intestinal–blood barrier. A non-absorbable, stable gaseous marker, 5% sulphur hexafluoride (SF_6), was added to the gas mixture infused during the first 10 min of infusion.

Measurement of anal gas evacuation

Intestinal gas evacuation was collected via the rectal tube connected to a computerized barostat (Fig. 2). The volume of gas evacuated was continuously recorded (Tensotat-Barostat; Sicie, Barcelona, Spain). A sample of gas evacuated during each 30-min period was stored in metallized containers for later analysis of SF_6 concentration by infrared absorbance after determination of standard curves.

Measurement of abdominal girth changes

Subjects were placed in bed (see Procedure below), and then a non-stretch 48-mm wide belt with a metric tape measure was adjusted around the abdomen over the umbilicus by means of two elastic bands. Girth measurements were taken at 15-min intervals while the subjects were breathing relaxed as the average of inspiratory and expiratory determinations over three consecutive respiratory excursions.

Duodenal nutrients infusion

The experiments were performed during a continuous infusion with either isotonic saline (Isotonische Natriumchlorid-Lösung, Boehringer Ingelheim Delta Pharma GmbH, 72793 Pfullingen, Germany); lipids (Lipovenös 20%, Fresenius Kabi Deutschland GmbH, D61346 Bad Homburg v.d.H, Germany) diluted in saline; proteins (Intrafusin 15%E, Baxter Deutschland GmbH, D85716 Unterschlißheim, Germany) or glucose (Glucose-Lösung 10% Boehringer Ingelheim Delta Pharma GmbH, 72793 Pfullingen, Germany) at a rate of 2 ml/min (1 kcal/min) using a volumetric pump (Asid Bonz PP 50-300; Lubratronics, Unterschleissheim, Germany).

Perception questionnaire

Subjective perception was measured at 15-min intervals using a graded questionnaire to measure the intensity and type of sensations perceived, and an anatomical questionnaire to measure the location and extension of the perceived sensations. The graded questionnaire included four graphic rating scales graded from 0 (no perception) to 6 (pain), specifically for scoring the following abdominal sensations: (a) pressure/bloating, (b) cramp/colicky sensation, (c) stinging sensation, and (d) other types of sensation (to be specified), respectively. The questionnaire included an additional rating scale for scoring rectal perception, and a tick box (yes/no) to mark belching. Participants were asked to score any perceived sensation (one or more perceived simultaneously) on the scales. The anatomical questionnaire incorporated a diagram of the abdomen divided into nine regions corresponding to epigastrium, periumbilical area, hypogastrium, both hypochondria, flanks, and iliac fossae. Participants were instructed to mark the location, i.e. abdominal region(s), where the sensations were perceived.

Procedure

During the 2 days preceding the study participants were instructed to follow a diet excluding gas-producing foodstuffs. Participants were required to have one bowel movement within the 12 h prior to the study; otherwise, the study was

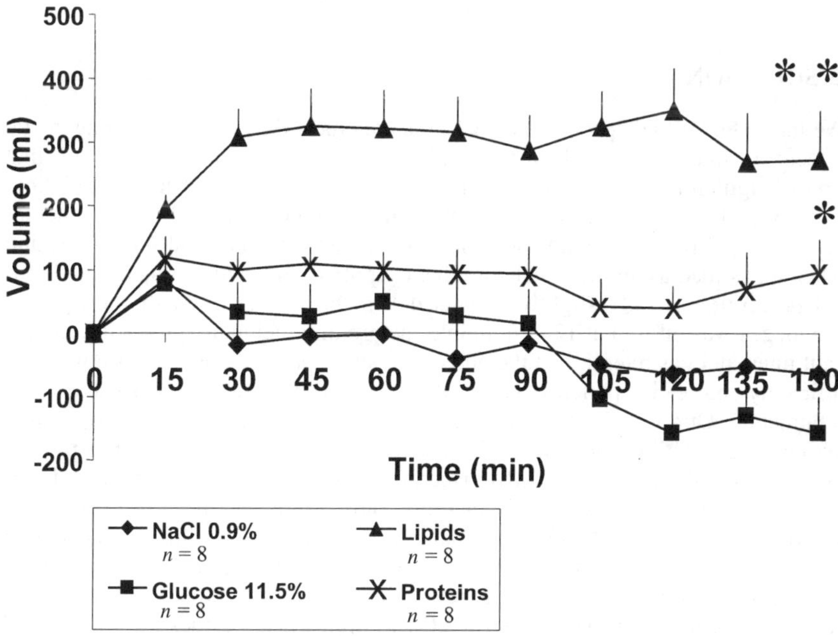

Fig. 3 Intestinal gas retention (volume of gas infused minus evacuated) during continuous intraduodenal nutrient infusion (1 kcal/min) and concomitant gas infusion (12 ml/min); $*p < 0.05$ vs. NaCl and glucose; $**p < 0.05$ vs. proteins; $\overline{\delta} \pm$ SE

postponed. On the day of the study participants were intubated after a 8-h fasting period. The intestinal tube assembly was orally introduced and was positioned under fluoroscopic control with the gas infusion port located 120 cm caudal to the angle of Treitz, and the nutrients infusion port in the proximal duodenum. The rectal tube was then introduced. The studies were conducted in a quiet, isolated room with the subjects placed supine in bed at an angle of 30°.

RESULTS

Both lipids and proteins led to significant abdominal gas retention (271 ± 78 ml and 96 ± 51 ml, $p < 0.05$ vs. control), whereas lipids had a more pronounced effect, also increasing significantly abdominal girth (3 ± 1 mm, $p < 0.05$ vs. control), and heightening abdominal (2.3 ± 0.6 score, $p < 0.05$ vs. control) as well as rectal perception (1.9 ± 0.5 score, $p < 0.05$ vs. control). Protein-induced abdominal gas retention was low (96 ± 51 ml) and no significant changes in abdominal girth (1 ± 1 mm) or abdominal or rectal perception were seen (1 ± 0.5 and 1 ± 0.3 score). In contrast, after intraduodenal glucose, negative gas retention similar to saline as control ($-157 ± 57$ ml and $-63 ± 29$ ml) was observed, without significant changes in abdominal girth (0 ± 1 mm and 0 ± 1 mm) and abdominal (1.1 ± 0.3 and 0.6 ± 0.2 score) or rectal perception (1.3 ± 0.7 and 0.1 ± 0.1 score) for glucose and saline, respectively (for gas retention see Fig. 3).

DISCUSSION

We have shown that specific meal components have different, even antagonistic effects on intestinal gas dynamics and tolerance in humans. It is known that lipids heighten intestinal sensitivity to mechanical but not electrical stimulation. The level of sensitization of mechanosensitive afferents induced by fat, whether central or peripheral, remains unclear[3]. Lipids increase intestinal sensitivity, and when a gas load as an intestinal stimulus is applied, in healthy subjects, abdominal perception is only slightly increased[9]. In the former work of the Spanish group, gas was infused at 12 ml/min into the proximal jejunum, producing significant intestinal gas retention at the end of the study period. Gas retention was significantly more in patients with IBS[7] and responded to pharmacological treatment[18]. Our aim was to investigate the role of intestinal gas for postprandial symptom generation, showing the influences of food composition on postprandial (a) intestinal gas dynamics, (b) visceral sensitivity, and (c) objective abdominal distension. We have shown that not only lipids but also proteins (at 1 kcal/min) induce significant intestinal gas retention in healthy humans with slightly increased abdominal perception while infusing lipids into the duodenum. Glucose failed to induce gas retention, in contrast, expediting gas transit from the beginning on. This opposite effect implies that, besides the volume and the caloric content of a meal, its composition plays an important role for specific postprandial effects on intestinal gas dynamics and tolerance. Abdominal and rectal symptoms depend only partly on the total volume of gas retained in the gut, initiated by the specific nutrient ingested. Underlying mechanisms and neurohormonal pathways need to be further investigated.

Acknowledgement

This work was supported in part by the 'Forschungsfonds der Fakultät für Klinische Medizin Mannheim der Universität Heidelberg'.

References

1. Maxton DG, Martin DF, Whorwell PJ, Godfrey M. Abdominal distension in female patients with irritable bowel syndrome: exploration and possible mechanisms. Gut. 1991;32:662–4.
2. Poynard T, Hernandez M, Xu P, Couturier D *et al*. French Cooperative Study Group. Visible abdominal distension and gas surface: description of an automatic method of evaluation and application to patients with irritable bowel syndrome and dyspepsia. Eur J Gastroenterol Hepatol. 1992;4:831–6.
3. Accarino AM, Azpiroz F, Malagelada J-R. Modification of small bowel mechanosensitivity by intestinal fat. Gut. 2001;48:690–5.
4. Accarino AM, Azpiroz F, Malagelada J-R. Gut perception in humans is modulated by interacting gut stimuli. Am J Gastroint Liver Physiol. 2002;282:G220–5.
5. Camilleri M. Therapeutic approach to the patient with irritable bowel syndrome. Am J Med. 1999;8:107:27–32S.
6. Serra J, Azpiroz F, Malagelada J-R. Mechanisms of intestinal gas retention in humans: impaired propulsion vs. obstructed evacuation. Am J Physiol. 2001;281:G138–43.
7. Serra J, Azpiroz F, Malagelada J-R. Impaired handling and tolerance of intestinal gas in the irritable bowel syndrome. Gut. 2001;48:14–19.
8. Serra J, Azpiroz F, Malagelada J-R. Abdominal symptoms, distension and intestinal gas retention induced by lipids. Gastroenterology. 1999;116:A1081.
9. Serra J, Azpiroz F, Malagelada J-R. Gastric distension and duodenal lipid infusion modulate intestinal gas transit and tolerance in humans. Am J Gastroenterol. 2002;97:2225–30.
10. Serra J, Azpiroz F, Malagelada J-R. Intestinal gas dynamics and tolerance in humans. Gastroenterology. 1998;115:542–50.
11. Harder H, Serra J, Azpiroz F, Malagelada J-R. Reflex control of intestinal gas dynamics and tolerance. Gastroenterology. 2000;118:A3778.
12. Harder H, Serra J, Azpiroz F, Malagelada J-R. Responses of intestinal gas loads: proximal versus distal source. Gastroenterology. 2001;122:A32987.
13. Levitt MD. Volume and composition of human intestinal gas determined by means of an intestinal washout technique. N Engl J Med. 1971;284:1394–8.
14. Levitt MD. Production and excretion of hydrogen gas in man. N Engl J Med. 1969;281:122–7.
15. Levitt MD, Bond JH. Volume, composition and source of intestinal gas. Gastroenterology. 1970;59:921–9.
16. Serra J, Salvioli B, Azpiroz F, Malagelada J-R. Lipid-induced intestinal gas retention in irritable bowel syndrome. Gastroenterology. 2002;123:700–6.
17. Serra J, Azpiroz F, Malagelada J-R. Modulation of gut perception in humans by spatial summation phenomena. J Physiol. 1998;506:579–87.
18. Caldarella M, Serra J, Azpiroz F, Malagelada J-R. Prokinetic effects in patients with intestinal gas retention. Gastroenterology. 2002;122:1748–55.

Section IV
Inflammation and nerve function

11
Vagal afferents and regulation of inflammation and hyperalgesia in remote body domains

W. JÄNIG and J. D. LEVINE

INTRODUCTION

The body is continuously threatened by stimuli originating in the external world and within the body. These challenges are met by multiple mechanisms for protection. The mechanisms involved are related to the immune system, the nociceptive system, the autonomic nervous systems (notably the sympathetic nervous system), the neuroendocrine systems and centrally organized programmes which orchestrate these systems. The protective mechanisms enable the organism to function in the confines of a dynamic and frequently challenging and dangerous environment. The mechanisms of protection are continuously active and therefore also continuously adapted to the actual situation of the organism. They function in the fast (seconds to hours) and slow (days to months) time domains. Unravelling these mechanisms is important to understand the principles of curative components in medicine which are based on biological processes. The use of these biologically operating mechanisms should theoretically lead to better therapeutic strategies for treating various diseases. Understanding the principles of the underlying mechanisms would also lead to the formulation of a better scientific basis of psychosomatic medicine.

This chapter concentrates on possible mechanisms which underlie the neural and neuroendocrine controls of inflammation and mechanical hyperalgesia (generated by sensitization of nociceptors). Both are protective mechanisms of the body which are represented and integrated in the brain (brainstem, hypothalamus, limbic system and neocortex). Perceptions of painful sensations, autonomic responses, endocrine responses and somatomotor responses occur principally in parallel, and are therefore parallel 'read-outs' of the central representations (Fig. 1). The central representations obtain continuous afferent neural, hormonal and other signals which monitor the state of the different tissues.

Inflammation and hyperalgesia following tissue trauma are protective reactions which further healing. Mechanisms of inflammation are commonly

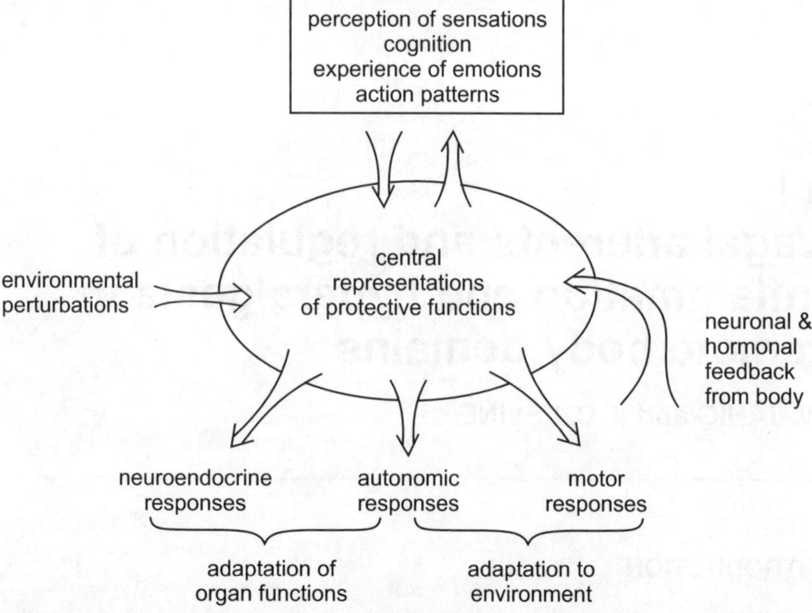

Fig. 1 Central representations of protective mechanisms, their output systems and afferent input systems. Activation of these representations leads to neuroendocrine, autonomic and somatomotor responses and to special perceptions. The central representations are adapted by the forebrain mechanisms (action patterns). They obtain continuously afferent feedback information from the different body domains. The afferent feedback is neuronal, hormonal and humoral (e.g. glucose concentration, osmolality) and of other nature (e.g. body core temperature). A powerful feedback from the viscera occurs via vagal afferent neurons. (Modified from ref. 1)

considered to be confined to the periphery involving immune-competent and related inflammatory cells as well as vascular cells. The main mechanism of hyperalgesia during inflammation in this view is confined to the sensitization of nociceptors by inflammatory mediators leading to central changes (central sensitization) and appropriate protective behaviour. However, using animal models of experimental inflammation of the knee joint synovia and mechanical hyperalgesic behaviour, it has recently been shown that both inflammation and nociceptor sensitization are potentially under the control of the sympatho-adrenal system (as well as probably of the hypothalamo-pituitary axis [HPA]), implying that the brain can influence both via this system. Although both animal models (bradykinin-induced plasma extravasation in the synovia of the rat knee; bradykinin-induced mechanical hyperalgesic behaviour) are rather artificial and specific, and although we have up to now no human models and no clinical situation which correspond to these animal models, it is of interest to learn from these animal models in which way neuroendocrine systems can principally influence peripheral mechanisms of inflammation and nociceptor sensitization.

This chapter will discuss results, obtained on these two animal models, which show that vagal afferents that innervate the small intestine can influence, via the sympatho-adrenal system, inflammatory processes in the knee synovia and

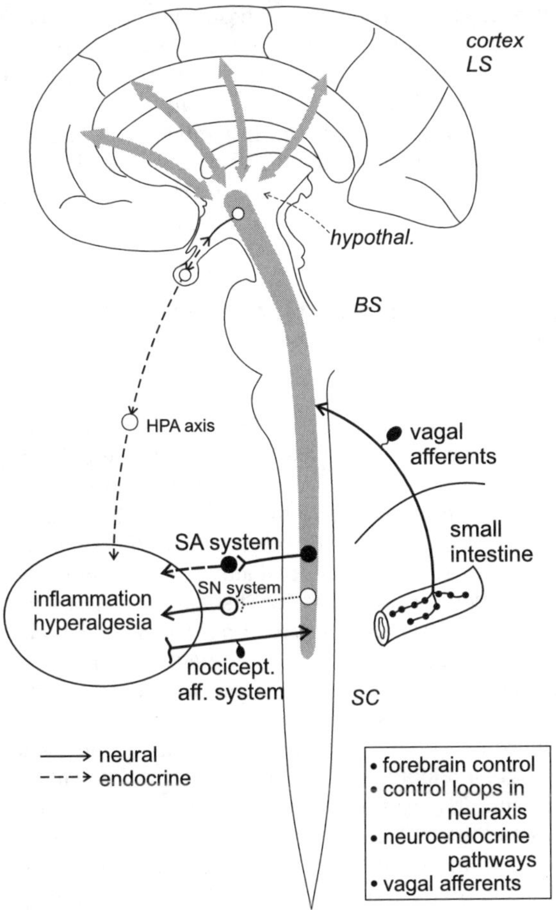

Fig. 2 The neuraxis contains neuronal circuits which control nociceptor sensitivity and inflammation in the periphery of the body via the sympatho-adrenal (SA) system and the hypothalamo-pituitary-adrenal (HPA) system. The sympathoneural (SN) system is also involved too (see footnote †). Feedback information from the peripheral inflammatory process occurs via nociceptive primary afferent neurons and cytokines. Vagal afferents from the gastrointestinal tract (and probably from other organs) modulate these central integrative processes. The forebrain controls the inflammation and sensitivity of nociceptors via the circuits in the neuraxis (see shaded double arrows). BS, brainstem; LS, limbic system; SC, spinal cord

sensitivity of cutaneous nociceptors.* The results imply indirectly that (Fig. 2):

1.   there exist a special set of vagal afferents which innervate the small intestine (including distal duodenum and proximal colon) and monitor events in the visceral domain related to (potentially damaging) stimuli (e.g. toxins);

---

* At the Falk Symposium 99 held in Titisee in the Black Forest 1997 I presented similar data[2]. In the meantime the story developed in a highly interesting direction which could not have been predicted at that time (see also footnote ‡).

2. the final pathway to the peripheral tissue is a neuroendocrine system;

3. the neuraxis has distinct neural circuits, probably related to the endogenous neural system controlling nociceptive impulse transmission[3], which link vagal afferent neurons and neuroendocrine system;

4. the sensitivity of nociceptors and inflammation in the somatic domain is potentially under remote control from the viscera via vagal afferents; and

5. the forebrain can modulate these neural circuits in the neuraxis and in this way has access to the peripheral protective mechanisms of the body.

ABDOMINAL VAGAL AFFERENTS AND PROTECTION OF THE BODY

The abdominal vagus nerves contain 80–85% visceral afferent fibres and 15–20% preganglionic parasympathetic fibres[4,5]. The vagal afferents innervate the gastrointestinal tract (GIT) and associated organs (e.g. liver, pancreas). The vagal afferents encode in their activity mechanical and chemical events of the GIT. They project viscerotopically to the nucleus of the solitary tract (NTS[6,7]). The second-order neurons in the NTS project to various sites in the lower brainstem, upper brainstem, hypothalamus and amygdala, establishing well-organized neural pathways which are the basis for distinct regulations of GIT functions. The *preganglionic parasympathetic axons* have their cell bodies in the dorsal motor nucleus of the vagus nerve. These efferent neurons are also topographically organized and establish final efferent pathways for the regulation of various functions of the GIT[8] (see refs 6 and 7).

The small intestine is a very vulnerable portal of entry into the body and therefore it is of great teleological advantage to have a potent local defence system as well as an early-warning system to the rest of the body for entry of microorganisms and toxins located there. This part of the GIT does, in fact, contain a powerful immune system (the gut-associated lymphoid tissue [GALT][9]). The small intestine is innervated by vagal afferents that project through the coeliac branches of the abdominal vagus nerve. Specific modulation of activity in these afferents in conjunction with the reaction of the GALT may act as an early-warning system to the rest of the body by transmitting important information to the brain concerning toxic events and agents in the intestine which are dangerous for the organism[10].

Recent experimental investigations support the idea that abdominal vagal afferents may be important for protective functions of the GIT and the body:

1. Electrical stimulation of abdominal vagal afferents exerts inhibition or excitation of the central nociceptive system and depresses nociceptive behaviour, depending on whether unmyelinated or myelinated afferents are stimulated[11,12].

2. When injected intraperitoneally in rats, illness-inducing agents, such as the bacterial cell wall endotoxin lipopolysaccharide (LPS), produce behavioural hyperalgesia. This is mediated by activity in subdiaphragmatic vagal afferents, specifically afferents running in the hepatic branch. It is suggested that LPS activates

hepatic macrophages (Kupffer cells) which release interleukin-1β (IL-1β) and tumour necrosis factor α (TNF-α). This in turn activates vagal afferents from the liver. By the same token, IL-1β and TNF-α injected intraperitoneally themselves generate behavioural hyperalgesia (enhancement of the thermal nociceptive tail-flick reflex) which is abolished by vagotomy[13–18]. These results suggest that vagal afferents innervating the liver (another internal defence line in the body) are activated by cytokines released by activated leucocytes and signal these events to the brain resulting in pain behaviour (i.e. an enhanced tail-flick reflex). Watkins and co-workers suggest that the IL-1 (and possibly TNF-α) released by the Kupffer cells binds specifically to glomus cells in the abdominal paraganglia which are innervated by vagal afferents; the vagal afferents are activated and signal the peripheral events to the brain, leading to hyperalgesia and other illness responses (see below).

3.   Recently it has been shown that the first (fast) phase of the fever response which can be generated in the rat and guinea-pig by intravenous injection of the endotoxin LPS is mediated by vagal afferents which possibly innervate the liver[19,20]. This fast component of fever generated by LPS is abolished after abdominal vagotomy. Activation of vagal afferents by LPS leads to activation of neurons in the nucleus tractus solitarius (NTS) and subsequently of noradrenergic neurons in the A1 and A2 areas of the brainstem which project to the hypothalamus.

4.   Pain behaviour mediated by vagal afferents, which are activated by intraperitoneal injection of LPS, is part of a general sickness behaviour characterized by various protective illness responses (e.g. immobility, decrease in food intake, formation of taste aversion to novel foods, decrease of digestion, loss of weight (anorexia), fever, increase of sleep, change in endocrine functions, malaise, etc.) and is correlated with marked alterations of brain function. For example, food aversions and anorexia are generated in rats by TNF (injected intraperitoneally) and subcutaneous implantation of Leydig LTW(m) tumour cells. Both sickness behaviours are abolished or attenuated by subdiaphragmatic vagotomy[21,22]. By the same token it has been shown that endotoxin injected intraperitoneally generates profound changes in various brain areas in rodents (such as c-fos expression in neurons of the NTS and in hypothalamic nuclei as well as induction of IL-1β mRNA in the pituitary gland, hypothalamus and hippocampus). These changes do not occur, or are significantly attenuated, in subdiaphragmatically vagotomized animals[23–25].

5.   Vagal afferents in the coeliac branches of the abdominal vagus nerve monitor chemical and mechanical events that occur in the intestine under physiological and pathophysiological conditions (for review see ref. 26), i.e. are related to meals, ingestion of toxic substances, inflammation, obstruction, etc. Neurophysiological recordings have shown that these afferents respond to distension or contraction of the small intestine and to intraluminal chemical stimulation. Cholecystokinin released locally, in response to chemical stimuli, may activate these afferents[27] and sensitize them for mechanical and other stimuli[28–30]. Cells of the mucosa may function as secondary sensory cells and modulate activity in vagal afferents via paracrine actions[31]. These afferents may be important for preabsorptive detection of energy-yielding molecules and probably

for other properties of nutrient solutions which may be toxic and deleterious for the GIT and for the body[32,33]. Additionally some vagal afferents which innervate the small intestine and the liver respond to cytokines (e.g. IL-1β); these afferents may encode events which are related to the immune system of the GIT and liver[34].

NOCICEPTIVE–NEUROENDOCRINE CONTROL OF EXPERIMENTAL INFLAMMATION MEDIATED BY THE SYMPATHO-ADRENAL SYSTEM IS ENHANCED AFTER VAGOTOMY

The synovia exhibits under resting conditions a baseline plasma extravasation. Bradykinin infused into the rat knee joint cavity increases plasma extravasation by about five times the baseline plasma extravasation (for details of knee joint perfusion, bradykinin concentrations and measurements of plasma extravasation

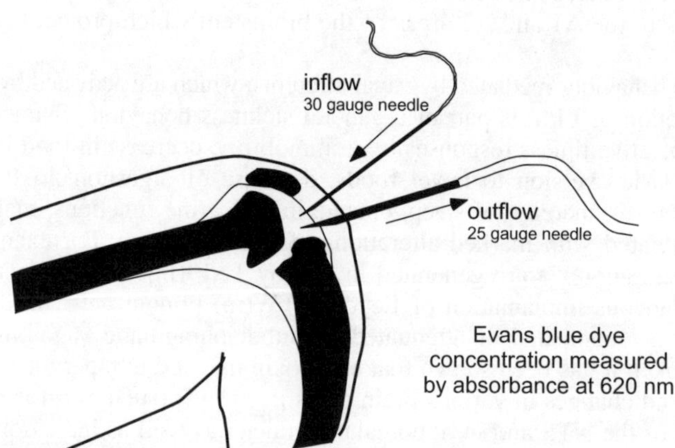

Fig. 3 The perfused knee joint of the rat as a model to study mechanisms of neurogenic inflammation and its control. After incision of the skin and connective tissue overlying the anterior aspect of the knee and the saphenous vein, Evans blue dye (50 mg kg^{-1}) is administered intravenously in the saphenous vein. Ten minutes after injection of the dye a 30-gauge needle is inserted into the cavity of the knee joint for the infusion of fluid (250 μl min^{-1}, controlled by a syringe pump from Sage Instruments, Model 351, Cambridge, MA). After infusion of an initial volume of 100–200 μl of vehicle, a second needle (25-gauge) is inserted into the knee joint, approximately 3 mm from the inflow needle. This second needle serves as an outflow cannula. Fluid is withdrawn from the joint through the outflow cannula using a second syringe pump. The fluid is infused and withdrawn at a constant rate of 250 μl min^{-1}. Perfusate samples are collected every 5 min for up to 120 min. Samples are analysed for the amount of Evans blue dye by spectrophotometric measurement of absorbance at 620 nm. The absorbance at this wavelength is linearly related to the dye concentration[37] and therefore to the degree of plasma extravasation of the synovia (see ordinate scale in Figs 4 and 6). After a baseline perfusion period of 15 min with vehicle (normal saline), plasma extravasation into the knee joint is stimulated by adding bradykinin (160 ng ml^{-1}, i.e. 0.15 μM) to the perfusion fluid[35]. The concentration of bradykinin in various inflamed tissues is in the range of 50 nM to 0.1 μM[38,39]. (Modified from Green, with permission; figure from P. Green).

see Fig. 3 and legend of Fig. 3, as well as the literature[35,36]). This increase in plasma extravasation lasts throughout the bradykinin infusion with a decay by about 10% by 90 min (crosses in Fig. 4A,B)[†].

Stimulation of cutaneous nociceptors in the hindpaw by injection of capsaicin at doses of 3–30 μg into the plantar skin of the contralateral hindlimb decreases the bradykinin-induced plasma extravasation only weakly but significantly at 30 μg (circles in Fig. 4A). Intra-plantar injection of capsaicin, in these doses, into the denervated plantar skin (sciatic and saphenous nerves cut) has no effect on bradykinin-induced plasma extravasation. Furthermore, intra-plantar injection of capsaicin has no effect on plasma extravasation generated by platelet-activating factor (10^{-7} M) in the rat knee joint (data not shown). Stimulation of nociceptors in the forepaw by intra-palmar injection of capsaicin decreases bradykinin-induced plasma extravasation significantly at doses of 3–30 μg. This depression is significantly stronger than that elicited from the hindpaw (circles in Fig. 4B). After denervation of the adrenal medullae, by bilateral severing of the preganglionic axons in the adrenal nerve, intra-plantar injection of capsaicin no longer significantly inhibits bradykinin-induced plasma extravasation at 30 μg (open triangles in Fig. 4A; not shown for the forepaw). Stimulation of spinal visceral afferents by intraperitoneal or intravesical injection of capsaicin also powerfully inhibits bradykinin-induced plasma extravasation[40,41].

After acute subdiaphragmatic vagotomy depression of bradykinin-induced plasma extravasation generated by intraplantar injection of capsaicin is strongly enhanced. This inhibition is now already significant at 3 μg and decreases to 20–30% of the maximal bradykinin-induced plasma extravasation at the dose of 30 μg (closed circles in Fig. 4A). For the forepaw stimulation the potentiating effect of vagotomy is smaller than for the hindpaw stimulation being most notable at 30 μg (closed circles in Fig. 4B). In vagotomized animals with denervated adrenal medullae stimulation of nociceptors by capsaicin injected in the hindpaw or forepaw does not significantly depress bradykinin-induced plasma extravasation (closed triangles in Fig. 4A,B). The degree of bradykinin-induced plasma extravasation in these animals is not significantly different from that in animals with denervated adrenal medullae but intact vagus nerves (compare open triangles with closed triangles in Fig. 4A) and is slightly reduced when compared to the controls (no capsaicin, compare crosses with closed triangles in Fig. 4A,B).

The following conclusions can be drawn from these experiments:

1.   Noxious stimulation of skin by intradermal capsaicin leads to depression of synovial plasma extravasation. This depression is mediated by the sympatho-adrenal system (adrenal medullae). The signal to the synovia is most likely

---

[†] Bradykinin-induced plasma extravasation of the knee joint synovia which occurs at the venular side of the vascular bed is reduced to about 30% after surgical sympathectomy (removal of the postganglionic neurons) but not after decentralization of the postganglionic neurons (cutting the preganglionic axons). Thus this synovial plasma extravasation is dependent on the innervation of the synovia by sympathetic postganglionic axons but not on activity (action potentials) in these axons and not on release of noradrenaline. The idea is that the varicosities of the sympathetic postganglionic axons mediate directly or indirectly the effect of bradykinin (see refs 35 and 36). Details regarding the underlying mechanism of this novel function of postganglionic sympathetic terminals have not been explored so far.

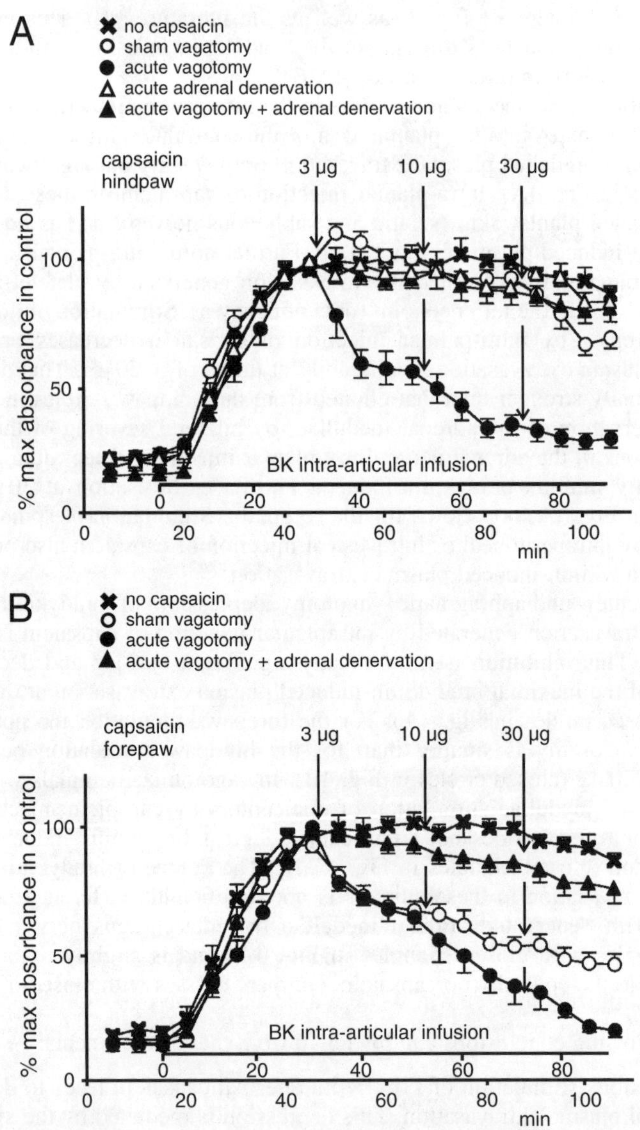

Fig. 4 Inhibition of bradykinin-induced plasma extravasation by stimulation of nociceptors by capsaicin (CAP) is mediated by the sympatho-adrenal axis and enhanced after vagotomy. Effect of intradermal injection of CAP (3–30 µg) into the plantar skin of hindpaw (**A**) or into the palmar skin of the forepaw (**B**) on bradykinin-induced plasma extravasation in the knee joint in sham-vagotomized rats (open circles), in vagotomized rats (closed circles), in rats with intact vagus nerves and denervated adrenal medullae (open triangles) and in vagotomized rats with denervated adrenal medullae (closed triangles). Crosses (in **A,B**): no stimulation of nociceptors by capsaicin (control). Ordinate scale, degree of plasma extravasation in the rat knee joint normalized with respect to maximum (before stimulation of nociceptors by capsaicin). For details see legend of Fig. 3. Mean ± SEM; $n = 8$ knees in animals with interventions; $n = 16$ knees in control. (Modified from ref. 42.)

epinephrine. The mechanism in the synovia by which epinephrine generates a depression of synovial plasma extravasation is unknown; but it is unlikely to be generated by decrease in blood flow since the synovial plasma extravasation produced by platelet-activating factor is *not* decreased by noxious stimulation![‡]

2.   The central pathway activated by the noxious input and leading to the reflex activation of the preganglionic neurons innervating the adrenal medullae is a spino-bulbo-spinal pathway and probably a spinal pathway (see circuit in bold and grey-shaded neurons in Fig. 5). Such spinal and spino-bulbo-spinal somato-sympathetic reflex pathways to sympathetic preganglionic neurons innervating the adrenal medullae, which are activated by noxious stimulation, have been shown to exist in experiments in which activity in the adrenal nerve (which contains the preganglionic axons innervating the chromaffin cells of the adrenal medullae) and release of catecholamines from the adrenal medullae have been measured. For example, stimulation of cutaneous nociceptive afferents activates the preganglionic neurons to the adrenal medullae and leads to release of catecholamines from the adrenal medullae in rats with intact spinal cord and in spinalized rats[45–47] (see refs 48 and 49). From the studies reported here[42,50], for the hindpaw-induced reflexes, a spinal pathway from the lumbar segments L_4 and L_5 (which receives the afferent input from the plantar skin of the hindpaw) to the preganglionic neurons in the segments T_4 to T_{12} which innervate the adrenal medullae[51] is postulated: spinalization at the segmental level T_{12}/L_1 (which separates the afferent inflow from hindpaw and the efferent outflow to the adrenal medullae) entirely abolishes the depression of bradykinin-induced plasma extravasation which is normally generated by noxious hindpaw stimulation. In animals spinalized at the segmental level T_1/T_2 some depression is present which is similar in degree to that in normal animals with intact vagus nerves[42].

3.   The nociceptive–neuroendocrine reflex pathways are normally inhibited by activity in vagal afferents. The vagal afferents involved project through the coeliac branches of the abdominal vagus nerves which innervate the small intestine, distal duodenum and proximal colon. Experiments have shown that section of the coeliac branches has the same effect as subdiaphragmatic vagotomy, but section of the gastric and/or hepatic branches has no effect[41].

Two experiments have shown that the ascending limb of the postulated spino-bulbo-spinal reflex pathway projects through the spinal cord contralateral to the afferent nociceptive input from the hindlimb and that the inhibition generated by activity in vagal afferents occurs at the spinal cord level and is mediated by a descending pathway ipsilateral to the afferent nociceptive input. After section of

[‡] Continuous transcutaneous *electrical* stimulation of cutaneous afferent nerve fibres innervating the plantar skin at C-fibre strength (but not at A-fibre strength) and at low stimulation frequencies ($\leq 4\,$Hz) leads to depression of bradykinin-induced plasma extravasation which is mediated by the hypothalamo-pituitary-adrenal (HPA) axis[43,44]. Also this depression generated by activation of the HPA axis is enhanced after subdiaphragmatic vagotomy[40]. These experiments principally show that inflammatory processes are under the control of both endocrine systems. The differential activation of both neuroendocrine systems, the HPA axis or the sympatho-adrenal system, generated by the two modes of afferent stimulation is interesting but puzzling. The mechanisms underlying this differential activation are unknown and are presently being explored.

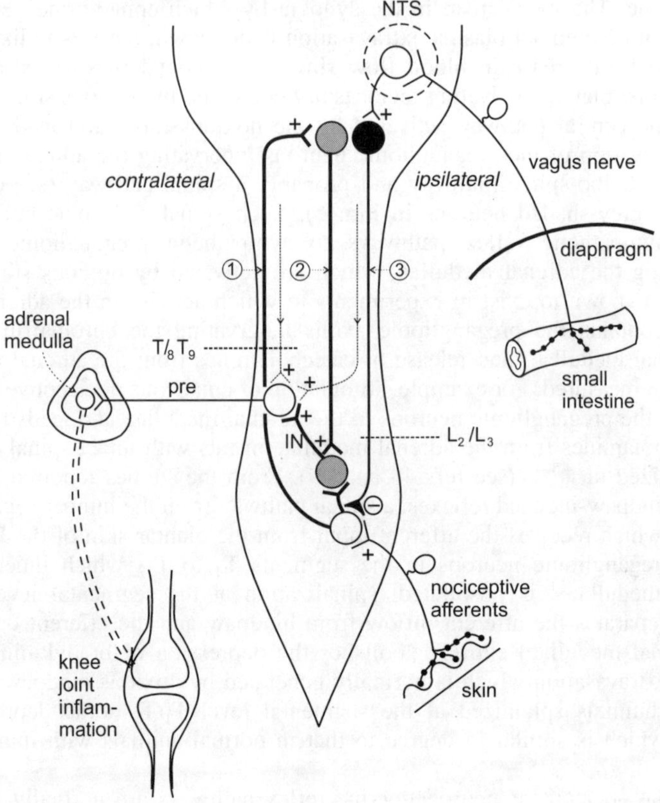

Fig. 5 Schematic diagram showing the proposed neural circuits in spinal cord and brainstem which modulate experimental inflammation in the rat knee joint via the sympatho-adrenal system (adrenal medullae). Experimental inflammation is generated by perfusion of the knee joint with saline containing the inflammatory mediator bradykinin (160 ng/ml; 1.51×10^{-7} M). Bradykinin generates plasma extravasation at the venules of the synovia into the knee joint cavity. Stimulation of cutaneous nociceptors by capsaicin (CAP) leads to depression of inflammation by activation of preganglionic neurons innervating the adrenal medullae via a spinal and a spino-bulbo-spinal excitatory circuit (grey neurons and circuit in bold). The ascending limb of this spino-bulbo-spinal reflex loop (①) projects through the contralateral dorsolateral funiculus of the spinal cord (DLF). The descending limb of this reflex loop (②) projects through the dorsal quadrants. This circuit is inhibited by activity in abdominal vagal afferents from the small intestine which is exerted at the level of the spinal cord (black neuron). The descending limb of this inhibitory pathway (③) projects through the ipsilateral DLF. Dotted thin lines: axons of sympathetic premotor neurons in the brainstem which project through the dorsolateral funiculi of the spinal cord to the preganglionic neurons of the adrenal medullae. Indicated are the levels of ipsi- and contralateral sections of the DLF in the experiments documented in Fig. 6. For details see text. +, excitation; −, inhibition. (Modified from refs 42 and 50.)

the dorsolateral funiculus of the spinal cord contralateral to the afferent nociceptive input (Fig. 6A left), the depression of bradykinin-induced plasma extravasation is almost totally abolished in rats with intact vagus nerves as well as in vagotomized rats (open triangles and open squares in Fig. 6C), showing that the reflex activation of the preganglionic neurons requires the spino-bulbo-spinal positive feedback

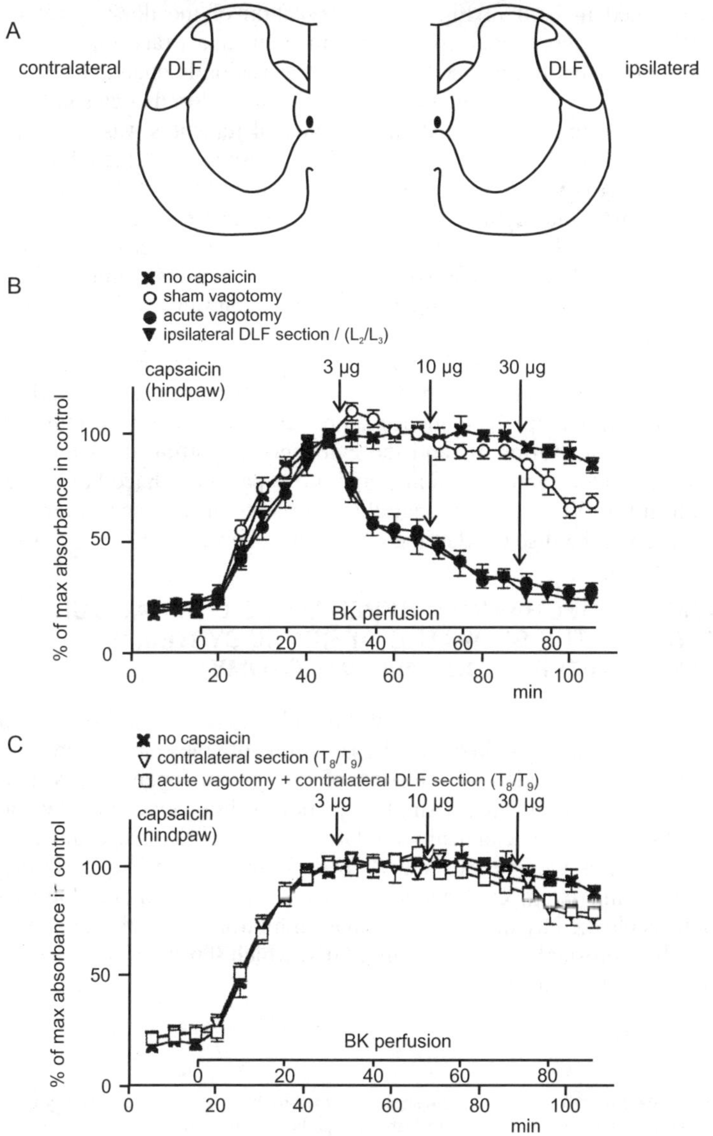

Fig. 6 Effect of section of the ipsilateral dorsolateral funiculus (DLF) at the segmental level of L2/L3 (B) or of the contralateral DLF at the segmental level of T8/T9 (C) on depression of bradykinin-induced plasma extravasation generated by intradermal injection of capsaicin (3, 10 and 30 µg) in the plantar skin of the hindpaw in sham-vagotomized and vagotomized rats. A: Diagrams of transverse spinal sections showing the DLF lesions. B: Ipsilateral DLF section (closed inverted triangles); closed circles: acute vagotomy; open circles: sham vagotomy. C: Contralateral DLF section without vagotomy (inverted open triangles) and with vagotomy (open squares). Crosses (in B,C): no stimulation of nociceptors by capsaicin (control). Ordinate scale, degree of plasma extravasation in the rat knee joint normalized with respect to maximum. For details see legend of Fig. 3. Mean ± SEM; $n = 8$ knees; $n = 16$ knees in control. (Modified from ref. 50)

89

circuit (outlined in bold in Fig. 5). After section of the dorsolateral funiculus ipsilateral to the afferent nociceptive input in vagus-intact rats (Fig. 6A right), the depression of bradykinin-induced plasma extravasation is quantitatively the same as in vagotomized rats (compare closed triangles with closed circles in Fig. 6B). In this type of experiment the ipsilateral dorsolateral funiculus was sectioned at the spinal segmental lumbar level L_2/L_3 (Fig. 5). This shows that the inhibition maintained by the activity in the vagal afferents occurs at the spinal level, possibly in the dorsal horn at the segmental level of the activated nociceptive afferent input (Fig. 5). Various other types of experiments were conducted (hemisection of the spinal cord, section of the dorsolateral funiculi at various segmental levels, section of the dorsal funiculi[50]) to support the key conclusions which are graphically illustrated in Fig. 5.

The hypothesis (as outlined in Fig. 5) explaining the results of the spinal lesion experiments, the evidence supporting the existence of the spino-bulbo-spinal reflex loop, the evidence supporting the descending inhibitory pathway linked to vagal afferents and the evidence supporting the lateralization of ascending excitatory and descending inhibitory pathways have been extensively discussed in ref. 50. The functional characteristics of the vagal afferents which are involved will be discussed at the end of this chapter.

CUTANEOUS MECHANICAL HYPERALGESIC BEHAVIOUR MEDIATED BY THE SYMPATHO-ADRENAL SYSTEM IS ENHANCED AFTER ABDOMINAL VAGOTOMY

Withdrawal threshold to stimulation of the rat hindpaw with a linearly increasing mechanical stimulus applied to the dorsum of the paw decreases dose-dependently after intradermal injection of bradykinin (open circles and closed squares in Fig. 7). Following a single injection of bradykinin this decrease lasts for more than 1 h for mechanical stimulation[52]. This type of mechanical hyperalgesic behaviour is mediated by the B_2 bradykinin receptor[53] and is not present when bradykinin is injected subcutaneously[54]. Bradykin-induced hyperalgesic behaviour is blocked by the cyclooxygenase inhibitor indomethacin and therefore mediated by a prostaglandin (probably PGE_2) which sensitizes the nociceptors for mechanical stimulation[§,¶].

[§] The decrease in paw-withdrawal threshold provided by bradykinin is significantly reduced after surgical sympathectomy. This shows that the sympathetic innervation of the skin is involved in the sensitization of the nociceptors to mechanical stimulation[55]. Interestingly, decentralization of the lumbar paravertebral sympathetic ganglia (denervating the postganglionic neurons by cutting the preganglionic sympathetic axons) does not abolish bradykinin-induced mechanical hyperalgesic behaviour. This indicates that the sensitizing effect of bradykinin is not dependent on activity in the sympathetic neurons innervating skin, and therefore not on release of norepinephrine. It is believed that bradykinin stimulates release of prostaglandin from the sympathetic varicosities; however, this has to be shown to occur[56].

[¶] Evidence for sensitization of cutaneous nociceptors to mechanical stimulation by bradykinin is poor or absent (see ref. 57). Some sensitization to mechanical stimulation by bradykinin has been demonstrated for afferents from the knee joint[58] and from skeletal muscle[59]. These discrepancies may be due to technical difficulties with this experimental approach.

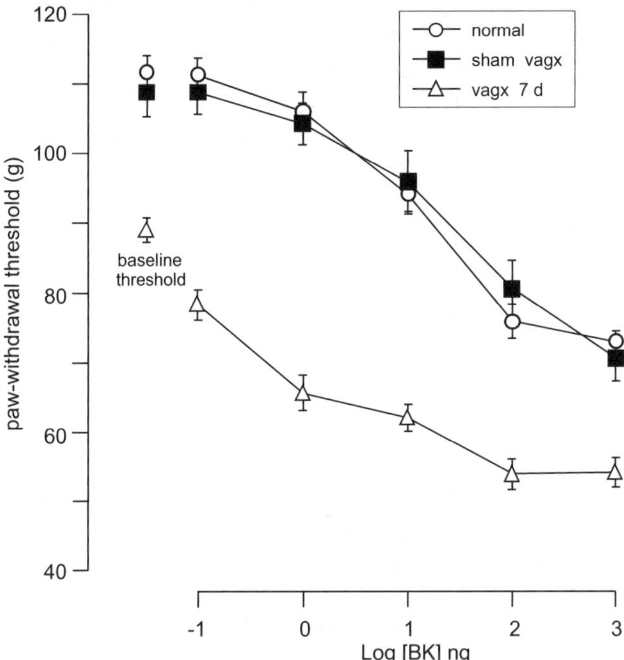

Fig. 7 Decrease of paw-withdrawal threshold to mechanical stimulation of the dorsum of the rat hindpaw induced by bradykinin (bradykinin-induced behavioural mechanical hyperalgesia) in normal control (squares, $n = 26$), vagotomized (triangles, $n = 16$) and sham-vagotomized (circles, $n = 18$) rats. Experiments conducted 7 days after vagotomy. *Post-hoc* test shows significant differences between vagotomized and normal ($p < 0.05$) as well as between vagotomized and sham vagotomized ($p < 0.05$) rats, in response to bradykinin. Cutaneous mechanoreceptors in the hairy skin are stimulated by a linearly increasing mechanical force using a Basile Algesimeter (Stoelting, Chicago, IL). Threshold is defined as the minimum force (g) at which the paw is withdrawn by a rat. Ordinate scale expresses paw-withdrawal threshold in grams. The abscissa scale is the log dose of BK (in ng) injected in a volume of 2.5 µg saline into the dermis of the skin of the dorsal aspect of the hindpaw. Vagx, subdiaphragmatic vagotomy. (Data from ref. 56 with permission.)

If inhibition maintained by activity in vagal afferents acts continuously on the central nociceptive pathway one would expect, on the basis of studies reported by Gebhart, Randich and co-workers (see refs 11 and 12), that subdiaphragmatic vagotomy might enhance the mechanical hyperalgesic behaviour, irrespective of the way the nociceptive afferents have been sensitized (e.g. by bradykinin or another hyperalgesic agent), and lower baseline threshold to mechanical stimulation.

Baseline paw-withdrawal threshold in normal (109 ± 2.1 g, mean $\pm$ SEM) and sham-vagotomized rats (107 ± 2.8 g) is significantly decreased 7 days after subdiaphragmatic vagotomy (89 ± 1.7 g; triangles in Fig. 7). Intradermal injection of bradykinin produces a dose-dependent decrease in mechanical nociceptive threshold (i.e. generates a mechanical hyperalgesic behaviour) in normal rats and in rats 7 days after subdiaphragmatic sham-vagotomy (open circles and squares in Fig. 7). Bradykinin-induced hyperalgesia was significantly enhanced 7 days

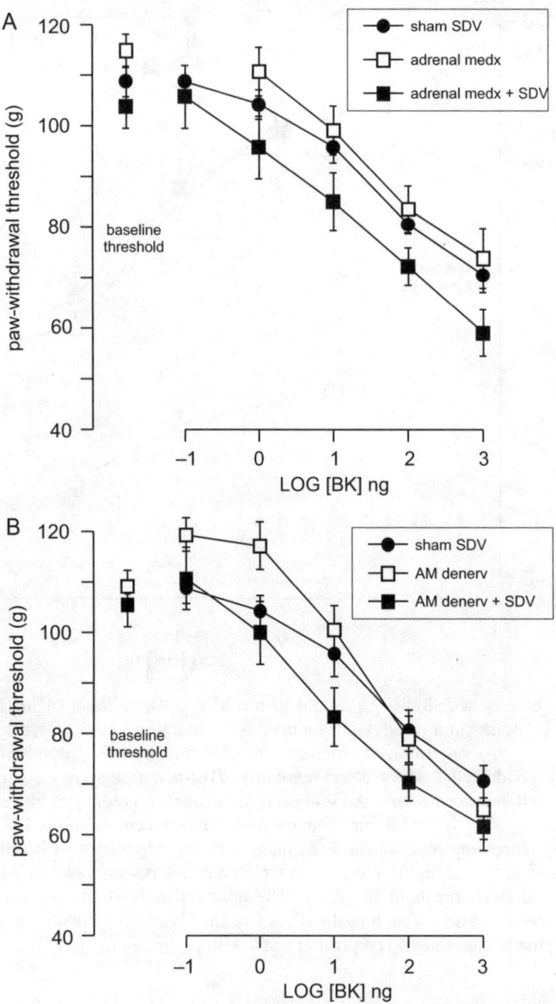

Fig. 8 Role of adrenal medulla in bradykinin-induced behavioural mechanical hyperalgesia and its enhancement after subdiaphragmatic vagotomy. A: Baseline and decrease of paw-withdrawal threshold to mechanical stimulation of the dorsum of the rat hindpaw, induced by bradykinin (bradykinin-induced behavioural mechanical hyperalgesia) in sham-vagotomized rats (closed circles, $n = 18$), in rats whose adrenal medullae are removed (Adrenal Medx, open squares, $n = 12$) and in rats with removed adrenal medullae and which are also vagotomized (closed squares, $n = 12$). Experiments conducted 5 weeks after removal of the adrenal medullae and 7 days after additional vagotomy. B: Data from experiments in which the adrenal medullae are denervated: rats with denervated adrenal medullae (AM denerv, open squares, $n = 6$); vagotomized rats with denervated adrenal medullae (AM denerv plus SDV, closed squares, $n = 10$). Experiments were conducted 7 days after surgery. Paw-withdrawal thresholds of vagotomized rats in which the adrenal medullae are removed or denervated are significantly higher than those of rats which are only vagotomized (see open triangles in Fig. 7; $p < 0.05$). Paw-withdrawal thresholds of rats in which the adrenal medullae are removed or denervated are significantly higher than those of rats which were additionally vagotomized ($p < 0.05$; compare open with closed squares). Data on sham-vagotomized rats in A and B are the same as in Fig. 7. (Modified from ref. 60.)

after subdiaphragmatic vagotomy (triangles in Fig. 8). There are three important characteristics of the effect of vagotomy on mechanical baseline threshold and on bradykinin-induced decrease of paw-withdrawal threshold to mechanical stimulation:

1.   The dramatic enhancement of bradykinin-induced mechanical hyperalgesic behaviour occurs also when only the *coeliac vagal branches* are interrupted, but not when the gastric and/or hepatic branches of the abdominal vagus nerves are interrupted. Thus, the vagal afferents involved project through the coeliac branches of the abdominal vagus nerves, which innervate the small intestine and proximal part of the large intestine, and not through the hepatic or gastric branches[56]. Surprisingly, the baseline paw-withdrawal threshold to mechanical stimulation does not decrease when only the coeliac vagal branches are interrupted[56].

2.   Both vagotomy-induced changes (decrease in baseline paw-withdrawal threshold, bradykinin-induced hyperalgesic behaviour) take about 2 weeks to reach maximum and remain stable over 5 weeks (Fig. 9[56,60]).

3.   Subdiaphragmatic vagotomy does not have a significant effect on cutaneous mechanical hyperalgesic behaviour produced by intradermal injection of prostaglandin E_2 (which is supposed to act directly to sensitize nociceptors)[56].

Thus, the effect of vagotomy is not a general effect of all abdominal vagal afferents and cannot readily be explained by an immediate removal of inhibition from the central nociceptive system (e.g. acting in the dorsal horn) as predicted by the experiments of Foreman, Gebhart, Randich and co-workers (see above)[11,12,61]. We therefore looked for an alternative explanation and discovered that the sympatho-adrenal system is the important link mediating these changes.

Enhancement of mechanical hyperalgesic behaviour after vagotomy is mediated by the sympatho-adrenal system

Effect of adrenal medullectomy or denervation of the adrenal medullae

Bilateral removal of the adrenal medulla or denervation of the adrenal medullae (cutting the sympathetic preganglionic axons) generates both a small increase in baseline paw-withdrawal threshold and paw-withdrawal threshold to intradermal injection of bradykinin compared to the controls (Fig. 8). Under this condition of defunctionalized adrenal medullae, subdiaphragmatic vagotomy is followed by only a small decrease in paw-withdrawal threshold (compare open and closed squares in Fig. 8) but not by the large changes seen in animals with functioning adrenal medullae. These small changes are significant, with the exception of the change of baseline threshold in animals with denervated adrenal medullae. They can fully be explained by removal of central inhibition of nociceptive impulse transmission occurring probably in the dorsal horn (see above).[60]

Effect of denervation of adrenal medullae 14 days following subdiaphragmatic vagotomy

If the decrease of baseline mechanical paw-withdrawal threshold and enhanced decrease of paw-withdrawal threshold to mechanical stimulation, generated by

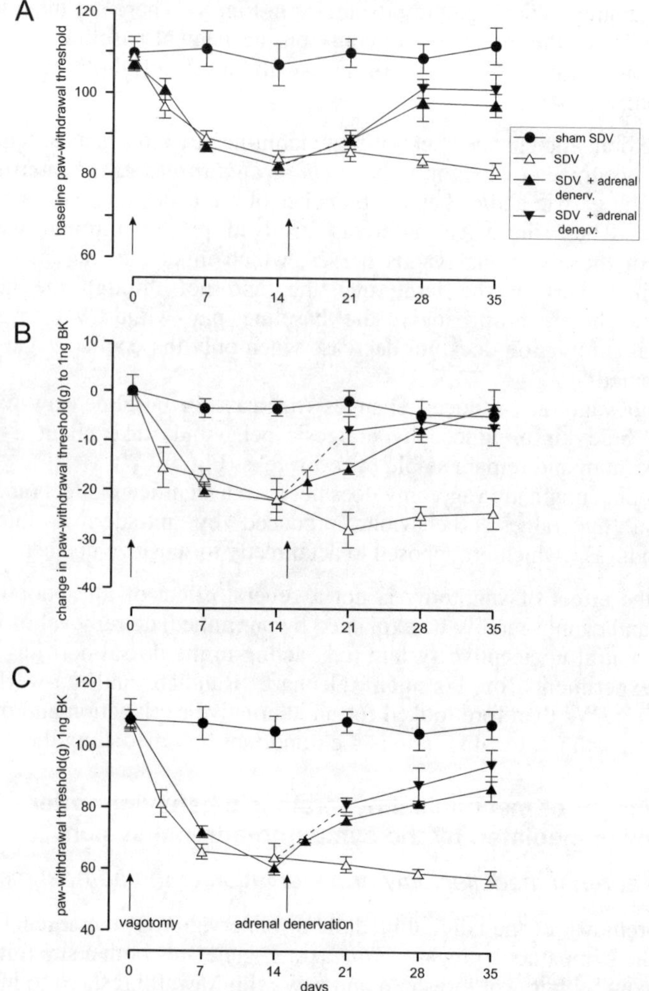

Fig. 9 Long-term enhancement of bradykinin-induced behavioural mechanical hyperalgesia after vagotomy and its disappearance after denervation of the adrenal medullae. Baseline paw-withdrawal threshold (A), difference between baseline paw-withdrawal threshold and paw-withdrawal threshold in response to 1 ng BK injected intradermally (B), and total change of paw-withdrawal threshold in response to intradermal injection of 1 ng bradykinin (C) in rats before and 7–35 days after vagotomy (open triangles, $n = 6$), before and 7–35 days after sham-vagotomy (closed circles, $n = 8$) and in rats which are first vagotomized and whose adrenal medullae (AM) are denervated 14 days after vagotomy and measurements taken up to 35 days after initial surgery. The latter group of animals consists of two subgroups: rats which are tested after vagotomy and after additional denervation of the adrenal medullae (closed normal triangles, $n = 6$) and rats which are only tested after additional denervation of the adrenal medullae (closed inverted triangles, $n = 4$). Ordinate scale is threshold in grams. Data of the sham-vagotomy and the vagotomy group of rats are significantly different 7 days after vagotomy ($p < 0.01$). Data of vagotomized rats with denervated AM and rats that are only vagotomized are significantly different on days 28 and 35 ($p < 0.01$). Data between sham-vagotomized rats and vagotomized rats in which the adrenal medullae are denervated are not significantly different on days 28 and 35 ($p > 0.05$). (Modified from ref. 60)

intradermal injection of bradykinin, are related to a signal released from the adrenal medullae, which is dependent on activity in sympathetic preganglionic axons, one would expect both changes to be reversed when the adrenal medullae are denervated. This is in fact the case.

To test this idea, groups of rats were repeatedly tested over 5 weeks for their mechanical paw-withdrawal threshold to 1 ng bradykinin injected intracutaneously (a dose which does not decrease the threshold to mechanical stimulation in normal rats with intact vagus nerves) (see Figs 7 and 8): (1) Rats in which the vagus nerves were severed subdiaphragmatically followed 14 days later by denervation of the adrenal medullae (this group consisted of two subgroups: one subgroup being tested throughout the period of 5 weeks and a second subgroup being tested before vagotomy, just before denervation of the adrenal medullae and repeatedly after denervation of the adrenal medullae). (2) Rats which were vagotomized only and repeatedly tested. (3) Control rats which were repeatedly tested without any surgical intervention. Figure 9 demonstrates the results for the baseline paw-withdrawal threshold (A), for the decrease in paw-withdrawal threshold to intradermal injection of 1 ng bradykinin alone (B) and for both effects together (C). After vagotomy the paw-withdrawal threshold slowly decreases, reaching its lowest values after 7–14 days. The reversal of the vagotomy effect after denervation of the adrenal medullae also has a slow time-course similar to the time-course of the decrease in baseline paw-withdrawal threshold following vagotomy (open triangles in Fig. 9) over a 5-week period. Repeated testing of sham-vagotomized control rats over the same period of time does not reveal a decrease in paw-withdrawal threshold produced by 1 ng bradykinin (closed circles in Fig. 9). The paw-withdrawal thresholds, 14 and 21 days after denervation of the adrenal medullae, are significantly higher than those measured in the animals which are only vagotomized (compare closed triangles with open triangles in Fig. 9). Furthermore, the paw-withdrawal thresholds in response to 1 ng bradykinin at 14 and 21 days after denervation of the adrenal medullae in vagotomized animals are not significantly different from those in sham-vagotomized animals which had repeatedly been tested over a period of 5 weeks after surgery (compare closed triangles with closed circles in Fig. 9).

Interpretation and implications

These results suggest that two mechanisms contribute to the decrease of baseline paw-withdrawal threshold to mechanical stimulation and to enhancement of the decrease of paw-withdrawal threshold generated by intracutaneous injection of bradykinin following vagotomy:

1. Ongoing central inhibition of nociceptive impulse transmission (occurring probably in the dorsal horn) which is normally maintained by spontaneous activity in vagal afferents is removed after vagotomy (Fig. 10), resulting in a small but significant enhancement of nociceptive behaviour to mechanical stimulation (see Fig. 8). This enhancement is in accordance with the idea that nociception and pain is centrally under inhibitory control from the visceral domain via vagal afferents (see refs 11, 12 and 61).

2. Vagotomy triggers the activation of sympathetic preganglionic neurons innervating the adrenal medullae (Fig. 10), probably by removing central inhibition

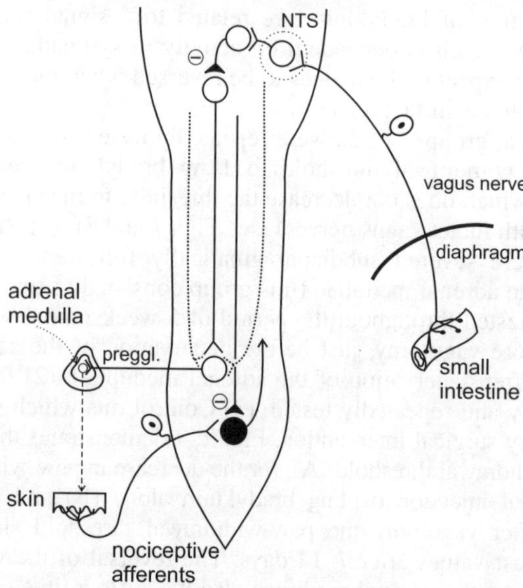

Fig. 10 Schematic diagram showing the proposed neural circuits in spinal cord and brainstem which modulate nociceptor sensitivity via the sympatho-adrenal system (adrenal medulla). Sensitivity of cutaneous nociceptors for mechanical stimulation is modulated by a signal (probably epinephrine) from the adrenal medulla. Activation of the adrenal medulla increases the sensitivity of the nociceptors. Activity in preganglionic neurons innervating the adrenal medullae depends on activity in vagal afferents from the small intestine which has an inhibitory influence on the central pathways to these preganglionic neurons. Thus, interruption of the vagal afferents leads to activation of the adrenal medullae. It is hypothesized that these neuronal (reflex) circuits in the brainstem are under the control of upper brainstem, hypothalamus and forebrain. Dotted thin lines: axons of sympathetic premotor neurons in the brainstem which project through the dorsolateral funiculi of the spinal cord to the preganglionic neurons of the adrenal medullae. For details see text. +, Excitation; −, inhibition. (Modified from ref. 60)

acting at this sympathetic pathway, thus leading to release of a hormonal signal (probably epinephrine) from the adrenal medullae. Interruption of these sympathetic preganglionic axons innervating the adrenal glands (Fig. 10), stops the release of this hormonal signal and therefore prevents or reverses the decrease of baseline mechanical paw-withdrawal threshold and the enhancement of bradykinin-induced decrease of paw-withdrawal threshold to mechanical stimulation. This novel finding could principally imply that the sensitivity of nociceptors to mechanical stimulation is under neuroendocrine control and that nociceptor sensitivity can be regulated from remote body domains and by the brain via this neuroendocrine pathway.

The second mechanism is novel and has several implications. In connection with the effect of vagotomy several interesting questions and problems are raised:

1. The vagal afferents which are involved in modulation of hyperalgesic behaviour project through the coeliac branches of the abdominal vagus nerves and supply small and large intestines, but not liver and stomach. These vagal afferents

are capsaicin-sensitive, whereas most of those vagal afferents which innervate stomach or liver are not[10,62,63]. Do these vagal afferents monitor toxic and other events at the inner defence line of the body (the 'gut-associated lymphoid tissue', GALT)? What are the physiological stimuli to activate these vagal afferents? Is it possible to increase mechanical paw-withdrawal threshold (baseline, to intradermally injected bradykinin) by physiological stimulation of these vagal afferents (by further increasing inhibition of nociceptive impulse transmission in the dorsal horn and inhibition of preganglionic neurons innervating the adrenal medullae)?

2.   The changes following vagotomy (decreased mechanical baseline threshold and enhanced bradykinin-induced mechanical hyperalgesic behaviour[56,60]) are generated by the *interruption* of vagal afferents. Therefore, the vagal afferents involved must be tonically active[28,29]. This conclusion is fully supported by experiments in which the influence of activity in vagal afferents on the nociceptive–neuroendocrine negative feedback pathway controlling neurogenic inflammation of the synovia of the rat knee joint has been studied (see above).

3.   Maier, Watkins and co-workers have shown, using the thermal tail-flick reflex, that behavioural hyperalgesia in rats produced by intraperitoneal injection of the illness-inducing bacterial cell wall endotoxin (LPS) is mediated by activity in subdiaphragmatic vagal afferents projecting through the hepatic vagal branch[13,17]. The results of these experiments imply that *stimulation* of vagal afferents generates thermal hyperalgesic behaviour, and are apparently at variance with the results reported here, showing that *removal* of activity in vagal afferents leads to hyperalgesic behaviour. However, it must be kept in mind that: (a) two different types of nociceptive behaviour (mechanical, thermal) have been tested; (b) two different groups of vagal afferents (innervating small/large intestine and liver, respectively) are involved; (c) induction and depression of the two hyperalgesic behaviours probably occur at different time-courses; (d) different (central and peripheral) mechanisms are probably involved in the modulation of both nociceptive behaviours from the visceral domain.

4.   The hormonal signal released by the adrenal medullae is most likely epinephrine (Khasar, personal communication). The decrease of paw-withdrawal threshold (baseline as well as after intradermal injection of bradykinin) following vagotomy takes several days to reach peak effect and the recovery following additional denervation of the adrenal medullae also takes several days.

5.   The mechanism of the slow time-course of the changes of paw-withdrawal threshold is not clear at the moment. Epinephrine has obviously to act over a long time to induce changes in the micromilieu of the nociceptor population which in turn leads to their sensitization. It does most likely act *not directly* on the nociceptors but on other cells (e.g. macrophages, mast cells, keratinocytes) which then release substances that generate the sensitization, this in particular since prostaglandin E_2-induced mechanical hyperalgesic behaviour is not changed after vagotomy[56].

6.   The change of sensitivity of a population of cutaneous nociceptors generated by epinephrine which is regulated by the brain would be a novel mechanism of sensitization. This novel mechanism of sensitization of the nociceptor population by epinephrine released by the sympatho-adrenal system would be different from mechanisms that lead to activation and/or sensitization of nociceptors by sympathetic–afferent coupling under pathophysiological conditions[64–66].

7. Which central pathways are involved leading to activation of preganglionic sympathetic neurons that innervate the adrenal medullae after subdiaphragmatic vagotomy? Are only sympathetic neurons which innervate the adrenal medulla activated after vagotomy or also other functional types of sympathetic neurons[67–71]?

8. Do the same changes, related to the abdominal vagal afferents and the adrenal medullae, also occur in other behavioural pain models? For example, do the changes, probably induced by epinephrine in the cutaneous nociceptor population, also occur in deep somatic and visceral nociceptive afferents? Finally, is it possible that these mechanisms operate in such ill-defined pain syndromes as irritable bowel syndrome, functional dyspepsia, fibromyalgia. etc.[72–74]? (see contributions by Locke, Chang and Mayer in this volume).

SYNOPSIS AND CONCLUSIONS

Overall, these findings mean that inflammatory processes and sensitivity of nociceptors can be changed via the sympatho-adrenal system (adrenal medullae) by interventions at remote body domains (here the visceral body domain and activity in vagal afferents). The changes are mediated by reflex circuits in the spinal cord and brainstem (see Figs 5 and 10) which connect the nociceptive afferent inputs and the vagal afferent inputs (via the NTS) with the sympathetic preganglionic neurons innervating the adrenal medullae. It is postulated, on the basis of the experimental results, that the reflex circuits consist of excitatory spinal and spino-bulbo-spinal pathways associated with the nociceptive afferent input and inhibitory bulbo-spinal pathways associated with the vagal afferent input (Figs 6 and 10[42,50]). Details of these reflex circuits have to be worked out. Experimental investigations performed on rats show that sympathetic preganglionic neurons innervating cells of the adrenal medullae which release epinephrine are connected to distinct neuronal circuits in the neuraxis. These circuits are different from those connected to preganglionic neurons innervating cells of the adrenal medullae which release norepinephrine and preganglionic neurons innervating postganglionic neurons supplying resistance vessels in skeletal muscle or viscera[75,76] or functionally other types of sympathetic preganglionic neurons.

It is not far-fetched to assume that the multiple reflex circuits connected to the adrenomedullary cells which release epinephrine and to the HPA axis, which also forms a nociceptive–neuroendocrine reflex circuit in the control of inflammation[43,44], are under the control of the hypothalamus and forebrain (see Fig. 2). Thus, these basic reflex circuits connected to both neuroendocrine systems could be 'used' by higher brain centres to control both inflammation and nociceptor sensitization. The detailed peripheral and central mechanisms by which this occurs have to be worked out.

SUMMARY

Inflammation and hyperalgesia are mechanisms which protect the organism against damage and naturally lead to healing. They may inflict secondary damage to the body, if uncontrolled in chronic conditions. The experimental rat models of bradykinin-induced synovial plasma extravasation of the knee joint (neurogenic inflammation) and bradykinin-induced cutaneous mechanical hyperalgesia have been used to study the control of inflammation and hyperalgesia and its modulation by activity in vagal afferents and by the brain.

1. Neurogenic inflammation is under inhibitory control of the sympatho-adrenal system (adrenal medulla) (and in certain conditions of the HPA axis). The final signal from the adrenal medullae is possibly epinephrine.

2. The sympatho-adrenal system can be activated by nociceptive afferents from the somatic and visceral body domains via spinal and spino-bulbo-spinal reflex pathways. The nociceptive system activated during inflammation constitutes an inhibitory feedback system via the sympatho-adrenal system to the inflammatory process.

3. Subdiaphragmatic vagotomy enhances this negative nociceptive neuroendocrine control of the peripheral inflammatory process. The vagal afferents involved pass through the coeliac branches. Ongoing activity in these vagal afferents inhibits the ascending pathway of the spino-bulbo-spinal reflex loop at the spinal cord level. Thus, the gain of the nociceptive–neuroendocrine negative feedback control of inflammation is determined by activity in vagal afferents from abdominal organs.

4. The paw-withdrawal threshold to mechanical stimulation of the dorsal skin of the hindpaw (baseline, after intradermal injection of bradykinin (bradykinin-induced mechanical hyperalgesic behaviour)) decreases significantly after subdiaphragmatic vagotomy. These vagotomy-induced changes develop slowly over 14 days. They are not present in rats with defunctionalized adrenal medullae and reversed when the adrenal medullae are denervated in vagotomized rats. This indicates that the sensitivity of cutaneous nociceptors is controlled by the sympatho-adrenal system and therefore by activity in preganglionic sympathetic neurons innervating the adrenal medullae. The signal is most likely epinephrine.

5. The vagal afferents which are involved in the modulation of the inhibitory feedback system (controlling experimental inflammation) and in the modulation of the Sympatho-adrenal system (controlling sensitivity of the nociceptor population) mainly supply the small intestines. These afferents possibly innervate the inner defence line of the gastrointestinal tract (the gut-associated lymphoid tissue) and monitor toxic events.

6. It is concluded from these experiments that: (a) experimental inflammation of the rat synovia and sensitivity of nociceptors to mechanical stimulation are under the control of the sympatho-adrenal system; (b) both can be influenced from the visceral domain by vagal afferents innervating the small intestines; (c) the central pathways involved are inhibitory and excitatory in the spinal cord and lower brainstem; and (d) the central nervous system can modulate the integrative protective actions involving visceral and somatic body domains.

Acknowledgement

This work was supported by grants from TRDRP (8RT-0032) and NIH (AR-32634).

References

1. Jänig W, Häbler HJ. Specificity in the organization of the autonomic nervous system: a basis for precise neural regulation of homeostatic and protective body functions. Prog Brain Res. 2000;122:351–67.
2. Jänig W, Green PG, Khasar SG, Miao FJ-P, Strausbaugh H, Levine JD. Role of vagal afferents in neuroendocrine control of joint inflammation and cutaneous mechanical hyperalgesia. In: Goebell H, Holtmann G, Talley N, editors. Functional Dyspepsia and Irritable Bowel Syndrome: Concepts and Controversies. Boston: Kluwer, 1998:41–54.
3. Mason P. Contributions of the medullary raphe and ventromedial reticular region to pain modulation and other homeostatic functions. Annu Rev Neurosci. 2001;24:737–77.
4. Berthoud HR, Carlson NR, Powley TL. Topography of efferent vagal innervation of the rat gastrointestinal tract. Am J Physiol. 1991;260:R200–7.
5. Precht JC, Powley TL. The fibre composition of the abdominal vagus in the rat. Anat Embryol. 1990;181:101–15.
6. Loewy AD, Spyer KM. Central Regulation of Autonomic Functions. New York: Oxford University Press, 1990.
7. Ritter S, Ritter RC, Barnes CD. Neuroanatomy and Physiology of Abdominal Vagal Afferents. Boca, Raton: CRC Press, 1992.
8. Kalia M, Mesulam MM. Brain stem projections of sensory and motor components of the vagus complex in the cat: II. Laryngeal, tracheobronchial, pulmonary, cardiac, and gastrointestinal branches. J Comp Neurol. 1980;193:467–508.
9. Shanahan F. The intestinal immune system. In: Johnson LR, editor. Physiology of the Gastrointestinal Tract. New York: Raven Press, 1994:643–84.
10. Berthoud HR, Neuhuber WL. Functional and chemical anatomy of the afferent vagal system. Auton Neurosci. 2000;85:1–17.
11. Gebhart GF, Randich A. Vagal modulation of nociception. Am Pain Soc J. 1992;1:26–32.
12. Randich A, Gebhart GF. Vagal afferent modulation of nociception. Brain Res Rev. 1992;17:77–99.
13. Watkins LR, Wiertelak EP, Goehler LE *et al*. Neurocircuitry of illness-induced hyperalgesia. Brain Res. 1994;639:283–99.
14. Watkins LR, Wiertelak EP, Goehler LE, Smith KP, Martin D, Maier SF. Characterization of cytokine-induced hyperalgesia. Brain Res. 1994;654:15–26.
15. Watkins LR, Goehler LE, Relton J, Brewer MT, Maier SF. Mechanisms of tumor necrosis factor-alpha (TNF-alpha) hyperalgesia. Brain Res. 1995;692:244–50.
16. Watkins LR, Goehler LE, Relton JK *et al*. Blockade of interleukin-1 induced hyperthermia by subdiaphragmatic vagotomy: evidence for vagal mediation of immune–brain communication. Neurosci Lett. 1995;183:27–31.
17. Watkins LR, Maier SF, Goehler LE. Immune activation: the role of pro-inflammatory cytokines in inflammation, illness responses and pathological pain states. Pain. 1995;63:289–302.
18. Watkins LR, Maier SF, Goehler LE. Cytokine-to-brain communication: a review and analysis of alternative mechanisms. Life Sci. 1995;57:1011–26.
19. Sehic E, Blatteis CM. Blockade of lipopolysaccharide-induced fever by subdiaphragmatic vagotomy in guinea pigs. Brain Res. 1996;726:160–6.
20. Blatteis CM, Sehic E. Fever: how may circulating pyrogens signal to the brain. News Physiol Sci. 1994;12:1–9.
21. Bernstein IL. Neutral mediation of food aversions and anorexia induced by tumor necrosis factor and tumors. Neurosci Biobehav Rev. 1996;20:177–81.
22. Bret-Dibat JL, Bluthe RM, Kent S, Kelley KW, Dantzer R. Lipopolysaccharide and interleukin-1 depress food-motivated behavior in mice by a vagal-mediated mechanism. Brain Behav Immun. 1995;9:242–6.
23. Ericsson A, Kovacs JC, Sawchenko PE. A functional anatomical analysis of central pathways subserving the effects of interleukin-1 on stress-related neuroendocrine neurons. J Neurosci. 1994;14:897–913.
24. Wan W, Wetmore L, Sorensen CM, Greenberg AH, Nance DM. Neural and biochemical mediators of endotoxin and stress-induced c-fos expression in the rat brain. Brain Res Bull. 1994;34:7–14.
25. Layé S, Bluthe RM, Kent S *et al*. Subdiaphragmatic vagotomy blocks induction of IL-1 beta mRNA in mice brain in response to peripheral LPS. Am J Physiol. 1995;268:R1327–31.

26. Grundy D, Scratcherd T. Sensory afferents from the gastrointestinal tract. In: Wood JD, editor. Handbook of Physiology, The Gastrointestinal System. Baltimore: American Physiological Society, 1989:593–620.

27. Richards W, Hillsley K, Eastwood C, Grundy D. Sensitivity of vagal mucosal afferents to cholecystokinin and its role in afferent signal transduction in the rat. J Physiol (Lond). 1996;497:473–81.

28. Schwartz GJ, Moran TH. CCK elicits and modulates vagal afferent activity arising from gastric and duodenal sites. Ann NY Acad Sci. 1994;713:121–8.

29. Schwartz GJ, Moran TH. Sub-diaphragmatic vagal afferent integration of meal-related gastro-intestinal signals. Neurosci Biobehav Rev. 1996;20:47–56.

30. Berthoud HR, Kressel M, Raybould HE, Neuhuber WL. Vagal sensors in the rat duodenal mucosa: distribution and structure as revealed by *in vivo* DiI-tracing. Anat Embryol. 1995;191:203–12.

31. Grundy D. Vagal afferent mechanisms of mechano- and chemoreception. In: Ritter S, Ritter RC, Barnes CD, editors. Neuroanatomy and Physiology of Abdominal Afferents. Boca Raton: CRC Press, 1992:181–91.

32. Walls EK, Phillips RJ, Wang FB, Holst MC, Powley TL. Suppression of meal size by intestinal nutrients is eliminated by celia vagal deafferentation. Am J Physiol. 1995;269:R1410–19.

33. Walls EK, Wang FB, Holst MC *et al.* Selective vagal rhizotomies: a new dorsal surgical approach used for intestinal deafferentations. Am J Physiol. 1995;269:R1279–88.

34. Niijima A. The afferent discharge from sensors for interleukin-1 beta in the hepatoportal system in the anesthetized rat. J Auton Nerv Syst. 1996;61:287–91.

35. Miao FJ-P, Jänig W, Levine JD. Role of sympathetic postganglionic neurons in synovial plasma extravasation induced by bradykinin. J Neurophysiol. 1996;75:715–24.

36. Miao FJ-P, Green P, Coderre TJ, Jänig W, Levine JD. Sympathetic-dependence in bradykinin-induced synovial plasma extravasation is dose-related. Neurosci Lett. 1996;205:165–8.

37. Carr J, Wilhelm DL. The evaluation of increased vascular permeability in the skin of guinea pigs. J Exp Biol Med Sci. 1964;42:511–22.

38. Hargreaves KM, Roszkowski MT, Swift JQ. Bradykinin and inflammatory pain. Agents Actions Suppl. 1993;41:65–73.

39. Swift JQ, Garry MG, Roszkowski MT, Hargreaves KM. Effect of flurbiprofen on tissue levels on immunoreactive bradykinin and acute postoperative pain. J Oral Max Surg. 1993;51:112–17.

40. Miao FJ-P, Jänig W, Green PG, Levine JD. Inhibition of bradykinin-induced synovial plasma extravasation produced by noxious cutaneous and visceral stimuli and its modulation by activity in the vagal nerve. J Neurophysiol. 1997;78:1285–92.

41. Miao FJ-P, Jänig W, Levine JD. Vagal branches involved in inhibition of bradykinin-induced synovial plasma extravasation by intrathecal nicotine and noxious stimulation in the rat. J Physiol (Lond). 1997;498:473–81.

42. Miao FJ-P, Jänig W, Levine JD. Nociceptive-neuroendocrine negative feedback control of neuro-genic inflammation activated by capsaicin in the skin: role of the adrenal medulla. J Physiol (Lond). 2000;527:601–10.

43. Green PG, Miao FJ-P, Jänig W, Levine JD. Negative feedback neuroendocrine control of the inflammatory response in rats. J Neurosci. 1995;15:4678–86.

44. Green PG, Jänig W, Levine JD. Sympathetic terminal: target for negative feedback neuro-endocrine control of inflammatory response in the rat. J Neurosci. 1997;17:3234–8.

45. Araki T, Ito K, Kurosawa M, Sato A. Responses of adrenal sympathetic nerve activity and catecholamine secretion to cutaneous stimulation in anesthetized rats. Neuroscience. 1984;12:289–99.

46. Ito K, Miura M, Furuse H *et al.* Voltage-gated Ca^{2+} channel blockers, omega-AgaIVA and $Ni2^{+}$, suppress the induction of theta-burst induced long-term potentiation in guinea-pig hippocampal CA1 neurons. Neurosci Lett. 1995;183:112–15.

47. Kurosawa M, Saito H, Sato A, Tsuchiya T. Reflex changes in sympatho-adrenal medullary functions in response to various thermal cutaneous stimulations in anesthetized rats. Neurosci Lett. 1985;56:149–54.

48. Sato A. Neural mechanisms of somatic sensory regulation of catecholamine secretion from the adrenal gland. Adv Biophys. 1987;23:39–80.

49. Sato A, Sato Y, Schmidt RF. The impact of somatosensory input on autonomic functions. Rev Physiol Biochem Pharmacol. 1997;130:1–328.

50. Miao FJ-P, Jänig W, Jasmin L, Levine JD. Spino-bulbo-spinal pathway mediating vagal modulation of nociceptive–neuroendocrine control of inflammation in the rat. J Physiol. 2001;532: 811–22.

51. Strack AM, Sawyer WB, Marubio LM, Loewy AD. Spinal origin of sympathetic preganglionic neurons in the rat. Brain Res. 1988;455:187–91.

52. Taiwo YO, Levine JD. Characterization of the arachidonic acid metabolites mediating bradykinin and noradrenaline hyperalgesia. Brain Res. 1988;458:402–6.

53. Khasar SG, Miao FJ-P, Levine JD. Inflammation modulates the contribution of receptor-subtypes to bradykinin-induced hyperalgesia in the rat. Neuroscience. 1995;69:685–90.

54. Khasar SG, Green PG, Levine JD. Comparison of intradermal and subcutaneous hyperalgesic effects of inflammatory mediators in the rat. Neurosci Lett. 1993;153:215–18.

55. Gonzales R, Goldyne ME, Taiwo YO, Levine JD. Production of hyperalgesic prostaglandins by sympathetic postganglionic neurons. J Neurochem. 1989;53:1595–8.

56. Khasar SG, Miao FJ-P, Jänig W, Levine JD. Modulation of bradykinin-induced mechanical hyperalgesia in the rat by activity in abdominal vagal afferents. Eur J Neurosci. 1998;10: 435–44.

57. Treede RD, Meyer RA, Raja SN, Campbell JN. Peripheral and central mechanisms of cutaneous hyperalgesia. Prog Neurobiol. 1992;38:397–421.

58. Neugebauer V, Schaible HG, Schmidt RF. Sensitization of articular afferents to mechanical stimuli by bradykinin. Pflügers Arch. 1989;415:330–5.

59. Mense S, Meyer H. Bradykinin-induced modulation of the response behaviour of different types of feline group III and IV muscle receptors. J Physiol (Lond). 1988;398:49–63.

60. Khasar SG, Miao FJ-P, Jänig W, Levine JD. Vagotomy-induced enhancement of mechanical hyperalgesia in the rat is sympathoadrenal-mediated. J Neurosci. 1998;18:3043–9.

61. Foreman RD. Organization of the spinothalamic tract as a relay for cardiopulmonary sympathetic afferent fiber activity. Prog Sensory Physiol. 1989;9:1–51.

62. Berthoud HR, Neuhuber WL. Distribution and morphology of vagal afferents and efferents supplying the digestive system. In: Tache Y, Wingate DL, Burks TF, editors. Innervation of the Gut. Pathophysiological Implications. Boca Raton: CRC Press, 1994:43–66.

63. Berthoud HR, Patterson LM, Willing AE, Mueller K, Neuhuber WL. Capsaicin-resistant vagal afferent fibers in the rat gastrointestinal tract: anatomical identification and functional integrity. Brain Res. 1997;746:195–206.

64. Jänig W, Levine JD, Michaelis M. Interactions of sympathetic and primary afferent neurons following nerve injury and tissue trauma. Prog Brain Res. 1996;112:161–84.

65. Jänig W. Pain and the sympathetic nervous system: pathophysiological mechanisms. In: Mathias CJ, Bannister R, editors. Autonomic Failure. New York: Oxford University Press, 1999: 99–108.

66. Jänig W, Häbler HJ. Sympathetic nervous system: contribution to chronic pain. Prog Brain Res. 2000;129:451–68.

67. Jänig W. Organization of the lumbar sympathetic outflow to skeletal muscle and skin of the cat hindlimb and tail. Rev Physiol Biochem Pharmacol. 1985;102:119–213.

68. Jänig W. Spinal cord reflex organization of sympathetic systems. Prog Brain Res. 1996;107:43–77.

69. Jänig W, Häbler HJ. Organisation of the autonomic nervous system: structure and function. In: Appenzeller O, editor. Handbook of Clinical Neurology 74, The Autonomic Nervous System, part I: Normal Functions. Amsterdam: Elsevier, 1999:1–52.

70. Jänig W, McLachlan EM. Characteristics of function-specific pathways in the sympathetic nervous system. Trends Neurosci. 1992;15:475–81.

71. Jänig W, McLachlan EM. Neurobiology of the autonomic nervous system. In: Mathias CJ, Bannister R, editors. Autonomic Failure. New York: Oxford University Press, 1999:3–15.

72. Goebell H, Holtmann G, Talley NJ. Functional Dyspepsia and Irritable Bowel Syndrome. Lancaster: Kluwer, 1998.

73. Mayer EA, Raybould HE. Basic and Clinical Aspects of Chronic Abdominal Pain. Amsterdam: Elsevier, 1993.

74. Wolfe F, Smythe HA, Yunus MB *et al*. The American College of Rheumatology 1990 Criteria for the Classification of Fibromyalgia. Report of the Multicenter Criteria Committee. Arthritis Rheum. 1990;33:160–72.
75. Morrison SF, Cao WH. Different adrenal sympathetic preganglionic neurons regulate epinephrine and norepinephrine secretion. Am J Physiol Regul Integr Comp Physiol. 2000;279:R1763–75.
76. Morrison SF. Differential control of sympathetic outflow. Am J Physiol Regul Integr Comp Physiol. 2001;281:R683–98.

12
Inflammation-induced changes in nerves as a basis for symptom generation in irritable bowel syndrome

S. M. COLLINS

INTRODUCTION

There are several lines of evidence that may be followed to support the argument that inflammation-induced changes in nerves is a basis for symptom generation in irritable bowel syndrome (IBS)[1].

INFLAMMATION IN IBS

First, there is growing evidence that inflammation plays a role in the pathophysiology of this syndrome. Several studies have demonstrated that there are increased numbers of inflammatory cells in the mucosa of the colorectum of patients with IBS. Initially, these studies focused on mast cells. Indeed, in the early literature, when surgery was an accepted treatment for severe forms of IBS, full-thickness surgical resections revealed evidence of mast cell infiltration throughout the muscularis as well as in the myenteric plexus of patients with IBS – 'spastic colitis'[2]. Since that time, other studies have continued to demonstrate increased cellularity of the lamina propria in IBS patients. As the gut is normally in a state of physiological inflammation, small increments in the cellularity of the lamina propria may be difficult to identify. Using a semiquantitative approach, Saltzmann et al.[3] showed a definite increase in cell number in the colon of patients with diarrhoea-predominant IBS. Weston et al.[4] showed increased numbers of mast cells in the terminal ileum of patients with IBS, and O'Sullivan et al. demonstrated increased mast cell numbers in the colon itself[5]. Taken together, these studies would support the notion that there is an increased number of inflammatory cells in the colon of IBS patients. However, these studies do not provide any evidence of altered function, as they are merely morphological demonstrations. O'Sullivan *et al.* have shown immunohistochemical evidence suggestive of increased immunohistochemical staining, for iNOS, and its product nitrotyrosine, were found in colonic mucosal biopsies in IBS patients[6]. More recently, Barbara *et al.* provided preliminary evidence that mast cells harvested from the colon of patients with IBS secrete more histamine than do mast cells harvested from non-IBS patients[7]. Finally, Chadwick *et al.* showed evidence of lymphocytic activity in biopsies taken from IBS patients[8]; they found an increased incidence of CD25 staining in these biopsies, suggesting immune activity mediated via the interleukin-2 receptor. Interestingly, these findings were not restricted to those patients who had an acute onset or short duration of IBS. These findings were also found in most patients with chronic insidious-onset IBS.

ROLE OF NERVES IN SYMPTOM GENERATION IN IBS

It is generally assumed that nerves play a role in symptom generation in the gastrointestinal tract. The major functional abnormalities documented in IBS patients include changes in gastrointestinal motility, changes in sensory perception and accommodation, and changes in epithelial transport in some cases. While the clinical heterogeneity of IBS is well recognized, it is unlikely that the pathogenetic mechanisms that may lead to a clinical syndrome of IBS involve dysfunction in such varied target organs as the smooth muscle cell, the enteric nerve and the interstitial cell of Cajal – collectively the cells that constitute the motility apparatus of the gut. By the same reasoning, it is unlikely that afferent nerves are singled out as targets in IBS. Similarly, in the absence of overt manifestations, the epithelial cell itself is unlikely to be intrinsically abnormal in IBS. To incorporate these cells into the pathophysiology of IBS one must invoke changes in their nerve supply. An example of this is the alteration in colonic motility postprandially (the gastrocolic reflex), which is often exaggerated in IBS patients[9]. This can be blocked by naloxone or by antimuscarinic drugs, implicating neural mediation of this reflex. In general, drug development by the pharmaceutical industry has been targeted on antagonists or agonists of neurotransmission. Thus, the case can be made that the brunt of the pathogenetic processes involved in IBS involve nerves, either afferent, efferent, intrinsic or extrinsic to the gut.

INFLAMMATION ALTERS NEURAL FUNCTION

It is now well accepted that inflammatory processes can alter neural function in a variety of organs including the gastrointestinal tract. Studies have shown that, in models of inflammation, the content as well as the release of neurotransmitter is altered. It has also been shown that these inflammation-induced changes in neural function persist following resolution of the inflammatory process. Moreover, such changes may also be seen at non-inflamed sites, and this could explain the widespread nature of the physiological disturbances seen in IBS patients[10].

PERIPHERAL VERSUS CENTRAL PATHOGENESIS IN IBS

The mechanisms leading to gut dysfunction in IBS may be classified as originating from the CNS (the top-down model of IBS) or may arise as a result of peripheral events (the bottom-up model of IBS)[10]. While the role of behaviour and stress in IBS is well established, and generally acknowledged, it remains unclear how such processes may alter gastrointestinal function in the long term. The vast majority of studies examining the impact of stressful stimuli on gastrointestinal function are acute. There are very few, if any, studies of chronic stress and their impact on gut function. The recently described model of maternal deprivation or neonatal trauma may provide some insight but, to date, demonstrations of robust persistent changes in gastrointestinal function following these events are lacking. Furthermore, the relevance of psychological or physical trauma in the neonatal period to the pathogenesis of IBS is not known.

ROLE OF INFECTION IN IBS

In contrast, there is now ample evidence that acute gastroenteritis may lead to IBS. This theory is based on several prospective studies and patients recovering from acute gastroenteritis following outbreaks of food contamination. The incidence of IBS in these circumstances may range from 7% to 33%[11–13]. A large cohort study performed on a computerized database in the United Kingdom demonstrated that acute gastroenteritis is the highest risk factor for the development of IBS recognized to date. Acute gastroenteritis is associated with a relative risk of 11.9 for the development of IBS[14]. Studies in patients with postinfective IBS reveal evidence of ongoing inflammation[15]. There is increased intestinal permeability that would promote access of luminal antigen to the gut wall. There is also evidence of increased lymphocytes in the lamina propria, suggesting an ongoing inflammatory process. The concept that transient inflammation can lead to persistent dysfunction in the gastrointestinal tract comes from the development of an animal model. This model is based on a primary nematode infection in mice[16,17]. Studies in this model show that, after full recovery from the infection and resolution of the inflammatory process in the small intestine, there is evidence of persistently abnormal enteric smooth muscle and nerve function. Interestingly, these persistent postinfective changes can be reversed following a short course of corticosteroid therapy administered after recovering from the infection. These findings therefore attest to the presence of inflammation-induced changes in enteric nerve function as a consequence of a previous enteric infection.

INFLAMMATORY CHANGES IN THE ENTERIC NERVOUS SYSTEM

It is difficult to establish causality between inflammation, the involvement of enteric nerves, and symptom generation in human subjects with IBS. However, there are now data identifying the involvement of inflammatory cells in the myenteric plexus of patients with severe IBS. Tornblum *et al.* obtained ethical approval to perform laparoscopic-assisted full-thickness biopsies on patients with severe IBS. Their results showed that in at least six specimens the myenteric plexus showed evidence of a ganglionitis with nerve cells surrounded by lymphocytes and showing some evidence of degeneration[18]. This study is the first of its kind to directly address changes in enteric neural pathology in IBS patients and it provides a clear demonstration of the involvement of inflammatory cells in this tissue. The work of Barbara *et al.*, in which they provide evidence of *altered function* of mast cells in IBS patients also shows an abnormal juxtaposition between nerves and mast cells, again supporting the notion that inflammation plays a role in altering nerves in IBS[7]. Taken together, these findings support the position that inflammation-induced changes in enteric nerve function provide a basis for symptom generation in IBS.

CONCLUSION

Definitive proof awaits controlled studies in which IBS patients, carefully selected on the basis of an abnormal inflammatory marker, are treated with an anti-inflammatory preparation such as prednisone. A recent preliminary report, co-authored by this author, failed to demonstrate improvement in patients with postinfective IBS following a short course of corticosteroids. These patients were recruited retrospectively and the interval between infection and treatment varied considerably. In addition, these patients had mild symptoms, and differences between the treatment and controlled groups were small. Thus, with a limited sample size, it was difficult to determine any changes in steroid responsiveness between these two groups. This study does not, therefore, constitute strong evidence against the role of inflammation in postinfective IBS.

References

1. Collins SM, Piche T, Rampal P. The putative role of inflammation in the irritable bowel syndrome. Gut. 2001;49:743–5.
2. Hiatt RB, Katz J. Mast cells in inflammatory conditions of the gastrointestinal tract. Am J Gastroenterol. 1962;37:541–8.
3. Salzmann JL, Peltier-Koch F, Bloch F, Petite JP, Camilleri JP. Methods in laboratory investigation: morphometric study of colonic biopsies: a new method of estimating inflammatory diseases. Lab Invest. 1992;60:847–51.
4. Weston AP, Biddle WL, Bhatia PS, Miner PB Jr. Terminal ileal mucosal mast cells in irritable bowel syndrome. Dig Dis Sci. 1993;38:1590–5.
5. O'Sullivan M. Increased mast cells in the irritable bowel syndrome. Neurogastroenterol Motil. 2000;12:449–57.
6. O'Sullivan M, Clayton N, Wong T, Bountra C, Buckley M, O'Morain C. Increased inos and nitrotyrosine expression in irritable bowel syndrome (Ibs). Gastroenterology. 2000;118(Suppl. 2): A702 (abstract).
7. Barbara G, *et al.* Tryptase positive mast cells in IBS. Gastroenterology. 2002 (abstract).
8. Chadwick VS, Chen W, Shu D *et al.* Activation of the mucosal immune system in irritable bowel syndrome. Gastroenterology. 2002;122:1778–83.
9. Bazzocchi G, Ellis J, Villanueva-Meyer J *et al.* Postprandial colonic transit and motor activity in chronic constipation. Gastroenterology. 1990;98:686–93.
10. Mayer EA, Collins SM. Evolving pathophysiologic models of functional gastrointestinal disorders. Gastroenterology. 2002;122:2032–48.
11. Gwee KA, Leong YL, Graham C *et al.* The role of psychological and biological factors in postinfective gut dysfunction. Gut. 1999;44:400–6.

12. McKendrick MW, Read NW. Irritable bowel syndrome – post-*Salmonella* infection (see comments). J Infect. 1994;29:1–33.
13. Neal KR, Hebden J, Spiller R. Prevalence of gastrointestinal symptoms six months after bacterial gastroenteritis and risk factors for development of the irritable bowel syndrome: postal survey of patients. Br Med J. 1997;314:779–82.
14. Rodriguez LA, Ruigomez A. Increased risk of irritable bowel syndrome after bacterial gastroenteritis: cohort study. Br Med J. 1999;318:565–6.
15. Spiller RC, Jenkins D, Thornley JP *et al*. Increased rectal mucosal enteroendocrine cells, T lymphocytes and increased gut permeability following acute *Campylobacter* enteritis and in post-dysenteric irritable bowel syndrome. Gut. 2000;47:804–11.
16. Barbara G, Vallance BA, Collins SM. Persistent intestinal neuromuscular dysfunction after acute nematode infection in mice. Gastroenterology. 1997;113:1224–32.
17. Barbara G, De Giorgio R, Deng Y, Vallance B, Blennerhassett P, Collins SM. Role of immunologic factors and cyclooxygenase 2 in persistent postinfective enteric muscle dysfunction in mice. Gastroenterology. 2001;120:1729–36.
18. Tornblom H, Lindberg G, Nyberg B, Veress B. Histopathological findings in the jejunum of patients with severe irritable bowel syndrome. Gastroenterology. 2000;118(Suppl.1):A140 (abstract).

13
Inflammation-induced altered nerve function in the gut – does it play a role in gastrointestinal symptom generation?

S. BRADESI, I. SCHWETZ and E. A. MAYER

INTRODUCTION

It is commonly assumed that chronic inflammation, irritation, or injury of the gut is associated with gastrointestinal symptoms such as abdominal pain or discomfort. More recently the finding of mild or proinflammatory changes in the colonic mucosa of individuals who meet current irritable bowel syndrome (IBS) symptom criteria (Rome criteria; see Table 1) has been implicated as a possible mechanism underlying chronic visceral hyperalgesia and altered bowel habits[1,2], and frequently examples from the literature are quoted to suggest the association of visceral hypersensitivity (assessed by controlled rectal distension) with mucosal pathology[2,3]. However, there are several problems with this concept. First, true alterations in the perception of visceral stimuli (experimental or spontaneous) associated with mucosal immune activation (or other mucosal abnormalities) have not been reported, and the reported evidence for 'visceral hypersensitivity' in these patients is generally related to changes in mechanoelastic properties of the rectum[4,5]. Secondly, the assumption of a relationship between chronic inflammatory events of the mucosa and visceral hypersensitivity is based on the clinical observations of pain associated with *acute* gut irritation (gastroenteritis, intermittent acid reflux, symptom flare in inflammatory bowel disease) and on findings of acute visceral hyperalgesia seen in animal models of *acute* visceral inflammation[6,7]. However, a series of clinical observations, as well as experimental findings in humans and in animals, suggest that chronic inflammatory changes of the gastrointestinal mucosa are frequently not associated with symptoms of chronic pain, enhanced perception of visceral stimuli, or evidence for visceral mechanical hyperalgesia[8]. Furthermore, there are ample clinical examples, which demonstrate that even extensive mucosal lesions, such as those associated with peptic ulcer disease, severe gastro-oesophageal reflux disease

"

Table 1   Rome Consensus criteria for the diagnosis of irritable bowel syndrome[31]

(a) Diagnostic criteria

At least 12 weeks, which need not be consecutive, in the preceding 12 months of abdominal discomfort or pain that has two of three features:

1. Relieved with defaecation; and/or
2. Onset associated with a change in frequency of stool; and/or
3. Onset associated with a change in form (appearance of stool).

> Where abnormal frequency is > 3/day and < 3/week.
> Where abnormal stool form is 'lumpy/hard' or 'loose/watery'.

(b) Supportive symptoms

1. Fewer than three bowel movements a week
2. More than three bowel movements a day
3. Hard or lumpy stools
4. Loose (mushy) or watery stools
5. Straining during a bowel movement
6. Urgency (having to rush to have a bowel movement)
7. Feeling of incomplete bowel movement
8. Passing mucus (white material) during a bowel movement
9. Abdominal fullness, bloating or swelling

> *'Diarrhoea-predominant'* = one or more of 2, 4, or 6 and none of 1, 3, or 5.
> *'Constipation-predominant'* = one or more of 1, 3, or 5 and none of 2, 4, 6.

(Barrett's oesophagus) or even neoplastic lesions of the gastrointestinal tract are commonly not associated with any symptoms. In the following, we will provide evidence from clinical and epidemiological studies, as well as from human experimental studies, to support the hypothesis that, in the absence of alterations in endogenous pain modulation systems and associated alterations in visceral perception, chronic inflammatory mucosal changes in the gut are *not* associated with the cardinal IBS symptom of abdominal pain. We also suggest that the failure of the current IBS diagnostic criteria to distinguish between abdominal pain and discomfort plays a major role in the erroneous labelling of various forms of 'organic' mucosal alterations associated with altered bowel habits (for example, lymphocytic colitis), as IBS.

WHAT ARE THE VARIOUS MECHANISMS UNDERLYING SYMPTOM GENERATION IN INFLAMMATORY AND FUNCTIONAL GASTROINTESTINAL DISORDERS?

As shown in Fig. 1, the symptom complex of abdominal pain and/or discomfort associated with alterations in bowel habits is made up of two fundamentally different categories of symptoms: (1) a category of symptoms which includes bowel habits, which is related primarily to alterations in enteric nervous system (ENS) activity, and which is not dependent on the conscious perception of visceral afferent information; (2) a category which is critically dependent on the subjective perception of visceral afferent events, and which is subject to extensive central modulatory influences.

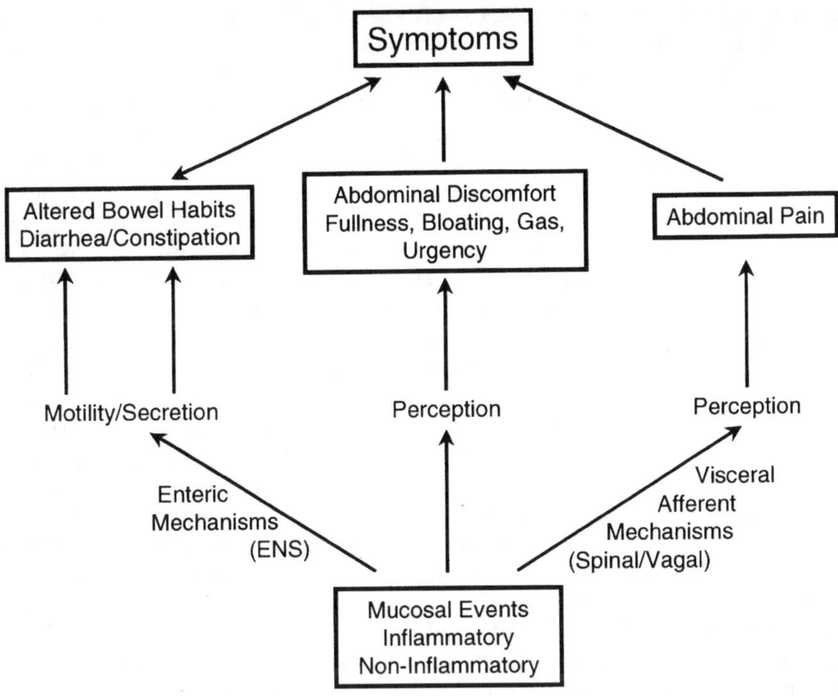

Fig. 1 Conceptual model illustrating differential roles of enteric nervous system (ENS) and central nervous system (CNS) involvement in gastrointestinal symptom generation

True alterations in bowel habits, such as changes in stool consistency and frequency, arise from alterations in gut motility and secretion, processes under the direct control of the ENS. Information regarding physiological and pathological mucosal events is encoded by intrinsic primary afferent neurons (IPANs) and transmitted via interneurons into myenteric and submucosal circuits which generate such stereotypic gut responses as the peristaltic and the secretomotor reflex. The encoding process involves enterochromaffine cells (ECCs) in the gut mucosa, and the sensitivity of IPAN terminals can be modulated by a variety of immune cell products, including proinflammatory cytokines and mast cell products such as tryptase and histamine[9]. Various changes in mucosal cell populations, including increases or decreases in ECCs[10], in mucosal mast cell numbers[11,12], or in mononuclear cells would be expected to result in altered responsiveness of basic ENS circuits, in particular of peristaltic and secretomotor reflex circuits. In addition, long-lasting alterations in the responsiveness of intestinal smooth muscle to inflammatory mediators have been demonstrated[13]. Thus, several different mucosal and transmural pathologies would be expected to alter basic gut functions via these mechanisms. In the case of response patterns resulting in diarrhoea, a sensation of urgency might be associated solely with the ENS-generated motility/secretory reflex alterations, without any need for an associated increase in perceptual sensitivity. Thus, even though the activity in basic ENS circuits can also be modulated by the sympathetic and parasympathetic branches of the autonomic nervous system based on information coming from the central nervous system (CNS), the subjective experience of symptoms of altered bowel habits in terms of consistency and frequency is not dependent on modulatory CNS mechanisms.

In contrast, symptoms of abdominal pain and abdominal discomfort regardless of their underlying aetiology are crucially dependent on central mechanisms of perception and modulation. Regardless of what neuronal changes and sensitization phenomena occur in ENS circuits, symptoms of pain and discomfort are not a linear reflection of events at the gut level, but the result of extensive modulation of afferent signals at the spinal, thalamic and suprathalamic level. Evidence for inhibitory as well as facilitatory modulation of visceral afferent signals has been reported[14]. Based on the observation that the majority of visceral events are not consciously perceived, one may postulate that under normal circumstances counter-regulatory inhibitory modulation of perception predominates, particularly in situations of chronic mucosal injury or inflammation. The uniqueness of interoception in the healthy organism (opposed to perception of somatic stimuli) is the fact that it is subliminal most of the time, e.g. it is not associated with conscious perception, even in the presence of pathology. Regarding the gut, this is probably essential to prevent a major disturbance of normal conscious processes by a constant barrage of visceral afferent signals arising from physiologically occurring high-amplitude contractions, distension by intake of fluid or food, exposure of vanilloid receptors to bile acids or capsaicin, and interaction of the mucosal immune system with the intestinal flora. On the other hand, the ability to modulate the perception of visceral signals makes it possible for a variety of emotional and cognitive factors to increase visceral perception acutely in the healthy individual. The ability to perceive upper gastrointestinal sensations, or sensations of fullness and urgency from the rectum and urinary bladder during states of acute anxiety are just two common examples which illustrate this point.

In summary, we propose that the symptom complex as defined by current IBS symptom criteria is non-specific since it can arise from at least two fundamentally different mechanisms:

1. Alterations in bowel habits in response to a variety of mucosal alterations mediated by sensitization and modulation of ENS circuitry underlying basic gut functions. In the absence of alterations in perception (e.g. inappropriate activation of endogenous pain-inhibitory systems, or exaggerated activation of pain-facilitatory systems), these ENS changes by themselves are probably not associated with symptoms of abdominal pain, but could cause a considerable amount of discomfort (e.g. urgency).
2. The experience of abdominal pain and discomfort which is crucially dependent on the brain's modulatory response to visceral signals. Unless there is an alteration in the normal response of the brain to prevent visceral signals from reaching conscious attention, a variety of mucosal alterations may never become symptomatic.

In the case of the common subjective symptom of 'constipation' (without alterations in intestinal transit), the second mechanism (altered perception) may play a prominent role as well: the patient's perception of being 'constipated' is commonly related to the perception of abdominal fullness, gas and the inability to get rid of these sensations of discomfort by passing a bowel movement. Thus, the general symptom of chronic constipation may arise from at least two fundamentally different mechanisms: one involving the ENS, another involving enhanced visceral perception. (A third mechanism not relevant to the current discussion is obviously related to modulation of gut function by the parasympathetic and sympathetic branches of the autonomic nervous system.)

TELEOLOGICAL REASONS AGAINST THE PHENOMENON OF CHRONIC GUT INFLAMMATION RESULTING IN VISCERAL HYPERALGESIA

Pain is an adaptive experience which ultimately aims to minimize tissue injury by promoting protective motor reflexes to avoid the injury, protecting the injured body part to maximize healing and recovery, and enhancing emotional learning to decrease the probability of future injuries. In the healthy organism these functions are assured by a well-controlled sequential engagement of endogenous mechanisms resulting first in sensitization followed by counterregulatory pain inhibition. Acute somatic as well as visceral pain is experienced following sensitization of pain pathways by an acute noxious stimulus. For example, acute acid perfusion in the oesophagus results in the transient acute burning pain of heartburn. Acute gastroenteric infections or toxin exposure result in acute, often severe abdominal pain and discomfort, which subsides following the resolution of the insulting agents. Acute inflammation or obstruction of the gallbladder or the pancreatic duct result in acute pain, which is relieved following resolution of the inflammation.

However, chronic pain is primarily a feature of *somatic* nociception and the resulting adaptive behavioural response (e.g. motor inhibition and protection of an injured body part) is aimed primarily at maximizing the chance for healing and recovery. For example, chronic joint pain associated with rheumatoid arthritis is aimed at immobilizing the affected joint and thereby avoiding physical strain on the affected joint. Chronic pain from a cut of the skin or a broken bone serves a similar purpose. On the other hand, chronic *visceral* pain generally does not have an adaptive value. Some of the most common causes of acute visceral pain (perforation, obstruction) are frequently associated with motor patterns aimed at clearing the digestive tract of its content (nausea/vomiting) and ultimately visceral motor inhibition (ileus), but do not generally result in chronic pain; if not surgically relieved they are not compatible with survival of the organism. One condition that has been suggested to be associated with chronic visceral pain is chronic mucosal inflammation. However, there are few behavioural responses in response to visceral pain (other than decreased food intake) which might be beneficial to promote a resolution of the underlying problem (e.g. mucosal inflammation) causing the chronic pain. In contrast to the somatic domain, visceral motor inhibition in response to visceral inflammation is involuntary and mediated by viscerovisceral reflexes. Long-term sensitization and enhancement of such ENS reflexes may be adaptive in order to expel potentially noxious agents from the gut, once the gut has been exposed to this insult. In contrast, visceral motor inhibition in form of ileus is a temporarily restricted strategy to protect the gut: contractions and distensions of the gut are essential for survival and voluntary inhibition of such motor activity in response to pain, if it were possible, would be highly maladaptive. Finally, and probably most importantly, a chronically inflamed state of the gastrointestinal mucosa related to recurrent infections and infestations with parasites is presumably the normal condition of the gastrointestinal tract in animals, including non-human primates, as well as in primal human societies. If inflammation-induced sensitization of primary afferents innervating the gastrointestinal tract played an important role in the development of functional gastrointestinal symptoms, including IBS, one would expect a greatly increased prevalence of these disorders in the population of developing countries (such as Africa, Mexico or India), an observation that has *not* been reported in the literature[15]. It is therefore fair to say that from an evolutionary standpoint it would be highly maladaptive to associate chronic pain with a chronically inflamed mucosa, a condition which may have been the norm for millions of years of human evolution.

EPIDEMIOLOGICAL REASONS ARGUING AGAINST A ROLE OF CHRONIC MUCOSAL INFLAMMATION PRODUCING MECHANICAL VISCERAL HYPERALGESIA

While mild inflammatory changes of the colonic mucosa may be considered a normal state of the intestinal immune system, pathological inflammation occurs primarily in situations of chronic infections, infestations or idiopathic inflammation as it is seen in inflammatory bowel disease. In the lower gastrointestinal tract chronic small intestinal and colonic inflammation occur primarily in the form of ulcerative colitis and Crohn's disease. In the upper gut some of the most common examples of chronic inflammation occur in the context of *Helicobacter pylori* infection. In the absence of complications (such as peptic ulcer disease or the development of strictures or abscesses) chronic abdominal pain and visceral hyperalgesia do not appear to be a hallmark of chronic inflammation of either the upper or lower gut. Several large multi-centre studies have addressed the question of whether *H. pylori* infection is associated with symptoms of functional dyspepsia, and if eradication of the organism in symptomatic patients results in resolution of the dyspepsia symptoms[16–18]. However, all published studies fairly consistently demonstrate that there is no significant relationship between *H. pylori* infection and symptoms of functional dyspepsia, despite the presence of well-characterized chronic inflammatory changes in the gastric mucosa of infected individuals. Thus, while it may be assumed that during chronic gastritis there are neuroplastic alterations in spinal afferents innervating the stomach, such as increase in substance P content, expression of TTX-resistant sodium channels and expression of novel receptors, counterregulatory mechanisms (presumably in the CNS) prevent these peripheral changes producing visceral hyperalgesia and associated symptoms.

EVIDENCE FROM HUMAN EXPERIMENTAL STUDIES ARGUING AGAINST THE ASSOCIATION OF CHRONIC MUCOSAL INFLAMMATION WITH VISCERAL HYPERALGESIA TO MECHANICAL STIMULI

Our group published a series of studies which support the concept that different types of chronic gut irritation/injury do not necessarily result in the development of visceral mechanical hyperalgesia and chronic abdominal pain. Fass and co-workers reported that patients with gastro-oesophageal reflux disease did not show evidence of visceral hypersensitivity during controlled oesophageal balloon distension[19]. Similarly, Mertz *et al.*[20] have shown that patients reporting symptoms of dyspepsia associated with organic lesions of the gastric mucosa (e.g. peptic ulcer disease) did not show evidence for visceral hypersensitivity to gastric distension, while those with functional dyspepsia and without any detectable lesions showed increased perceptual response. Holtmann and co-workers[21] performed controlled duodenal distension in patients with *H. pylori* infection and chronic gastritis, and did not find evidence for visceral hypersensitivity to the distending stimulus. Bernstein and co-workers used a similar distension technique in the rectum of patients with Crohn's disease limited to the small bowel. It was hypothesized that chronic inflammation of the small bowel would result in sensitization of spinal cord segments receiving converging afferent input from the rectosigmoid. However, no evidence of rectal hypersensitivity to phasic rectal distension was found, while discomfort thresholds to slow ramp distension were higher compared to healthy controls[22]. Finally, Chang and colleagues published a study comparing the perceptual response of three subject groups (healthy controls, patients with mild IBD, and IBS patients) to rectal distension before and following a train of noxious sigmoid distensions[23]. The sigmoid distensions were aimed to induce a state of central sensitization[24]. The authors hypothesized that both IBS and inflammatory bowel disease (IBD) patients would develop sensitization resulting in an enhanced perceptual response to rectal distension. While the sigmoid conditioning stimulus had no significant effect in healthy controls on perception of the rectal distension, it *decreased* the perception threshold in IBS patients, while IBD patients became less sensitive. The findings in IBD patients strongly suggest the presence of powerful counterregulatory pain modulation mechanisms which not only prevent the development of visceral hyperalgesia, but which can produce a transient state of visceral hypoalgesia.

THE NON-LINEAR MODEL OF VISCERAL PERCEPTION: ENDOGENOUS PAIN MODULATION

Based on the model shown in Fig. 2 it is suggested that, in the otherwise healthy individual, a variety of different mucosal pathologies will not result in a state of enhanced visceral perception, even in the presence of sensitization of peripheral pain pathways. This is presumably due to the activity of endogenous pain-inhibition systems. These systems can be active tonically, or can be activated only in response to phasic noxious stimuli[25]. Since the corticopontine circuitry

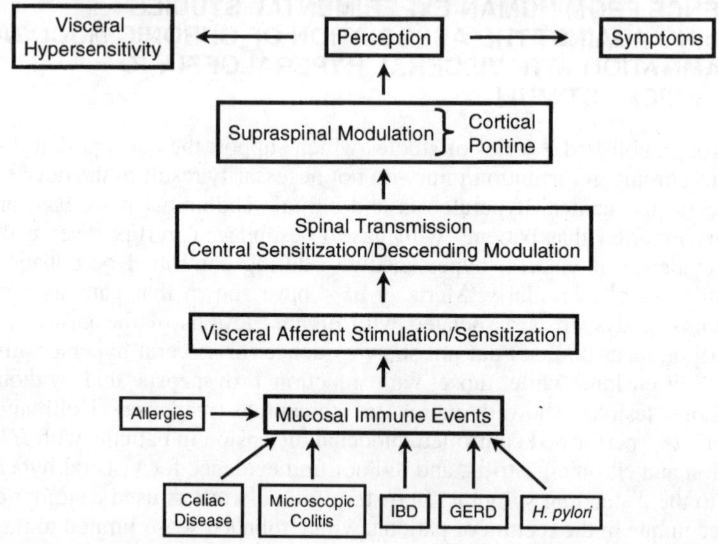

Fig. 2 A schematic emphasizing the non-linear nature of processing of visceral afferent signals by the CNS. Regardless of the various inflammatory changes at the mucosal level associated with different conditions, the perception of symptoms and the enhanced responsiveness to experimental gut stimulation is crucially dependent on the activity of several related pain-modulation systems, including the corticospinal pain-modulation systems

also receives input from cortical regions, emotional and cognitive influences can modulate the activity of these pain-modulation systems[26].

PROBLEMS WITH THE ROME CLASSIFICATION OF IBS WHICH MIGHT UNDERLIE THE DEBATE BETWEEN PERIPHERAL AND CENTRAL MODELS OF IBS

Most attempts to develop symptom-based diagnostic criteria for IBS, including the Rome criteria (see Table 1), have not differentiated between abdominal pain and abdominal discomfort as a necessary symptom. Interestingly, the majority of IBS patients seen at a tertiary referral centre for functional gastrointestinal disorders refer to their most bothersome symptom as discomfort and not pain, even though the great majority lists pain as one of the symptoms[27,28]. The difference between those who refer to their symptoms as painful and those who do not, does not appear to be a fundamental difference in clinical presentation or psychological characteristics. A plausible explanation may be differences in the way patients refer to the altered sensations they perceive from the gut: while some refer to them primarily in terms of discomfort, others refer to them as pain. Another possible explanation might be differences in the modulatory effect of endogenous pain-modulation systems, with less effective pain inhibition in patients with pain-predominant symptoms. Regardless of the reliability of patients' reports of their symptoms as pain or discomfort, it should easily be apparent that any patient with altered bowel habits due to alterations in intestinal motility and secretory function, who experiences discomfort in the form of either urgency or a sensation of incomplete evacuation, will meet the current diagnostic criteria for IBS (e.g. altered bowel habits associated with abdominal discomfort). The majority of patients with chronic diarrhoea (including such 'organic' entities as lymphocytic and collagenous colitis) should therefore meet the current Rome criteria. Thus, a referral centre for patients with chronic diarrhoea will presumably see a large proportion of patients who will meet the Rome criteria for IBS-D (by reporting chronic abdominal *discomfort* associated with change in bowel habits), while a referral centre for patients with IBS and abdominal pain will predominantly see patients who meet the same diagnostic criteria by reporting chronic abdominal pain associated with a change in bowel habits. For example, the most bothersome symptom in patients enrolled in a large multi-centre study for IBS patients with diarrhoea-predominant bowel habit was urgency[29]. Even though the sensation of urgency could result from an enhanced perception of rectal afferent signals, it is more likely to result from a combination of altered mechanoelastic properties of the rectosigmoid (reduced rectosigmoid compliance), a more rapid transit of colonic contents into a non-compliant rectum due to enhanced propulsive motility (increased number of migrating motor complexes, or hyperactive peristaltic reflexes) and to a more liquid stool due to altered water and electrolyte secretion. Many of these changes could result from alterations in mucosal immune or entero-chromaffine cell physiology, without any need for associated extracolonic patho-physiology, including CNS modulation. Such changes in colonic motility and secretion have been observed in a variety of acute and chronic inflammatory conditions of the colon, including collagenous and microscopic colitis, ulcerative and Crohn's colitis, acute gastroenteritis, coeliac sprue, etc. It is likely that many of the mucosal immune alterations recently reported in Rome-positive IBS patients[11,12,30] are simply a reflection of misclassification of a group of patients with well-characterized mucosal immune alterations as IBS patients.

SUMMARY AND CONCLUSIONS

In principle we have provided several lines of evidence suggesting that chronic intestinal inflammation is not typically associated with chronic visceral mechanical hyperalgesia, and that recently reported patterns of epithelial cell abnormalities in the human colonic mucosa by themselves are not a plausible cause of visceral mechanical hyperalgesia and chronic pain, unless accompanied by alterations in central pain-modulatory systems. The debate regarding symptoms, mucosal pathology, enhanced visceral perception and functional gastrointestinal disorders points out a fundamental problem with the current symptom-based classification of functional disorders, in particular IBS. Based on the above considerations we would like to point out several shortcomings in the existing way of diagnosing and classifying IBS using the Rome criteria.

1.   Symptom criteria that do not differentiate between discomfort and pain, if not accompanied by sophisticated histological tissue evaluations, will automatically include a range of disorders with clearly identifiable mucosal alterations

(immune, enterochromaffine, interstitial cells). The relative percentage of such patients with organic colonic lesions will depend on the referral setting. These mucosal alterations are likely to produce symptoms primarily via alterations in gastrointestinal motor and secretory function secondary to changes in ENS function, and do not require the presence of enhanced visceral perception or altered stress responsiveness. Patients with 'post-infectious IBS' may fall into this category. If a clear causative role between symptoms of diarrhoea and urgency can be established for any of these 'organic' abnormalities, this group of disorders should no longer be referred to as 'functional' gastrointestinal disorders, but rather should be included in the growing list of microscopic forms of colitis, presenting as subforms of organic diarrhoea.

2. Patients with enhanced stress responsiveness can develop symptoms by a fundamentally different mechanism, which does not require alterations in mucosal immune cells or other cell populations, even though the central alterations may also co-occur in such patients. Patients with the primary CNS-driven syndromes develop symptoms of altered bowel movements, pain and discomfort primarily by altered central autonomic regulation and alterations in the perception of visceral events. It is this latter, presumably larger, group of patients for which the diagnosis of IBS should be restricted. The central alterations responsible for symptom generation in IBS patients can also be present in patients with demonstrated mucosal abnormalities, resulting in such well-described clinical entities as post-infectious IBS, in a subset of patients with IBD who continue to have symptoms during full clinical remission in patients with coeliac disease, etc. These considerations have important implications for the development of effective IBS therapies. We hypothesize that peripherally targeted drugs, including laxatives, antidiarrhoeals, prokinetics and possibly anti-inflammatory drugs, will provide significant symptomatic relief by aiming to normalize altered ENS function and thereby normalizing altered bowel habits. However, they will have a relatively small effect in patients in whom symptoms arise primarily as a consequence of enhanced perception, resulting in abdominal pain, fullness and bloating and a 'sensory' form of constipation. In the latter group of patients one would predict much greater effectiveness of centrally targeted drugs aimed at normalizing stress hyperresponsiveness and altered central modulation of visceral sensations.

References

1. Mayer EA, Collins SM. Evolving pathophysiologic models of functional gastrointestinal disorders. Gastroenterology. 2002;122:2032–48.
2. Collins SM, Piche T, Rampal P. The putative role of inflammation in the irritable bowel syndrome. Gut. 2001;49:743–5.
3. Talley NJ, Spiller R. Irritable bowel syndrome: a little understood organic bowel disease? Lancet. 2002;360:555–64.
4. Gwee KA, Leong YL, Graham C et al. The role of psychological and biological factors in postinfective gut dysfunction. Gut. 1999;44:400–6.
5. Chan CL, Facer P, Davis JB et al. Sensory fibres expressing capsaicin receptor TRPV1 in patients with rectal hypersensitivity and faecal urgency. Lancet. 2003;361:385–91.
6. Ozaki N, Bielefeldt K, Sengupta JN, Gebhart GF. Models of gastric hyperalgesia in the rat. Am J Physiol Gastrointest Liver Physiol. 2002;283:G666–76.

7. Ness TJ, Gebhart GF. Inflammation enhances reflex and spinal neuron responses to noxious visceral stimulation in rats. Am J Physiol Gastrointest Liver Physiol. 2001;280:G649–57.
8. Bradesi S, McRoberts JA, Anton PA, Mayer EA. Inflammatory bowel disease and irritable bowel syndrome: separate or unified? Curr Opin Gastroenterol. 2003 (in press).
9. Bueno L, Fioramonti J. Visceral perception: inflammatory and non-inflammatory mediators. Gut. 2002;51:i19–23.
10. Spiller RC, Jenkins D, Thornley JP *et al.* Increased rectal mucosal enteroendocrine cells, T-lymphocytes, and increased gut permeability following acute *Campylobacter* enteritis and in post-dysenteric irritable bowel syndrome. Gut. 2000;47:804–11.
11. Weston AP, Biddle WL, Bhatia PS, Miner PBJ. Terminal ileal mucosal mast cells in irritable bowel syndrome. Dig Dis Sci. 1993;38:1590–5.
12. O'Sullivan M, Clayton N, Breslin NP *et al.* Increased mast cells in the irritable bowel syndrome. Neurogastroenterol Motil. 2000;12:449–57.
13. Wang XY, Berezin I, Mikkelsen HB *et al.* Pathology of interstitial cells of Cajal in relation to inflammation revealed by ultrastructure but not immunohistochemistry. Am J Pathol. 2002;160:1529–40.
14. Porreca F, Ossipov MH, Gebhart GF. Chronic pain and medullary descending facilitation. Trends Neurosci. 2002;25:319–25.
15. Drossman DA, Camilleri M, Mayer EA, Whitehead WE. AGA technical review on irritable bowel syndrome. Gastroenterology. 2002;123:2108–31.
16. Pantoflickova D, Blum AL, Koelz HR. *Helicobactor pylori* and functional dyspepsia: a real causal link? Baillieres Clin Gastroenterol. 1998;12:503–32.
17. McColl KE. *Helicobacter pylori* 1988–1998. Eur J Gastroenterol Hepatol. 1999;11:13–16.
18. Talley NJ, Janssens J, Lauritsen K, Racz I, Bolling-Sternevald E. Eradication of *Helicobacter pylori* in functional dyspepsia: randomised double blind placebo controlled trial with 12 months' follow up. The Optimal Regimen Cures Helicobacter Induced Dyspepsia (ORCHID) Study Group. Br Med J. 1999;318:833–7.
19. Fass R, Naliboff B, Higa L *et al.* Differential effect of long-term esophageal acid exposure on mechanosensitivity and chemosensitivity in humans. Gastroenterology. 1998;115:1363–73.
20. Mertz H, Fullerton S, Naliboff B, Mayer EA. Symptoms and visceral perception in severe functional and organic dyspepsia. Gut. 1998;42:814–22.
21. Holtmann G, Talley N, Goebell H. Association between *H. pylori*, duodenal mechanosenosory thresholds, and small intestinal motility in chronic and unexplained dyspepsia. Dig Dis Sci. 1996;41:1285–91.
22. Bernstein CN, Niazi N, Robert M *et al.* Rectal afferent function in patients with inflammatory and functional intestinal disorders. Pain. 1996;66:151–61.
23. Chang L, Munakata J, Mayer EA *et al.* Perceptual responses in patients with inflammatory and functional bowel disease. Gut. 2000;47:497–505.
24. Munakata J, Naliboff B, Harraf F *et al.* Repetitive sigmoid stimulation induces rectal hyperalgesia in patients with irritable bowel syndrome. Gastroenterology. 1997;112:55–63.
25. Fields HL, Basbaum AI. Endogenous pain control mechanisms. In: Wall PD, Melzack R, editors. Textbook of Pain. New York: Churchill Livingstone, 1989:206–19.
26. Petrovic P, Ingvar M. Imaging cognitive modulation of pain processing. Pain. 2002;95:1–5.
27. Lembo T, Naliboff B, Munakata J *et al.* Symptoms and visceral perception in patients with pain-predominant irritable bowel syndrome. Am J Gastroenterol. 1999;94:1320–6.
28. Sach J, Bolus R, FitzGerald L, Naliboff BD, Chang L, Mayer EA. Is there a difference between abdominal pain and discomfort in moderate to severe IBS patients? Am J Gastroenterol. 2002;97:3131–8.
29. Mangel AW, Hahn BA, Heath AT *et al.* Adequate relief as an endpoint in clinical trials in irritable bowel syndrome. J Int Med Res. 1998;26:76–81.
30. Chadwick VS, Chen W, Shu D *et al.* Activation of the mucosal immune system in irritable bowel syndrome. Gastroenterology. 2002;122:1778–83.
31. ROME II. The Functional Gastrointestinal Disorders. Diagnosis, Pathophysiology and Treatment: A Multinational Consensus, 2nd edn. McLean, VA: Degnon Associates, 2000.

14
Colonic spinal primary afferents: mechanosensory and chemosensory subtypes and effects of inflammation

S. M. BRIERLEY, J. R. COLDWELL, N. J. COOPER,
G. S. HOWARTH and L. A. BLACKSHAW

INTRODUCTION

Irritable bowel syndrome (IBS) is characterized by symptoms of bloating, frequent urge to defaecate, and pain. Many of these IBS symptoms are considered on the basis of provocative studies to arise from mechanical events in the colon, such as distension and contraction. Sensory pathways from the colon are conducted via sacral pelvic and hypogastric or lumbar splanchnic nerves to the spinal cord[1]. It is not yet established if these two pathways carry similar or different mechanosensory information, although it has been suggested that lumbar splanchnic afferents convey phasic, rather than tonic, signals that provide information to the central nervous system regarding transient events rather than maintained distension[2]. One of our aims was to test this hypothesis in isolated tissue where precise control over mechanical forces is possible.

Colonic sensory pathways, in addition to conveying mechanosensory information regarding distension and contraction, probably also convey chemosensory information regarding luminal content and release of mediators. In this respect it has been demonstrated that, in subpopulations of IBS patients (diarrhoea-predominant), the release of 5-hydroxytryptamine (5-HT) after a meal is exaggerated, and that this correlates with symptoms[3,4]. It is also evident that the source of 5-HT is increased in the form of enterochromaffin cells in the colonic mucosa[5]. This suggests an important role for chemosensitivity in generation of symptoms in IBS. We have determined the sensitivity of colonic afferents to 5-HT and performed preliminary studies on effects of whether this is affected by acute inflammation. Our model of choice was the rat dextran sulphate sodium model, which has been demonstrated to exhibit a mild colitis comparable to human forms of the disease[6]. Although this is not a model of IBS *per se*, it may mimic the perturbation of sensory function and increased release of mediators characteristic of the disease[6].

In addition to 5-HT, a number of other chemical mediators may be candidates in activation of colonic sensory pathways in health or disease. These include histamine (derived from mast cells), bradykinin and adenosine triphosphate (ATP) (both derived from tissue damage)[7]. We have investigated the direct effects of these stimuli on colonic afferents, and compared sensitivity with that to capsaicin, an activator of subpopulations of primary afferent fibres[8]. One of our major aims in this case was to determine if afferent endings in the colon co-express receptors to more than one of these stimuli.

METHODS

Electrophysiological preparation

Details of electrophysiological methods are available from our previous publications on the rat colonic afferent preparation[9,10]. All experiments were carried out with the approval of, and according to guidelines of, the Animal Ethics Committees of the Institute of Medical and Veterinary Science.

Dissection of the colon

Distal colon was removed along with the lumbar colonic nerves and the bundle containing the inferior mesenteric artery, abdominal aorta, inferior mesenteric ganglion, intermesenteric nerve (IMN) and lumbar splanchnic nerves (LSN), and hypogastric nerves (HGN) according to the classification of Baron *et al.*[11], and transferred into cold carbogenated modified Krebs' bicarbonate buffer. The distal colon was opened longitudinally, off-centre to the antimesenteric border so that lumbar colonic nerve insertions lay along the edge of the opened preparation. Connective tissue was dissected away from the neural bundle; the bundle was cut and tied 2–15 mm rostral to the junction of the inferior mesenteric artery and abdominal aorta. The colon was then pinned flat in the perfusion chamber, and the neurovascular bundle was passed through a small hole into an adjacent paraffin-filled recording chamber.

Perfusion chamber and perfusate

The organ bath consisted of two adjacent compartments machined from clear acrylic. One organ compartment was superfused with Krebs' solution and the recording compartment containing the nerve and electrodes was filled with paraffin oil. The floor of both compartments was covered with Sylgard® (Dow Corning). The serosal and mucosal surfaces of the colon were superfused with different media. This was achieved either by creating a basement chamber that was separated from the upper chamber by nylon mesh over which the colon was pinned, or by pinning the colon over a perforated tube through which Krebs' solution was perfused. For the serosal chamber, modified Krebs' solution containing (mM) 117.9 NaCl, 4.7 KCl, 25 NaHCO$_3$, 1.3 NaH$_2$PO$_4$, 1.2 MgSO$_4$

$(H_2O)_7$, 2.5 $CaCl_2$, and 11.1 D-glucose was used. For the mucosal chamber, glucose was replaced by the short-chain fatty acids butyrate (2 mM), and acetate (20 mM). In all preparations the prostaglandin synthesis inhibitor indomethacin (3 μM) was added to suppress potential inhibitory actions of endogenous prostaglandins. The L-type calcium channel antagonist nifedipine (1 μM) was added to suppress smooth muscle activity that may otherwise give rise to indirect responses secondary to contractile effects of 5-HT. Nifedipine was also used to inhibit degranulation of mast cells and enterochromaffin cells that could similarly give rise to secondary effects. The perfusion media were bubbled with carbogen (O_2 95%, CO_2 5%). After identification of receptive fields at room temperature, the perfusion solutions were warmed to 32–34 °C in a heating coil, and the flow rate was set at 15 ml/min.

Protocol for recordings from colon

Receptive fields were identified by systematically probing with a blunt glass probe (tip contact area 6 mm^2) with a transmural pressure of approximately 50 kPa. They were classified according to their responses to three mechanical stimuli as previously described. Drugs were added to both superfusion media or were locally applied by means of a metal cylinder of 10 mm diameter placed around a specific receptive field. Care was taken to expose serosal receptors directly to drugs by reflecting the colon and applying locally or superfusing the drug. No differences in the strength and pattern of response were evident between the two application methods. Drugs were applied for approximately 2 min then washed out and normal superfusion resumed for at least 10 min before further drug treatment.

Electrophysiological data collection and analysis

The signal from the recording electrode was amplified and filtered. The analogue signal was sampled at a rate of 20 kHz in a 1401 data interface (CED, Cambridge, UK) and stored on PC. Action potentials were discriminated as single units on the basis of distinguishable waveform, amplitude and duration. Responses to drugs were counted if a reproducible $> 25\%$ increase in discharge occurred with the maximum concentration used.

Inflammation model

We followed protocols previously shown to induce a mild colitis in rats[6]. Dextran sulphate sodium (DSS) was added to drinking water for 5 days as a 2% solution, which was found to induce a mild colitis with moderate indices of *in-vivo* disease activity. This was confirmed histologically in paraffin sections stained with haematoxylin and eosin.

Drugs

Drugs applied to tissue for investigation of chemosensitivity were capsaicin (10^{-6}–3×10^{-6} M), bradykinin (10^{-6} M), P_{2X} purinoceptor agonist αβmeATP (10^{-3} M), serotonin (10^{-10}–10^{-4} M), and histamine (10^{-10}–10^{-4} M).

RESULTS

Mechanosensitivity of colonic afferents

Afferents that respond to probing of the colon but not to stretch or mucosal stroking were classed as serosal receptors. Many of their receptive fields were located in the mesentery. Afferents that responded to $\geq 5\,\text{mm}$ circular stretch and probing but not to mucosal stroking were classed as muscular receptors. These all had receptive fields within the wall of the colon. Afferents that responded to mucosal stroking with a 0.1 mN von Frey hair and probing, but not to stretch, were classed as mucosal receptors. We found serosal/mesenteric, muscular and mucosal afferents in both splanchnic and hypogastric nerves, with the majority in both being serosal/mesenteric.

Mechanosensitive properties of serosal and mucosal afferents were indistinguishable between the two pathways, but muscular afferents behave differently. Splanchnic muscular afferents were rapidly adapting to stretch (e.g. Fig. 1), whereas our preliminary data showed that hypogastric muscular afferents were slowly adapting.

Chemosensitivity of colonic afferents

Approximately 30% of splanchnic and hypogastric serosal afferents responded to capsaicin (10^{-6}–$3 \times 10^{-6}\,\mu\text{M}$) and bradykinin ($10^{-6}\,\text{M}$), but only hypogastric afferents responded to the P_{2X} purinoceptor agonist $\alpha\beta\text{meATP}$ ($10^{-3}\,\text{M}$). In hypogastric afferents, responses were always seen to all three stimuli, but in splanchnic afferents this clustering of chemosensitivity was not evident.

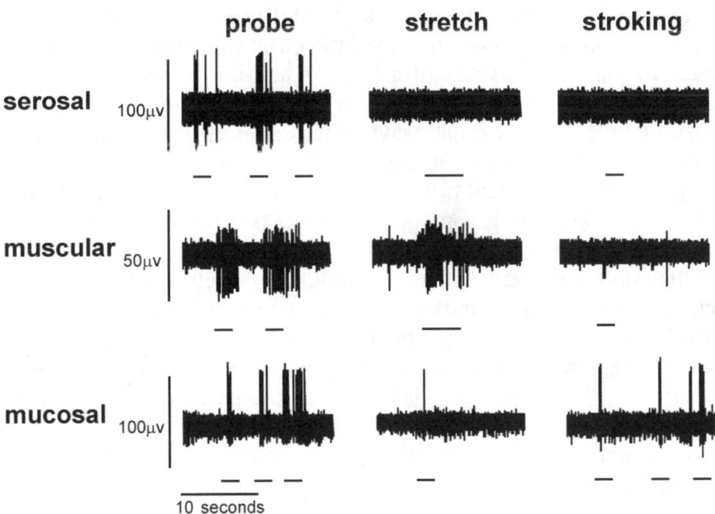

Fig. 1 Mechanosensory properties of three types of lumbar splanchnic afferents. Stretch corresponds to a 5 g load placed across the receptive field, and mucosal stroking corresponds to brief movement of a 0.1 mN von Frey hair over the receptive field. Stimuli are applied for the periods indicated by the bar

Splanchnic serosal afferents were studied for co-sensitivity to serotonin and histamine (10^{-10}–10^{-4} M); 56% of afferents in all three subclasses responded to both serotonin and histamine in a concentration-dependent manner. All afferents responsive to one stimulus were also responsive to the other, indicating clustering of chemosensitivity to these two stimuli on splanchnic afferents

Effects of inflammation on sensitivity to 5-HT

Colonic inflammation with oral DSS caused a shift in the concentration–response relationship for 5-HT, so that responses were seen at nanomolar, rather than micromolar, levels, indicating a sensitization. These data are from four serosal afferents so far.

DISCUSSION

Our data indicate that three mechanosensory subtypes of colonic afferent are present in the splanchnic and hypogastric nerves. Hypogastric and splanchnic muscular afferents convey different information to the spinal cord on maintained distension and activation by purines. Our data provide evidence also for distinct chemosensory and non-chemosensory populations of afferents according to sensitivity to five different stimuli. Inflammation induces a marked sensitization of afferents to 5-HT.

Symptoms in IBS include both maintained and episodic sensations, which can be mimicked by colorectal balloon distension. Our data indicate that the hypogastric/pelvic pathway would be the most likely to convey signals relating to maintained stimuli such as presence of stool or gas, whereas the splanchnic pathway would be better tuned to signal the onset of events such as contraction or passage of material. A study of colonic distension in patients arrived at this conclusion some time ago[12]; however, it was not until this study that a direct comparison between the two pathways in the same setting has been performed. Other than the differences in sensitivity of muscular afferents to maintained strain, there were no apparent differences in mechanosensitivity of the other two types of afferent, indicating homogeneity in the two pathways. However, differences in chemosensitivity may be more relevant in serosal and mucosal fibres because they do not encode distension stimuli in the setting of our experiments.

When we investigated chemosensitivity of hypogastric afferents to three well-established sensory stimuli – αβ-methylene ATP, bradykinin and capsaicin, it was notable that fibres responded either to all three or to none of these. This indicates that chemosensitivity is not specific to a particular chemical stimulus, but is clustered on a subpopulation of fibres. This means that signalling of mechanical events can be directed to different processing pathways in the spinal cord compared with signalling of chemical stimuli. Splanchnic fibres were insensitive to αβ-methylene ATP, but some responded to bradykinin and/or capsaicin, although the clustering was not evident as seen with hypogastric afferents. In a more thorough study of co-sensitivity which was done only on splanchnic afferents, we found a strong clustering of 5-HT and histamine sensitivity on a subpopulation of fibres. This may relate to the fact that both of these may be released by mast cells in pathophysiological situations[7]. We have yet to establish, however, if the response to one may be mediated through release of the other, which would explain co-sensitivity as well as co-expression of 5-HT and histamine receptors on afferent endings.

In a preliminary study of effects of inflammation on colonic afferent endings we found a remarkable sensitization of the response to 5-HT. However, the mechanism of this remains to be evaluated, as well as its relationship to induced release of 5-HT or other mediators. As 5-HT release is exacerbated in subpopulations of IBS patients[3,4], and this correlates with symptoms, there are interesting parallels with our findings and those possibly active in disease. The concentrations of 5-HT with which we were able to evoke a response were well within the range of those that would be circulating postprandially in IBS patients. Whether our model of DSS colitis compares with IBS in humans is of course a difficult question, but it suggests that further investigation of 5-HT sensitivity in both situations is warranted, especially studies on chronic sensitivity after resolution of inflammation.

In conclusion, our data are beginning to reveal a picture of mechanosensitive and chemosensitive subtypes of afferents in two pathways from the colon that may have direct relevance in the signalling of symptoms.

References

1. Cervero F. Sensory innervation of the viscera: peripheral basis of visceral pain. Physiol Rev. 1994;74:95–138.
2. Lembo T, Munakata J, Mertz H et al. Evidence for the hypersensitivity of lumbar splanchnic afferents in irritable bowel syndrome. Gastroenterology. 1994;107:1686–96.
3. Bearcroft CP, Perrett D, Farthing MJ. Postprandial plasma 5-hydroxytryptamine in diarrhoea-predominant irritable bowel syndrome: a pilot study. Gut. 1998;42:42–6.
4. Houghton LA, Whitaker P, Atkinson W et al. Increased platelet stores of 5-hydroxytryptamine (5-HT) in female patients with diarrhoea-predominant irritable bowel syndrome. Gastroenterology. 2001;120:A–636.
5. Spiller RC, Jenkins D, Thornley JP et al. Increased rectal mucosal enteroendocrine cells, T lymphocytes, and increased gut permeability following acute *Campylobacter* enteritis and in post-dysenteric irritable bowel syndrome. Gut. 2000;47:804–11.
6. Howarth GS, Xian CJ, Read LC. Insulin-like growth factor I partially attenuates colonic damage in rats with experimental colitis induced by oral dextran sulphate sodium. Scand J Gastroenterol. 1998;33:180–90.
7. Kirkup AJ, Brunsden AM, Grundy D. Receptors and transmission in the brain–gut axis: potential for novel therapies. I. Receptors on visceral afferents. Am J Physiol Gastrointest Liver Physiol. 2001;280:G787–94.
8. Blackshaw LA, Page AJ, Partosoedarso ER. Acute effects of capsaicin on gastrointestinal vagal afferents. Neuroscience. 2000;96:407–16.
9. Berthoud HR, Lynn PA, Blackshaw LA. Vagal and spinal mechanosensors in the rat stomach and colon have multiple receptive fields. Am J Physiol Regul Integr Comp Physiol. 2001;280:R1371–81.
10. Lynn PA, Blackshaw LA. *In vitro* recordings of afferent fibres with receptive fields in the serosa, muscle and mucosa of rat colon. J Physiol (Lond). 1999;518:271–82.
11. Baron R, Janig W, Kollmann W. Sympathetic and afferent somata projecting in hindlimb nerves and the anatomical organization of the lumbar sympathetic nervous system of the rat. J Comp Neurol. 1988;275:460–8.
12. Lembo T, Munakata J, Mertz H et al. Evidence for the hypersensitivity of lumbar splanchnic afferents in irritable bowel syndrome. Gastroenterology. 1994;107:1686–96.

15
Regulation of vagal afferent sensitivity to gastric acid

P. HOLZER, M. DANZER, R. SCHICHO and I. TH. LIPPE

IMPLICATION OF GASTRIC ACID IN DYSPEPTIC SYMPTOMS

The term 'dyspepsia' refers to chronic or recurrent pain and discomfort centred in the upper abdomen. If these prolonged symptom patterns occur in the absence of an identifiable organic cause, the disorder may be classified as functional dyspepsia[1-3]. Although the causes and mechanisms behind this symptom profile are still largely unknown, it seems obvious that the signalling of information from the gut to the brain and/or its processing within the brain are disturbed. Conceptually, the pain of dyspeptic patients may reflect pathological alterations in gut function and/or signify that events in the gastrointestinal tract are represented in the brain in a distorted fashion because the sensory gain of afferent neurons or the central gain of afferent input from the gut is set abnormally high[4]. Thus, if the threshold of the sensors is tuned down below normal, dyspeptic symptoms may occur even when the reported events are within the physiological range[5]. It is appropriate to assume, therefore, that in dyspeptic patients the primary afferent or central pathways of gastric nociception have become hypersensitive. It need in addition be considered that summation effects may be of relevance, given that unperceived electrical stimulation of mechano-*in*sensitive jejunal afferents can increase the perception of background distension to an uncomfortable level[6].

There is ample evidence that patients suffering from functional dyspepsia are hypersensitive to gastric distension[7-10], as are patients with irritable bowel syndrome to colonic distension[11-14]. Importantly, patients with functional dyspepsia are also hypersensitive to chemical stimuli such as fat and acid. Thus, lipid infusion into the duodenum contributes to the meal-like fullness and nausea which dyspeptic patients experience during gastric distension[15,16]. Although gastric acid secretion is in the normal range[17], the stomach and duodenum of dyspeptic patients are hypersensitive to acid and the duodenum fails to clear exogenous acid as quickly as the duodenum of healthy subjects[18-21]. In addition, acid seems to be able to sensitize mechanosensitive afferents in the stomach[22].

These observations, and the ability of antisecretory therapy to alleviate symptoms in some dyspeptic patients[23], suggest that acid hypersensitivity, but not acid hypersecretion, is a factor in functional dyspepsia[24]. It should not go unnoticed in this context that acid also contributes to gastric and duodenal ulcer pain[25–27] and that gastro-oesophageal reflux disease is associated with an enhanced oesophageal sensitivity to acid, but not distension[28].

RISK FACTORS FOR THE INDUCTION OF AFFERENT NEURON HYPERSENSITIVITY IN DYSPEPSIA

If it is held that hypersensitivity of afferent pathways from the gut to the brain is a factor in dyspeptic pain, the question arises as to which pathological circumstances cause the afferent nervous system to increase its sensory gain. It is now recognized that gastroenteritis, which may have subsided long ago, is a major risk factor for irritable bowel syndrome and the associated discomfort and pain[29–34]. These observations have led to the hypothesis that immunological and inflammatory processes initiate long-lasting changes in bowel function and afferent neuron sensitivity (Fig. 1). Indeed, acetic acid-induced ulceration of the rat stomach increases the excitability of nodose and dorsal root ganglion neurons and enforces tetrodotoxin-resistant sodium currents in these afferent neurons[35]. Gastritis

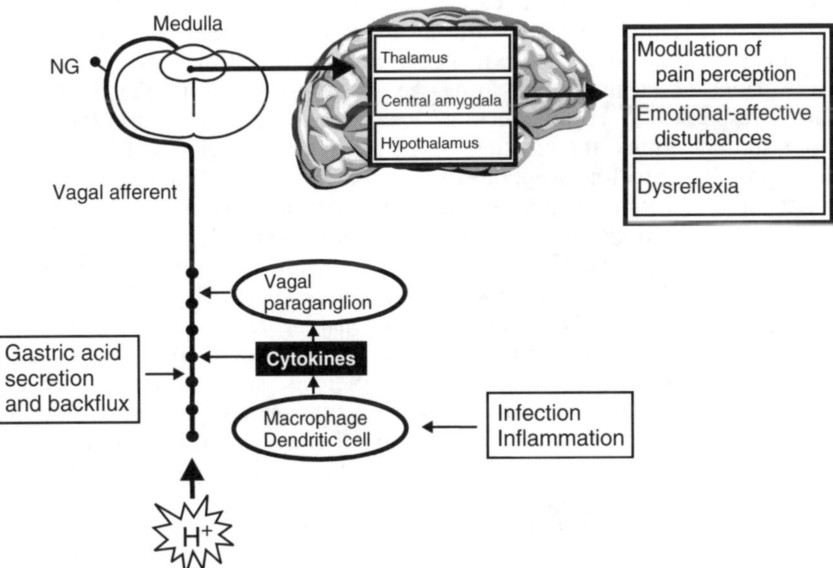

Fig. 1 Diagrammatic overview of some factors that enhance vagal afferent sensitivity to gastric acid and in this way contribute to gastric hyperalgesia. The figure illustrates that cytokines and endogenous acid can boost the nociceptive sensitivity of vagal afferents, and highlights some functional consequences of exaggerated vagal afferent input to the brainstem: modulation of pain perception, emotional–affective disturbances and dysregulation of digestive function (dysreflexia)

elicited by chronic exposure to iodoacetamide likewise enhances tetrodotoxin-resistant sodium currents in spinal, but not nodose, ganglia projecting to the rat stomach, and these molecular alterations are associated with hypersensitivity to gastric distension[36]. The enforcement of tetrodotoxin-resistant sodium currents may be brought about by nerve growth factor, because acetic acid-induced gastric ulcers are associated with excess production of nerve growth factor in the gastric wall and nerve growth factor can up-regulate tetrodotoxin-resistant sodium channels in spinal afferents innervating the stomach[37].

Of particular interest is the finding that *Helicobacter pylori*-induced gastritis in mice is associated with a long-lasting increase in the sensitivity to gastric distension as measured by the distension-evoked increase in heart rate[38]. However, the relevance of this finding to functional dyspepsia is not clear because clinical studies do not unequivocally support a role of *H. pylori* in the aetiology of functional dyspepsia[5,39,40]. It needs to be taken into account, though, that dyspeptic patients with a very intense immune reaction to *H. pylori* infection, as measured by the *H. pylori* antibody titre, exhibit a significantly lowered sensory threshold to duodenal distension[41]. This subgroup of patients may therefore be at particular risk to develop functional dyspepsia after infection by *H. pylori*[34,42].

ROLE OF VAGAL AFFERENTS IN GASTRIC ACID SURVEILLANCE AND NOCICEPTION

After it had long been maintained that vagal sensory neurons do not play a role in abdominal pain, there is now growing awareness that these neurons can make a distinct contribution to disease-related alterations in visceral sensation[43,44]. The participation of vagal afferents in nausea and emesis[45] and in cytokine-evoked illness responses[46,47] corroborates the view that sensory neurons in the vagus nerve may determine the emotional-affective, neuroendocrine and behavioural aspects of abdominal nociception[48]. Furthermore, it is worth noting that strong electrical stimulation of the vagus nerve for the treatment of medically intractable epilepsy can even give rise to the sensation of pain[49].

That the vagus nerve plays a major role in communication between the gut and the brain is beyond doubt. Thus, the vast majority (80–90%) of the axons in the vagus nerves are afferent nerve fibres[4,45], making the vagus nerve the largest visceral sensory nerve in the body[50]. Information from the alimentary canal is delivered tonically to the brain via vagal afferents, and this massive sensory input is thought to be relevant not only to the autonomic regulation of gastrointestinal function but also to the interpretation of external sensory inputs, attitude and behaviour[50]. In this context the afferent part of the vagus nerve has even been suggested to mediate the 'sixth sense'[50].

A role of vagal afferents in the affective, behavioural and autonomic, rather than perceptive, aspects of gastric nociception (Fig. 1) has been confirmed in our own studies of the afferent processing of gastric acid noxae by functional c-fos neuroanatomy. Exposure of the rat gastric mucosa to minimally injurious concentrations of hydrochloric acid leads to rapid expression of c-fos in the brainstem, but not spinal cord[51]. It follows that vagal afferents respond promptly to acid challenge of the rat gastric mucosa and carry this information to the nucleus tractus solitarii and area postrema of the brainstem. The vagal afferent input from the acid-threatened stomach is processed in the medullary brainstem such that the information is passed on to the lateral parabrachial nucleus, the thalamic and hypothalamic paraventricular nuclei, the supraoptic nucleus, the central amygdala and the mediolateral habenula[52]. There is, however, no activation of the insular cortex, the major cerebral representation area of afferent input from the stomach. Thus, vagal afferent signalling of gastric acid challenge does not give rise to perception of pain, but leads to activation of subcortical brain nuclei that are involved in emotional, behavioural, autonomic and neuroendocrine reactions to noxious stimuli[52].

Although vagal afferents in the stomach have long been known to discharge action potentials when their peripheral terminals are exposed to acid[53,54], their molecular sensors of H^+ ions remain unknown. Since the acid-evoked afferent signalling is not altered by capsaicin pretreatment[51] it appears improbable that acid transduction is accomplished by the acid-sensitive vanilloid receptor of type 1[55]. Whether acid-sensing ion channels present on vagal afferent neurons[56] are involved has not yet been explored. It likewise awaits to be examined whether P2X purinoceptor ion channels are transducers of gastrointestinal mucosal damage. The P2X receptors on nodose ganglion neurons are preferentially homomeric $P2X_2$ and heteromeric $P2X_2/P2X_3$ receptors[57–59]. Vagal afferents expressing these receptors are activated or sensitized by adenosine triphosphate[60,61] which in the injured gut may be released from damaged mucosal cells and a variety of other cells including enteric, sensory and sympathetic nerve endings[62,63]. Acidification can, in addition, sensitize the $P2X_2$ subunit to the excitatory effect of adenosine triphosphate[64,65].

A further mediator of the excitatory action of acid on vagal afferents could be 5-hydroxytryptamine, given that in the rat stomach considerable quantities of 5-hydroxytryptamine are released from the acid-injured mucosa[66], most probably from enterochromaffin cells but possibly also from platelets and mucosal mast cells. A contribution by 5-hydroxytryptamine to the sensory neuron-stimulating effect of acid is unlikely, though, because this amine does not seem to contribute to the acid-evoked excitation of vagal afferents[67]. It also remains to be explored whether cytokines which can be induced by acid injury in the gastric mucosa[68,69] play a mediator role.

The ability of sensory neurons to signal various types of mucosal noxae to the brain is further exemplified by reports of c-fos expression in the brainstem or higher brain areas in response to gastric mucosal injury elicited by aspirin[70], cinchophen[71], ethanol[72], formalin[73] or cold-restraint stress[74]. Activation of neurons in prevertebral ganglia and spinal cord has been noted following intracolonic administration of formalin[75] or acetic acid[76].

REGULATION OF VAGAL AFFERENT SENSITIVITY
TO GASTRIC ACID

Clinical observations of the algesic effect of gastric acid[18–20,25–27] and the ability of antisecretory treatment to alleviate dyspeptic symptoms[23] attest to the implication of gastric acid in nociceptive processes of the upper gastrointestinal tract.

However, the precise role of endogenous gastric acid in the vagal afferent signalling of gastric mucosal noxae awaits to be explored. Preliminary experiments indicate that inhibition of gastric acid secretion by cimetidine or omeprazole attenuates the ability of exogenous acid to induce c-Fos expression in the nucleus tractus solitarii of the rat brainstem (M. Danzer and P. Holzer, unpublished). Further work has shown that stimulation of endogenous gastric acid secretion by pentagastrin is *per se* able to induce c-Fos expression in the brainstem, an effect that is in part inhibited by omeprazole (M. Danzer and P. Holzer, unpublished). From these findings it would appear that endogenous gastric acid enhances the sensitivity of vagal afferents to an exogenous acid stimulus (Fig. 1), much as acid is able to sensitize mechanosensitive afferent neurons to distension[22]. Furthermore, massive stimulation of gastric acid secretion can by itself activate afferent neurons that signal to the brainstem.

This and other findings corroborate the view that the sensitivity of vagal afferents to gastric acid and other stimuli is dynamically regulated and can be enhanced under particular circumstances, which is an aspect relevant to visceral hypersensitivity (Fig. 1). Importantly, we have also found experimental evidence that vagal afferent pathways can be markedly sensitized by proinflammatory cytokines. Thus, systemic administration of interleukin-1β and tumour necrosis factor-α leads to a prolonged increase in the gastric acid-evoked expression of c-Fos in the brainstem[77]. Furthermore, antigen challenge of allergic guinea-pigs or stimulation with 5-hydroxytryptamine 5-HT$_3$ receptor agonists unmasks tachykinin NK$_2$ receptors in nodose ganglia for a prolonged period of time[78,79], which may be interpreted as a sensitization equivalent.

VAGAL AFFERENTS AS INTERFACE BETWEEN IMMUNE SYSTEM AND BRAIN

The ability of proinflammatory cytokines to sensitize vagal afferent pathways to gastric acid[77] is in keeping with the prominent position which vagal afferents take in the communication between the peripheral immune system and the brain[4,46,47]. Analysis of this implication has revealed that, following intraperitoneal administration, bacterial lipopolysaccharide (endotoxin) is primarily transported to the liver where it induces the release of interleukin-1β from Kupffer cells (macrophage-like cells to screen blood and lymph) and thereby causes stimulation of afferents in the hepatic branch of the vagus nerve[80,81]. Furthermore, the abdominal vagus is associated with paraganglia and connective tissue containing macrophages and dendritic cells (Fig. 1) that respond to intraperitoneal administration of endotoxin with synthesis of interleukin-1β[82,83]. The abdominal paraganglia of the vagus nerve contain glomus-like cells which have interleukin-1 receptors[84], are innervated by vagal afferents[85] and may hence serve as chemosensory accessory cells[46]. In addition, vagal afferents innervate abdominal lymph nodes which represent another interface with the visceral immune system[46].

Electrophysiological recordings demonstrate that peripheral administration of interleukin-1β leads to increased firing in vagal afferents[86,87] and induces c-Fos expression in the nucleus tractus solitarii, the central termination area of vagal sensory neurons[77,88]. Since interleukin-1 receptors of type I are expressed by nodose ganglion cells, it appears as if the cytokine excites vagal afferents by a direct action on the axons, although prostaglandins acting via EP_3 receptors and cholecystokinin acting via CCK_1 receptors may also contribute[87,89]. Moreover, interleukin-1β is able to increase the sensitivity of gastric vagal afferents to fire in response to PGE_2 and CCK[87,90]. Being responsive to peripheral interleukin-1ß, vagal afferents participate in the behavioural *illness responses* to infection and inflammation, which comprise fever, anorexia, somnolence, decrease in locomotor activity, decrease in social exploration and hyperalgesia[46,47]. Accordingly, certain features of this *sickness behaviour* are attenuated by subdiaphragmatic vagotomy, although circulating proinflammatory cytokines can access the brain via circumventricular organs that are devoid of a blood–brain barrier[46,47].

The ability of proinflammatory cytokines to sensitize vagal afferent pathways to acid and other noxae is of relevance to understanding the upper abdominal hyperalgesia associated with dyspepsia. It seems that, at least in cases of postinfectious and postinflammatory dyspepsia, cytokines participate in the establishment of persistent changes in afferent pathways that are responsible for the increased pain sensitivity (Fig. 1). Apart from the question as to how sustained hyperalgesia is evoked by certain antecedent events, it is an equally intriguing question why this altered state of sensitivity does not revert to normal after resolution of the initial trigger. One clue to this problem may come from the observation that some patients with irritable bowel syndrome have a genetic background that is associated with a diminished production of anti-inflammatory cytokines such as interleukin-10[91].

Acknowledgements

This work was supported by the Austrian Research Foundation (FWF grants P14295-MED and P15452-MED) and the Jubilee Foundation of the Austrian National Bank (grant 9296). Thanks are due to Evelin Painsipp for drawing the graph.

References

1. De Ponti F, Malagelada J-R. Functional gut disorders: from motility to sensitivity disorders. A review of current and investigational drugs for their management. Pharmacol Ther. 1998;80: 49–88.
2. Tack J, Bisschops R, DeMarchi B. Causes and treatment of functional dyspepsia. Curr Gastroenterol Rep. 2001;3:503–8.
3. Talley NJ, Phung N, Kalantar JS. ABC of the upper gastrointestingal tract. Indigestion: when is it functional? Br Med J. 2001;323:1294–7.
4. Holzer P. Sensory neurone responses to mucosal noxae in the upper gut: relevance to mucosal integrity and gastrointestinal pain. Neurogastroenterol Mot. 2002;14:1–17.
5. Malagelada J-R. The continuing dilemma of dyspepsia. Aliment Pharmacol Ther. 2001; 15(Suppl. 1):6–9.
6. Accarino AM, Azpiroz F, Malagelada J-R. Gut perception in humans is modulated by interacting gut stimuli. Am J Physiol. 2002;282:G220–5.
7. Bradette M, Paré P, Douville P, Morin A. Visceral perception in health and functional dyspepsia. Crossover study of gastric distension with placebo and domperidone. Dig Dis Sci. 1991; 36:52–8.

8. Lémann M, Dederding JP, Flourie B, Franchisseur C, Rambaud J, Jian R. Abnormal perception of visceral pain in response to gastric distension in chronic idiopathic dyspepsia: the irritable stomach. Dig Dis Sci. 1991;36:1249–54.

9. Mearin F, Cucala M, Azpiroz F, Malagelada J-R. The origin of symptoms on the brain gut axis in functional dyspepsia. Gastroenterology. 1991;101:999–1006.

10. Coffin B, Azpiroz F, Guarner F, Malagelada J-R. Selective gastric hypersensitivity and reflex hyporeactivity in functional dyspepsia. Gastroenterology. 1994;107:1345–51.

11. Bradette M, Delvaux M, Staumont G, Fioramonti J, Bueno L, Frexinos J. Evaluation of colonic sensory thresholds in IBS patients using a barostat. Definition of optimal conditions and comparison with healthy subjects. Dig Dis Sci. 1994;39:449–57.

12. Lembo T, Munakata J, Mertz H et al. Evidence for the hypersensitivity of lumbar splanchnic afferents in irritable bowel syndrome. Gastroenterology. 1994;107:1686–96.

13. Accarino AM, Azpiroz F, Malagelada JR. Selective dysfunction of mechanosensitive intestinal afferents in irritable bowel syndrome. Gastroenterology. 1995;108:636–43.

14. Mertz H, Naliboff B, Munakata J, Niazi N, Mayer EA. Altered rectal perception is a biological marker of patients with irritable bowel syndrome. Gastroenterology. 1995;109:40–52.

15. Barbera R, Feinle C, Read NW. Abnormal sensitivity to duodenal lipid infusion in patients with functional dyspepsia. Eur J Gastroenterol Hepatol. 1995;7:1051–7.

16. Feinle C, Meier O, Otto B, D' Amato M, Fried M. Role of duodenal lipid and cholecystokinin A receptors in the pathophysiology of functional dyspepsia. Gut. 2001;48:347–55.

17. Collen MJ, Loebenberg MJ. Basal gastric acid secretion in nonulcer dyspepsia with or without duodenitis. Dig Dis Sci. 1989;34:246–50.

18. Son HJ, Rhee PL, Kim JJ, Koh KC, Paik SW, Rhee JC. Hypersensitivity to acid in ulcer-like functional dyspepsia. Korean J Intern Med. 1997;12:188–92.

19. Rhee PL, Kim YH, Son HJ et al. The etiologic role of gastric hypersensitivity in functional dyspepsia in Korea. J Clin Gastroenterol. 1999;29:332–5.

20. Samsom M, Verhagen MA, vanBerge Henegouwen GP, Smout AJ. Abnormal clearance of exogenous acid and increased acid sensitivity of the proximal duodenum in dyspeptic patients. Gastroenterology. 1999;116:515–20.

21. Schwartz MP, Samsom M, Van Berge Henegouwen GP, Smout AJ. Effect of inhibition of gastric acid secretion on antropyloroduodenal motor activity and duodenal acid hypersensitivity in functional dyspepsia. Aliment Pharmacol Ther. 2001;15:1921–8.

22. Coffin B, Chollet R, Flourié B et al. Intraluminal modulation of gastric sensitivity to distension: effects of hydrochloric acid and meal. Am J Physiol. 2001;280:G904–9.

23. Talley NJ, Lauritsen K. The potential role of acid suppression in functional dyspepsia: the BOND, OPERA, PILOT, and ENCORE studies. Gut. 2002;50(Suppl. 4):iv36–41.

24. Read NW. Functional dyspepsia: a case of indecision. Gastroenterology. 1999;116:761–2.

25. Kang JY, Yap I, Guan R, Tay HH. Acid perfusion of duodenal ulcer craters and ulcer pain: a controlled double blind study. Gut. 1986;27:942–5.

26. Kang JY, Yap I, Guan R, Tay HH, Math MV. Acid induced duodenal ulcer pain: the influence of symptom status and the effect of an antispasmodic. Gut. 1989;30:166–70.

27. Kang JY, Yap I. Acid and gastric ulcer pain. J Clin Gastroenterol. 1991;13:514–16.

28. Fass R, Naliboff B, Higa L et al. Differential effect of long-term esophageal acid exposure on mechanosensitivity and chemosensitivity in humans. Gastroenterology. 1998;115:1363–73.

29. Collins SM. The immunomodulation of enteric neuromuscular function: implications for motility and inflammatory disorders. Gastroenterology. 1996;111:1683–99.

30. Neal KR, Hebden J, Spiller R. Prevalence of gastrointestinal symptoms six months after bacterial gastroenteritis and risk factors for development of the irritable bowel syndrome: postal survey of patients. Br Med J. 1997:314:779–82.

31. Gwee KA, Leong YL, Graham C et al. The role of psychological and biological factors in postinfective gut dysfunction. Gut. 1999;44:400–6.

32. Pimintel M, Chow EJ, Lin HC. Eradication of small intestinal bacterial overgrowth reduces symptoms of irritable bowel syndrome. Am J Gastroenterol. 2000;95:3503–6.

33. Spiller RC, Jenkins D, Thornley JP et al. Increased rectal mucosal enteroendocrine cells, T lymphocytes, and increased gut permeability following acute Campylobacter enteritis and in post-dysenteric irritable bowel syndrome. Gut. 2000;47:804–11.

34. Holtmann G. (Post) inflammatory visceral hyperalgesia: don't we believe what we don't see? Gastroenterology. 2002;122:823–5.

35. Bielefeldt K, Ozaki N, Gebhart GF. Experimental ulcers alter voltage-sensitive sodium currents in rat gastric sensory neurons. Gastroenterology. 2002;122:394–405.
36. Bielefeldt K, Ozaki N, Gebhart GF. Mild gastritis alters voltage-sensitive sodium currents in gastric sensory neurons in rats. Gastroenterology. 2002;122:752–61.
37. Bielefeldt K, Ozaki N, Gebhart GF. Nerve growth factor and sensitization of gastric afferent neurons. Digestion. 2001;63:267–8.
38. Bercik P, De Giorgio R, Wang L *et al*. Neural changes during chronic *H. pylori* (Hp) infection in mice: role of the immune system. Neurogastroenterol Motil. 2001;13:374.
39. Moayyedi P, Soo S, Deeks J *et al*. Systematic review and economic evaluation of *Helicobacter pylori* eradication treatment for non-ulcer dyspepsia. Dyspepsia Review Group. Br Med J. 2000; 321:659–64.
40. Laine L, Schoenfeld P, Fennerty MB. Therapy for *Helicobacter pylori* in patients with nonulcer dyspepsia. A meta-analysis of randomized, controlled trials. Ann Intern Med. 2001;134:361–9.
41. Holtmann G, Talley NJ, Goebell H. Association between *H. pylori*, duodenal mechanosensory thresholds, and small intestinal motility in chronic unexplained dyspepsia. Dig Dis Sci. 1996;41: 1285–91.
42. Holtmann G, Gschossmann J, Holtmann M, Talley NJ. *H. pylori* and functional dyspepsia: increased serum antibodies as an independent risk factor? Dig Dis Sci. 2001;46:1550–7.
43. Gebhart GF. Pathobiology of visceral pain: molecular mechanisms and therapeutic implications. IV. Visceral afferent contributions to the pathobiology of visceral pain. Am J Physiol. 2000; 278:G834–8.
44. Holzer P, Michl T, Jocic M, Heinemann A, Schuligoi R. Essential role of vagal afferents in the central signalling of a gastric mucosal acid insult. In: Krammer HJ, Singer MV, editors. Neurogastroenterology. From the Basics to the Clinics. Dordrecht: Kluwer, 2000:697–707.
45. Andrews PLR. 5-HT3 receptor antagonists and antiemesis. In: King FD, Jones BJ, Sanger GJ, editors. 5-Hydroxytryptamine-3 Receptor Antagonists. Boca Raton: CRC Press, 1994:255–317.
46. Goehler LE, Gaykema RPA, Hansen MK, Anderson K, Maier SF, Watkins LR. Vagal immune-to-brain communication: a visceral chemosensory pathway. Auton Neurosci Basic Clin. 2000;85:49–59.
47. Konsman JP, Parnet P, Dantzer R. Cytokine-induced sickness behaviour: mechanisms and implications. Trends Neurosci. 2002;25:154–9.
48. Traub RJ, Sengupta JN, Gebhart GF. Differential c-fos expression in the nucleus of the solitary tract and spinal cord following noxious gastric distention in the rat. Neuroscience. 1996; 74:873–84.
49. Liporace J, Hucko D, Morrow R *et al*. Vagal nerve stimulation: adjustments to reduce painful side effects. Neurology. 2001;57:885–6.
50. Zagon A. Does the vagus nerve mediate the sixth sense? Trends Neurosci. 2001;24:671–3.
51. Schuligoi R, Jocic M, Heinemann A, Schöninkle E, Pabst MA, Holzer P. Gastric acid-evoked c-fos messenger RNA expression in rat brainstem is signaled by capsaicin-resistant vagal afferents. Gastroenterology. 1998;115:649–60.
52. Michl T, Jocic M, Heinemann A, Schuligoi R, Holzer P. Vagal afferent signaling of a gastric mucosal acid insult to medullary, pontine, thalamic, hypothalamic and limbic, but not cortical, nuclei of the rat brain. Pain. 2001;92:19–27.
53. Iggo A. Gastric mucosal chemoreceptors with vagal afferent fibres in the cat. Q J Exp Physiol Cogn Med Sci. 1957;42:398–409.
54. Clarke GD, Davison JS. Mucosal receptors in the gastric antrum and small intestine of the rat with afferent fibres in the cervical vagus. J Physiol (Lond). 1978;284:55–67.
55. Tominaga M, Caterina M, Malmberg AB *et al*. The cloned capsaicin receptor integrates multiple pain-producing stimuli. Neuron. 1998;21:531–43.
56. Waldmann R, Champigny G, Lingueglia E, De Weille JR, Heurteaux C, Lazdunski M. H^+-gated cation channels. Ann NY Acad Sci. 1999;868:67–76.
57. Cockayne DA, Hamilton SG, Zhu QM *et al*. Urinary bladder hyporeflexia and reduced pain-related behaviour in $P2X_3$-deficient mice. Nature. 2000;407:1011–15.
58. Chizh BA, Illes P. P2X receptors and nociception. Pharmacol Rev. 2001;53:553–68.
59. Dunn PM, Zhong Y, Burnstock G. P2X receptors in peripheral neurons. Prog Neurobiol. 2001;65:107–34.
60. Kirkup AJ, Booth CE, Chessell IP, Humphrey PP, Grundy D. Excitatory effect of P2X receptor activation on mesenteric afferent nerves in the anaesthetised rat. J Physiol (Lond). 1999;520: 551–63.

61. Page AJ, O'Donnell TA, Blackshaw LA. P2X purinoceptor-induced sensitization of ferret vagal mechanoreceptors in oesophageal inflammation. J Physiol (Lond). 2000;523:403–11.

62. Ralevic V, Burnstock G. Receptors for purines and pyrimidines. Pharmacol Rev. 1998;50:413–92.

63. Di Virgilio F, Borea PA, Illes P. P2 receptors meet the immune system. Trends Pharmacol Sci. 2001;22:5–7.

64. North RA, Surprenant A. Pharmacology of cloned P2X receptors. Annu Rev Pharmacol Toxicol. 2000;40:563–80.

65. Burnstock G. Purine-mediated signalling in pain and visceral perception. Trends Pharmacol Sci. 2001;22:182–8.

66. Wachter CH, Heinemann A, Donnerer J, Pabst MA, Holzer P. Mediation by 5-hydroxytryptamine of the femoral vasoconstriction induced by acid challenge of the rat gastric mucosa. J Physiol (Lond). 1998;509:541–50.

67. Hillsley K, Grundy D. Sensitivity to 5-hydroxytryptamine in different afferent subpopulations within mesenteric nerves supplying the rat jejunum. J Physiol (Lond). 1998;509:717–27.

68. Gislason H, Rokke O, Svanes K. Release of cytokines associated with gastric mucosal injury. Eur Surg Res. 1996;28:278–86.

69. Montuschi P, Tringali G, Mirtella A *et al*. Interleukin-1β release from rat gastric fundus. Am J Physiol. 1996;271:G275–81.

70. Takahashi A, Miura M. Neuronal expression of FOS protein in the nucleus tractus solitarii and the dorsal motor nucleus of the vagus nerve after i.p. injection of ulcerogenic aspirin. Neurosci Lett. 1995;185:214–16.

71. Takayama K, Xiong Y, Miura M. Neuronal expression of Fos protein in the paraventricular nucleus of the hypothalamus after i.p. injection of ulcerogenic cinchophen. Neurosci Lett. 1994;172:55–8.

72. Yamamoto T, Sawa K. c-Fos-like immunoreactivity in the brainstem following gastric loads of various chemical solutions in rats. Brain Res. 2000;866:135–43.

73. Dong YX, Han ZA, Xiong KH, Rao ZR. Fos expression in serotonergic midbrain neurons projecting to the paraventricular nucleus of hypothalamus after noxious stimulation of the stomach: a triple labeling study in the rat. Neurosci Res. 1997;27:155–60.

74. Bonaz B, Taché Y. Induction of Fos immunoreactivity in the rat brain after cold-restraint induced gastric lesions and fecal excretion. Brain Res. 1994;652:56–64.

75. Miampamba M, Sharkey KA. c-Fos expression in the myenteric plexus, spinal cord and brainstem following injection of formalin in the rat colonic wall. J Auton Nerv Syst. 1999;77:140–51.

76. Sharkey KA, Parr EJ, Keenan CM. Immediate–early gene expression in the inferior mesenteric ganglion and colonic myenteric plexus of the guinea pig. J Neurosci. 1999;19:2755–64.

77. Danzer M, Schicho R, Lippe IT, Holzer P. Interleukin-1β-induced sensitization of vagal afferent pathways to intragastric acid challenge: a novel experimental model of functional dyspepsia? Gastroenterology. 2002;122:A34.

78. Weinreich D, Moore KA, Taylor GE. Allergic inflammation in isolated vagal sensory ganglia unmasks silent NK-2 tachykinin receptors. J Neurosci. 1997;17:7683–93.

79. Moore KA, Taylor GE, Weinreich D. Serotonin unmasks functional NK-2 receptors in vagal sensory neurons of the guinea-pig. J Physiol (Lond). 1999;514:111–24.

80. Watkins LR, Wiertelak EP, Goehler LE, Smith KP, Martin D, Maier SF. Characterization of cytokine-induced hyperalgesia. Brain Res. 1994;654:15–26.

81. Simons CT, Kulchitsky VA, Sugimoto N, Homer LD, Szekely M, Romanovsky AA. Signaling the brain in systemic inflammation: which vagal branch is involved in fever genesis? Am J Physiol. 1998;275:R63–8.

82. Berthoud H-R, Kressel M, Raybould HE, Neuhuber WL. Vagal sensors in the rat duodenal mucosa: distribution and structure as revealed by *in vivo* DiI-tracing. Anat Embryol. 1995;191:203–12.

83. Goehler LE, Gaykema RPA, Nguyen KT *et al*. Interleukin-1β in immune cells of the abdominal vagus nerve: a link between the immune and nervous systems? J Neurosci. 1999;19:2799–806.

84. Goehler LE, Relton JK, Dripps D *et al*. Vagal paraganglia bind biotinylated interleukin-1 receptor antagonist: a possible mechanism for immune-to-brain communication. Brain Res Bull. 1997;43:357–64.

85. Berthoud H-R, Kressel M, Neuhuber WL. Vagal afferent innervation of the rat abdominal paraganglia as revealed by anterograde DiI-tracing and confocal microscopy. Acta Anat. 1995;152:127–32.

86. Niijima A. The afferent discharges from sensors for interleukin 1β in the hepatoportal system in the anesthetized rat. J Auton Nerv Syst. 1996;61:287–91.

87. Kurosawa M, Uvnäs-Moberg K, Miyasaka K, Lundeberg T. Interleukin-1 increases activity of the gastric vagal afferent nerve partly via stimulation of type A CCK receptor in anesthetized rats. J Auton Nerv Syst. 1997;62:72–8.

88. Ericsson A, Kovács KJ, Sawchenko PE. A functional anatomical analysis of central pathways subserving the effects of interleukin-1 on stress-related neuroendocrine neurons. J Neurosci. 1994;14:897–913.

89. Ek M, Kurosawa M, Lundeberg T, Ericsson A. Activation of vagal afferents after intravenous injection of interleukin-1β: role of endogenous prostaglandins. J Neurosci. 1998;18:9471–9.

90. Kreis MF, Haupt W, Grundy D. Interleukin-1β (IL-1β) selectively augments mesenteric afferent sensitivity to prostaglandin E₂. Gastroenterology. 2000;118:A431.

91. Chan J, Gonsalkorale WM, Perrey C *et al*. IL-10 and TGF-β genotypes in irritable bowel syndrome: evidence to support an inflammatory component? Gastroenterology. 2000;118:A184.

16
Alterations of the enteric nervous system and interstitial cells of Cajal in functional colorectal motility disorders

T. WEDEL, J. SPIEGLER, S. SÖLLNER, U. J. ROBLICK,
T. H. K. SCHIEDECK, H.-P. BRUCH and H.-J. KRAMMER

INTRODUCTION

A variety of functional intestinal motility disorders has been attributed to alterations of interstitial cells of Cajal (ICC) and malformations of the enteric nervous system (ENS). This study evaluates both the distribution of ICC and the structural texture of the ENS in two severe human colorectal motility disorders – slow-transit constipation (STC) and megacolon.

The crucial role of a morphologically intact ENS for the mediation of normal motility patterns is best illustrated if enteric ganglia are completely missing. After the first description of intestinal aganglionosis in Hirschsprung's disease[1], there is convincing evidence that non-aganglionic alterations of the ENS, such as hypoganglionosis or hyperganglionosis, may also lead to severe disturbances of colonic motor functions including the development of megacolon[2,3]. In regard to patients with STC several qualitative as well as quantitative changes of the ENS have been described. The neuropathologies included an abnormal enteric neuro-chemistry[4–7], a decrease of argyrophilic neurons[8], a reduction of intraganglionic neurofilaments[9] and hypoganglionosis of the myenteric plexus[10].

In identifying a further histopathological correlate for colorectal motility disorders apart from neuronal malformations, more recently the ICC have been considered a promising candidate. ICC are regarded as intestinal pacemakers due to their ability to generate slow-wave activity[11,12]. In addition, they have been considered to function as intermediaries in the neural control of the gut by transducing inhibitory and excitatory signals from the ENS[13,14]. The recognition of these physiological properties has led to the study of ICC in several gastrointestinal motility disorders.

As for the human colon, first evidence of a relative loss of ICC was given by Yamataka *et al.*[15] and Vanderwinden *et al.*[16], who studied colonic specimens from children with congenital aganglionosis. In a case report Faussone-Pelligrini *et al.*[17] described an adult patient with megacolon due to acquired intestinal hypoganglionosis associated with a relative loss of ICC. He *et al.*[18] addressed the distribution of ICC by means of a volumetric analysis in adult patients with STC. The data showed a significantly decreased volume of ICC in all layers of the colonic muscularis propria compared to controls. However, the assessment of neuronal structures was confined to nerve fibres within the circular muscle layer and did not include the ganglionated nerve plexus layers.

The present study combines a morphological assessment of both ICC and the ENS in order to characterize the extent and severity of abnormalities regarding distributional and structural patterns.

MATERIAL AND METHODS

Patients

Patients with slow-transit constipation (STC)

All patients ($n = 11$, mean age 49.8 years; range 19–70 years; all females) had a history of long-standing intractable constipation with defaecatory frequencies ranging between once per 10 and once per 20 days. Medical therapy failed to improve their bowel habits and defaecation frequently had to be achieved by manual emptying or the application of clysmata. The colonic transit time studied by radio-opaque markers was markedly increased and ranged between 140 and 220 h. Secondary causes of constipation as well as motor dysfunctions of the upper gastrointestinal tract had been previously excluded. Rectal manometry did not reveal abnormal findings. Upon defaecography analysis the patients showed neither an outlet obstruction nor a megacolon. The patients underwent subtotal colectomy with ileorectostomy performed either by laparotomy ($n = 6$) or by laparoscopy ($n = 5$).

Patients with megacolon

All patients ($n = 6$, mean age 44.6 years; range 17–67 years; three females, three males) had been suffering from chronic constipation and abdominal distension dating back to childhood. However, a definitive diagnosis has not been carried out until adolescence or adulthood. Barium enemas showed a megacolon which extended from the upper rectum to the sigmoid and descending colon. At rectal manometry the inhibitory rectoanal reflex was absent in four patients. These patients had shown an absence of nerve cells and a positive acetylcholinesterase reaction in submucosal rectal biopsies highly suggestive for Hirschsprung's disease. Submucous biopsies obtained from the other two patients had shown a normal histology. The dilated colonic segments were removed by deep anterior resection and transversorectostomy.

Control group

Patients of the control group ($n = 13$, mean age 61.1 years; range 23–83 years; seven females, six males) underwent partial colectomy for non-obstructive carcinoma (T1–T2) or adenoma not suitable for endoscopic resection. All control patients reported normal bowel habits with stool frequencies at regular intervals. Radiographic studies showed a normal anatomy of the colon and rectum. Rectal manometry did not reveal abnormal findings.

From all groups specimens were obtained immediately after the resection from corresponding sites of the rectosigmoid colon and were processed for immunohistochemical visualization of ICC and the ENS. The study of human tissue received approval from the Local Ethical Committee of the Medical University of Luebeck (002/97).

Interstitial cells of Cajal

Immunocytochemistry

The specimens were cut into blocks (20 mm length) and fixed in a solution containing 2% paraformaldehyde in 0.1 M phosphate-buffered saline (PBS) supplemented with 0.2% picric acid. After dehydration and cryoprotection with 10% sucrose, serial cryosections (10 µm thickness) were cut perpendicular to the intestinal axis. ICC were visualized by indirect immunocytochemical demonstration of the c-kit receptor. The intensity of the immunoreaction was enhanced by the application of a tyramide signal amplification system (TSA Indirect, NEN Life Science Products, USA) according to the manufacturer's instructions. The sections were pretreated with 0.5% blocking reagent and incubated in polyclonal rabbit antiserum (1 : 500 dilution) directed against the c-kit receptor (C-19, Santa Cruz Biotechnology, USA). After incubation in biotinylated goat-anti-rabbit IgG (1 : 100 dilution) and streptavidin-peroxidase (1 : 100 dilution) the biotinyl tyramide amplification reagent was applied. Prior to the chromogenic visualization with amino-ethylcarbazole the slides were again treated with streptavidin-peroxidase (1 : 100 dilution). In order to identify the nuclei of the red-stained ICC the sections were counterstained with Meyer's haematoxylin. No staining of ICC was observed, when the antibody had been omitted.

Morphometric analysis

A morphometric analysis was carried out to determine both the number and the process length of ICC per area. The stereological determination of the process length was achieved by means of an intersection counting method. The measuring grid (350 × 350 µm) consisted of eight horizontal and eight vertical lines, with the lines being 50 µm apart. The following equation was used to calculate the process length of ICC per area:

$$\text{Process length/area (mm/mm}^2\text{)} = \text{distance between grid lines} \times \text{counted intersections} \times \text{grid area}^{-1}$$

To determine the number of ICC per area the nuclei observed within the grid were counted according to the following equation:

$$\text{number of ICC/area (no./mm}^2\text{)} = \text{counted nuclei} \times \text{grid area}^{-1}$$

The different subpopulations of ICC described within the human colon[19] were taken into account by dividing the muscularis propria into four layers: (1) inner circular muscle layer including the submucosal border, (2) outer circular muscle layer adjacent to the myenteric plexus, (3) inner longitudinal muscle layer adjacent to the myenteric plexus, and (4) outer longitudinal muscle layer adjacent to the serosa. In each of these layers 20 areas were examined with a $25\times$ objective using the above-described measuring grid (total area measured $= 7000 \times 350\,\mu m$). A $63\times$ objective was used to identify those ICC processes which were less readily discernible at lower magnification. The data obtained for ICC processes and nuclei were averaged and expressed as mean values $\pm$ SD for each group. Statistical comparison between the different groups was carried out using the Mann–Whitney U test with $p \le 0.05$ considered as an indicator of significance.

Enteric nervous system

To comprehensively visualize the structural architecture of the intramural nerve plexus the colonic wall was dissected into wholemounts as described previously[20]. Briefly, rectangular segments (40 mm length, 20 mm width) were excised from the resected colonic specimens, stretched (60 mm length, 30 mm width) and fixed in a solution containing 2% paraformaldehyde in PBS supplemented with 0.2% picric acid for 24 h. After treatment with 50% ethanol (1 h) the specimens were treated with 0.05% thimerosal (24 h) and 0.1% $NaCNBH_3$ (30 min). Under stereomicroscopic control the intestinal wall was separated into its different layers to expose the myenteric and submucosal plexus compartments. To dissolve connective tissue components the wholemounts were subjected to a maceration procedure with 30% KOH for 20 min. After pretreatment with 10% normal goat serum the samples were incubated in a polyclonal rabbit antiserum (1 : 800 dilution) directed against protein gene product 9.5 (PGP 9.5, Ultraclone, GB). Incubation in goat anti-rabbit IgG (1 : 100 dilution) was followed by the application of an anti-rabbit-peroxidase–anti-peroxidase complex (1 : 100 dilution). The immunoreaction was visualized with the chromogen chloronaphthol.

RESULTS

Interstitial cells of Cajal

Control group

ICC were readily discernible throughout the entire smooth muscle coat. ICC processes running within the circular and longitudinal muscle layer were orientated preferably parallel to the axis of the smooth muscle cells. At the submucosal border ICC formed a specialized network which extended from the inner circular muscle layer into the submucosa. The myenteric ganglia were surrounded from both sides by ICC which frequently contacted the ganglionic borders. The highest density of ICC was found within the outer circular muscle layer (32.1 per mm^2) followed by the inner circular muscle layer (24.6 per mm^2). Within the longitudinal muscle layer the density of ICC decreased towards the serosa, yielding 15.1 per mm^2 in the inner portion and 3.6 per mm^2 in the outer portion (Table 1). The total process length of ICC per mm^2 measured 9.7 mm in the inner circular muscle layer, 13.4 mm in the outer circular muscle layer,

Table 1 Density of ICC

ICC-nuclei (number per mm^2)	Control	Slow-transit constipation		Megacolon	
Circular muscle					
Inner portion	24.6 ± 11.9	11.6 ± 4.5	$p < 0.05$	10.0 ± 6.8	$p < 0.05$
Outer portion	32.1 ± 13.7	14.0 ± 6.7	$p < 0.05$	8.4 ± 7.5	$p < 0.05$
Longitudinal muscle					
Inner portion	15.1 ± 7.9	8.4 ± 3.4	$p < 0.05$	4.8 ± 2.8	$p < 0.05$
Outer portion	3.6 ± 2.4	2.4 ± 1.0	n.s.	1.1 ± 1.0	$p < 0.05$
Entire tunica muscularis	18.8 ± 3.3	9.2 ± 2.8	$p < 0.05$	6.1 ± 3.2	$p < 0.05$

Data are presented as mean ± standard deviation; n.s. = not significant.

Table 2 Process length of ICC

ICC processes (total length, mm per mm^2)	Control	Slow-transit constipation		Megacolon	
Circular muscle					
Inner portion	9.7 ± 3.7	7.9 ± 2.5	n.s.	5.3 ± 4.2	n.s.
Outer portion	13.4 ± 5.0	10.8 ± 4.3	n.s.	4.7 ± 5.5	$p < 0.05$
Longitudinal muscle					
Inner portion	9.5 ± 1.9	8.5 ± 3.3	n.s.	2.8 ± 3.1	$p < 0.05$
Outer portion	2.2 ± 1.4	2.7 ± 2.4	n.s.	0.6 ± 0.5	$p < 0.05$
Entire tunica muscularis	8.7 ± 2.4	7.5 ± 2.7	n.s.	3.4 ± 3.2	$p < 0.05$

Data are presented as mean ± standard deviation; n.s. = not significant.

9.5 mm in the inner longitudinal muscle layer and 2.2 mm in the outer longitudinal muscle layer (Table 2).

Patients with STC

The topographical organization of ICC in patients with STC basically resembled the structural features of ICC observed in the control group. All ICC subpopulations (located at the submucosal border, adjacent to the myenteric plexus and within the muscularis propria) were present. However, the morphometric assessment revealed a significant numerical decrease of ICC in all layers examined except for the outer longitudinal muscle layer. The mean number of ICC per mm^2 was reduced to 11.7 in the inner circular muscle layer, 14.1 in the outer circular muscle layer and 8.4 in the inner longitudinal muscle layer (Table 1). Although, in general, the mean values of the process length were lower, they did not differ significantly from the control group in any of the four layers examined (Table 2). On histological examination some ICC exhibited a blunting of their processes and the network appeared disrupted.

Patients with megacolon

ICC were present in all layers of the muscularis propria including the regions at the submucosal border and adjacent to the myenteric plexus. Nevertheless, the histological assessment showed an obvious decrease of both the number and the process length of ICC in comparison to the control group. This observation was confirmed at morphometric analysis: whereas the numerical reduction was statistically significant within all layers examined (Table 1), the process length was decreased significantly except for the inner circular muscle layer (Table 2).

Enteric nervous system

Control group

All patients showed a normally configured ENS. The most prominent intramural nerve network was the myenteric plexus composed of densely distributed ganglia and interganglionic nerve fibre strands delimited by the circular and long-itudinal muscle layer (Fig. 1a). Whereas primary and secondary nerve fibre strands established the connections between the ganglia, tertiary nerve fibre

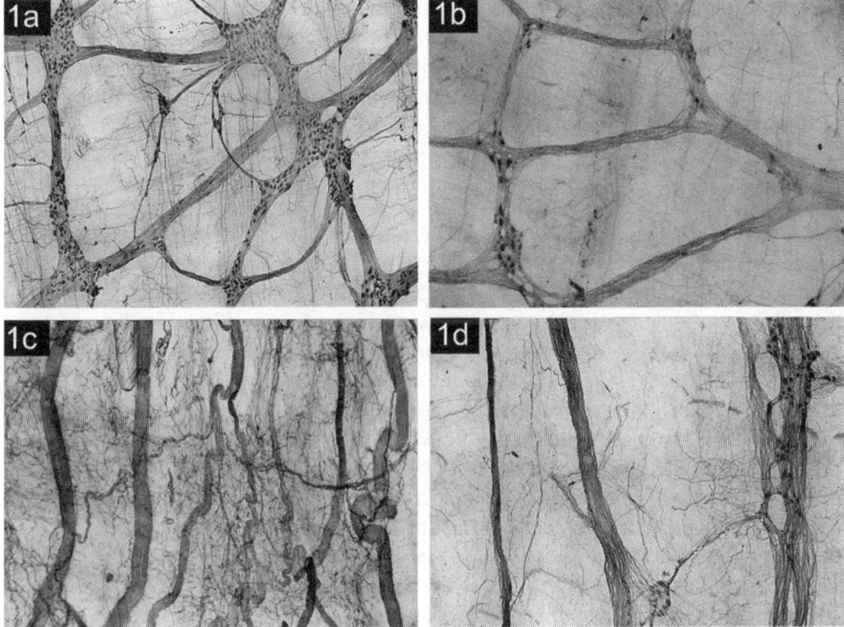

Fig. 1 Architecture of the ENS (myenteric plexus). Control group (a): the nerve network is composed of ganglia and interconnecting nerve fibre strands. Although the majority of neurons is located within the ganglia, some nerve cell bodies are also observed within the nerve fibre strands. Slow-transit constipation (b): in comparison to controls the meshes of the nerve network are widened and the ganglia are reduced in size containing a decreased amount of nerve cells. Megacolon (c): thickened nerve fibre strands run within the intermuscular plane and extend parallel to each other in caudocranial direction. The affected bowel wall is completely bare of ganglia (aganglionosis). Megacolon (d): two of the six patients exhibited severe oligoneuronal hypoganglionosis. Few nerve cells are encountered within the hypertrophied nerve fibre strands and form small intrafascicular ganglia. However, the structural features are similar to those observed in aganglionosis, e.g. parallel ori-entated nerve fibre strands (compare 1c). PGP 9.5 immunohistochemistry applied to wholemount preparations; original magnifications ×5

strands constituted a fine structured network ramifying into the adjacent muscle layers. The submucosal plexus comprised three separate nerve networks which could be distinguished by its different topography and architecture (plexus submucosus extremus, externus and internus).

Patients with STC

The general features of the ENS from patients with STC were similar to those observed in the control group. Both the myenteric and the submucosal plexus layers showed the typical network character and were equipped with ganglia located at the intersections of nerve fibre strands. However, in comparison to the control group, the myenteric plexus of patients with STC revealed a notable decrease in ganglionic density and size. The meshes of the nerve network were widened and the ganglia contained a reduced number of nerve cells (Fig. 1b). According to a consensus conference on innervational disorders of the colon[21] these alterations were classified as moderate oligoneuronal hypoganglionosis. The structural architecture of the submucosal plexus layers did not differ substantially from the control group. Only one patient showed a hypoganglionic submucosal nerve network with a decreased number of ganglia. None of the patients exhibited hyperplastic changes (e.g. giant ganglia) of the submucosal plexus, thereby excluding the diagnosis of intestinal neuronal dysplasia.

Patients with megacolon

Patients with megacolon showed severe malformations of the ENS. In those patients who were suspected as having Hirschsprung's disease on preoperative biopsies ($n = 4$), the diagnosis of complete intramural aganglionosis was confirmed. The affected colonic segments were bare of intramural ganglia and were characterized by thickened nerve fibre strands extending between the longitudinal and circular muscle layer and throughout the submucosa. Whereas in the intermuscular plane the hypertrophied nerve fibre strands were oriented in caudocranial direction (Fig. 1c), in the submucosa they formed an irregular network. A similar spatial arrangement of the ENS was found in the other two patients: myenteric nerve fibre strands extended in caudocranial direction and did not form a normal network. However, in contrast to the cases with complete aganglionosis, the specimens contained disseminated nerve cells within the thickened nerve fibre strands (intrafascicular ganglia) (Fig. 1d). As the number of nerve cells was highly decreased in comparison to both the control group and patients with STC, this innervational disorder was classified as severe oligoneuronal hypoganglionosis.

DISCUSSION

Alterations of interstitial cells of Cajal

It has been established that, apart from the ENS, ICC are actively involved in the mediation of intestinal motility. The scientific 'renaissance' of ICC originally described about 100 years ago[22] is based on the observations that ICC generate electrical slow-wave activity[11,12], and are capable of mediating neuronal input[13,14,19]. Evidence for these two main roles has mostly derived from animal experiments in which ICC have been removed mechanically[23], damaged chemically[24], or in which the kit tyrosine kinase receptor has been inactivated either by blocking antibodies[25] or loss of function due to spontaneous mutation of the c-kit gene[11,12,26]. The loss of ICC function abolishes electrical slow waves and leads to a decreased contractile response resulting in a delayed intestinal transit. Alterations of ICC, either structural or quantitative in nature, have been reported in a variety of human gastrointestinal motility disorders such as in achalasia, pyloric stenosis, chronic intestinal pseudo-obstruction or Hirschsprung's disease, suggesting a functional impact of ICC on the maintenance of normal gastrointestinal motility patterns[27–29].

Slow-transit constipation

The morphometric analysis in patients with STC ($n = 11$) yielded a significantly decreased density of ICC. Similar findings have been reported in a recent study[18] carried out on six cases with STC by calculating the volume of immunoreactive ICC in relationship to the surrounding non-immunoreactive tissue. Despite the different morphometric approaches both the present study and the study by He *et al.*[18] could reveal statistically significant alterations of ICC in patients with STC. The numerical decrease of ICC also included those ICC located at the submucosal border which have been considered to represent the pacemaker region within the human colon[30]. The relative loss of intestinal pacemaker cells may represent an underlying morphological substrate for the decreased smooth muscle contractile activity, thereby contributing to the prolonged colonic transit time. Nevertheless, in both studies there is no clear cut-off between controls and patients with STC: the values of the control group overlap with those obtained from patients with STC, suggesting that a lowered number of ICC *per se* does not necessarily lead to symptoms of chronic constipation. The exact amount of ICC required for a clinically satisfactory propelling function is not known, and a certain degree of redundancy seems to be likely.

The overall-process length of ICC did not differ significantly between patients with STC and the control group. However, at histological evaluation it was apparent that ICC of patients with STC exhibited considerably shortened but more numerous processes – an observation that was obviously missed by the intersection counting method, but had been described previously in the study by He *et al.*[18] It may be suggested that ICC have compensated their numerical decline by developing more processes, albeit of smaller size.

Megacolon

One of the first theories that ICC are altered in human gastrointestinal motility disorders has derived from studies examining the distribution of ICC in congenital megacolon[15,16,31,32]. Up to now there is only one case report of acquired megacolon[17] and a series of six adult patients with chagasic megacolon[33] in which ICC have been examined. Moreover, all studies used either a mere descriptive or semiquantitative approach to determine quantitative alterations of ICC, which might explain the contradictory findings regarding the distribution of ICC in patients with megacolon.

In contrast to patients with STC, in patients with megacolon both the number and the process length of ICC were significantly reduced. The substantial decrease of ICC demonstrated in the present study is in accordance with previous reports[15,16,32], but not with the study of Horisawa *et al.*[31], who found unchanged ICC populations within the aganglionic bowel segment. Surprisingly, the highest density of remaining ICC was found at the submucosal border of the circular muscle layer – the area in which the pacemaker activity has been mapped for the human colon[30]. This observation may throw doubt on whether the pacemaker region is exclusively confined to ICC located at the submucosal border. On the other hand, on histological examination the network of ICC at the submucosal border appeared to be disrupted and discontinuous (more than 50% decrease of ICC) resembling similar features as reported by Vanderwinden *et al.*[16]

In both groups (patients with megacolon and with STC) the ICC populations were not totally depleted. Given the long-standing history of chronic constipation dating back to childhood, the reduced amount of ICC is most likely due to congenital developmental disorder. However, as the present data only reflect the actual distribution of c-kit-immunoreactive ICC at the time of operation, it cannot be excluded that ICC may have redifferentiated into non-c-kit-expressing cells or cells of smooth muscle phenotype during postnatal life prior to the histological assessment.

Malformations of the enteric nervous system

Slow-transit constipation

The neuronal decrease demonstrated in the present study is in accordance with previous studies which reported a loss of argyrophilic myenteric neurons[8], a reduction of intraganglionic neurofilaments[9] and a reduced number of PGP 9.5-immunoreactive neurons within myenteric ganglia[10]. Although the meshes of the myenteric plexus were widened and exhibited a reduced ganglionic density, the network was not disrupted and basically displayed similar architectural features as observed in controls. This might explain that a recent study using PGP 9.5 immunohistochemistry for the determination of the myenteric fraction on conventional cross-sections yielded no significant differences between patients with STC and controls[34].

Megacolon

In patients with megacolon the intramural nerve networks had completely disintegrated and were replaced by hypertrophic nerve fibre strands. The fact that two of the six patients did not show a complete lack of intramural neurons clearly demonstrates that, apart from aganglionosis (classic Hirschsprung's disease), non-aganglionic innervational disorders (e.g. severe hypoganglionosis) are capable of causing megacolon. This concept is supported by an early contribution of Howard and Garret[2] and two more recently published case reports of a newborn infant[35] and of an adult patient[17] with myenteric hypoganglionosis who developed a megacolon. In both cases the neuronal malformations were accompanied by a complete loss respectively a decrease of ICC.

Concomitant alterations of enteric nervous system and interstitial cells of Cajal

There is increasing evidence that many gastrointestinal motility disorders caused by neuronal malformations are associated with concomitant alterations of ICC, e.g. pyloric stenosis, achalasia, Hirschsprung's disease, chagasic megacolon, chronic intestinal pseudo-obstruction[28,29]. Furthermore, from the present data it can be deduced that the severity of neuronal malformations correlates with the extent of ICC alterations: the loss of nerve cells appears to parallel the loss of ICC. This observation may suggest mutual influences between the ENS and ICC during development. Animal experiments have provided clear evidence that, unlike enteric neurons, ICC are of mesenchymal origin and do not derive from neural crest cells[36,37]. However, although ICC and the progenitor cells of the ENS are of different origin, during embryogenesis enteric neurons provide a source of the natural ligand for the c-kit receptor, the stem cell factor (SCF)[38]. SCF/kit-signalling is required for maintenance of the ICC phenotype[37], and withdrawal of SCF leads to re-differentiation of ICC into a mesenchymal smooth muscle phenotype[39]. Thus, a complete or a relative lack of enteric neurons (aganglionic and hypoganglionic conditions respectively) would abolish or reduce the neuronal source of SCF and may lead to a decreased population of phenotypically differentiated ICC.

Although this model fits well into the present findings it remains speculative whether a deficient colonization of the bowel wall by neural crest-derived neurons causes a depletion of the ICC population. It must be acknowledged that, in addition to neurons, the gut provides other sources of SCF. Smooth muscle cell lineages also express SCF; hence enteric nerve cells are not necessarily required for the development of ICC[37,40]. Experimental studies have shown that in aneural explants of murine[36] and chick[41] gut ICC develop normal morphology. It is not yet clear if their function is fully maintained in the absence of enteric neurons which under normal conditions are intimately associated with ICC and considered to be their 'physiological partners'. Even if developments of both cell systems can take place independently, the topographical and functional refinement between ICC and neuronal structures might be impaired during postnatal maturation[29,37].

CONCLUSIONS

In summary, the present study suggests an aetiological link between severe disorders of colorectal motility and alterations of both the intestinal pacemaker cell system and the enteric nervous system. Our own and previous data[18] would speak in favour of a combined immunological assessment of c-kit and PGP 9.5 expression in patients with idiopathic STC and megacolon. A meaningful histopathological examination requires a standardized morphometric analysis and can be carried out either postoperatively on resected colonic specimens or preoperatively on full-thickness biopsies. This approach, if applied to a larger number of carefully selected patients, may further elucidate the underlying pathophysiology of functional gastrointestinal motility disorders still considered to be 'idiopathic' in nature.

References

1. Dalla-Valle. Ricerche istologiche su di un casi megacolon congenito. Pediatria. 1920;28:740–52.
2. Howard ER, Garrett JR, Kidd A. Constipation and congenital disorders of the myenteric plexus. J R Soc Med. 1984;77(Suppl. 3):13–19.
3. Holschneider AM, Meier-Ruge W, Ure BM. Hirschsprung's disease and allied disorders – a review. Eur J Pediatr Surg. 1994;4:260–6.
4. Koch TR, Carney JA, Go L, Go VL. Idiopathic chronic constipation is associated with decreased colonic vasoactive intestinal peptide. Gastroenterology. 1988;94:300–10.
5. Milner P, Crowe R, Kamm MA, Lennard-Jones JE, Burnstock G. Vasoactive intestinal polypeptide levels in sigmoid colon in idiopathic constipation and diverticular disease. Gastroenterology. 1990;99:666–75.
6. Cortesini C, Cianchi F, Infantino A, Lise M. Nitric oxide synthase and VIP distribution in enteric nervous system in idiopathic chronic constipation. Dig Dis Sci. 1995;40:2450–5.
7. Sjolund K, Fasth S, Ekman R et al. Neuropeptides in idiopathic chronic constipation (slow transit constipation). Neurogastroenterol Motil. 1997;9:143–50.
8. Krishnamurthy S, Schuffler MD, Rohrmann CA, Pope CE. Severe idiopathic constipation is associated with a distinctive abnormality of the colonic myenteric plexus. Gastroenterology. 1985;88:26–34.
9. Schouten WR, ten Kate FJ, de Graaf EJ, Gilberts EC, Simons JL, Kluck P. Visceral neuropathy in slow transit constipation: an immunohistochemical investigation with monoclonal antibodies against neurofilament. Dis Colon Rectum. 1993;36:1112–17.
10. Wedel T, Roblick UJ, Ott V et al. Oligoneuronal hypoganglionosis in patients with idiopathic slow-transit constipation. Dis Colon Rectum. 2002;45:54–62.
11. Ward SM, Burns AJ, Torihashi S, Sanders KM. Mutation of the proto-oncogene c-kit blocks development of interstitial cells and electrical rhythmicity in murine intestine. J Physiol. 1994;480:91–7.
12. Huizinga JD, Thuneberg L, Kluppel M, Malysz J, Mikkelsen HB, Bernstein A. W/kit gene required for interstitial cells of Cajal and for intestinal pacemaker activity. Nature. 1995;373:347–9.
13. Burns AJ, Lomax AE, Torihashi S, Sanders KM, Ward SM. Interstitial cells of Cajal mediate inhibitory neurotransmission in the stomach. Proc Natl Acad Sci USA. 1996;93:12008–13.
14. Ward SM, Beckett EA, Wang X, Baker F, Khoyi M, Sanders KM. Interstitial cells of Cajal mediate cholinergic neurotransmission from enteric motor neurons. J Neurosci. 2000;20:1393–403.
15. Yamataka A, Kato Y, Tibboel D et al. A lack of intestinal pacemaker (c-kit) in aganglionic bowel of patients with Hirschsprung's disease. J Pediatr Surg. 1995;30:441–4.
16. Vanderwinden JM, Rumessen JJ, Liu H, Descamps D, De Laet MH, Vanderhaeghen JJ. Interstitial cells of Cajal in human colon and in Hirschsprung's disease. Gastroenterology. 1996;111:901–10.
17. Faussone-Pellegrini MS, Fociani P, Buffa R, Basilisco G. Loss of interstitial cells and a fibromuscular layer on the luminal side of the colonic circular muscle presenting as megacolon in an adult patient. Gut. 1999;45:775–9.
18. He CL, Burgart L, Wang L et al. G. Decreased interstitial cell of Cajal volume in patients with slow-transit constipation. Gastroenterology. 2000;118:14–21.
19. Sanders KM. A case for interstitial cells of Cajal as pacemakers and mediators of neurotransmission in the gastrointestinal tract. Gastroenterology. 1996;111:492–515.
20. Wedel T, Roblick U, Gleiss J et al. Organization of the enteric nervous system in the human colon demonstrated by wholemount immunohistochemistry with special reference to the submucous plexus. Anat Anz. 1999;181:327–37.
21. Borchard E, Meier-Ruge W, Wiebecke B et al. Innervationsstörungen des Dickdarms – Klassifikation und Diagnostik. Pathologe. 1991;181:171–4.
22. Cajal S. Sur les ganglions et plexus nerveux de l'intestine. CR Soc Biol (Paris). 1893;45:217–23.
23. Smith TK, Reed JB, Sanders KM. Origin and propagation of electrical slow waves in circular muscle of canine proximal colon. Am J Physiol. 1987;252:C215–24.
24. Liu LW, Thuneberg L, Huizinga JD. Selective lesioning of interstitial cells of Cajal by methylene blue and light leads to loss of slow waves. Am J Physiol. 1994;266:G485–96.
25. Maeda H, Yamagata A, Nishikawa S et al. Requirement of c-kit for development of intestinal pacemaker system. Development. 1992;116:369–75.

26. Isozaki K, Hirota S, Nakama A *et al.* Disturbed intestinal movement, bile reflux to the stomach, and deficiency of c-kit-expressing cells in Ws/Ws mutant rats. Gastroenterology. 1995;109: 456–64.
27. Huizinga JD, Thuneberg L, Vanderwinden JM, Rumessen JJ. Interstitial cells of Cajal as targets for pharmacological intervention in gastrointestinal motor disorders. Trends Pharmacol Sci. 1997;18:393–403.
28. Vanderwinden JM, Rumessen JJ. Interstitial cells of Cajal in human gut and gastrointestinal disease. Microsc Res Tech. 1999;47:344–60.
29. Sanders KM, Ordog T, Koh SD, Torihashi S, Ward SM. Development and plasticity of interstitial cells of Cajal. Neurogastroenterol Motil. 1999;11:311–38.
30. Rae MG, Fleming N, McGregor DB, Sanders KM, Keef KD. Control of motility patterns in the human colonic circular muscle layer by pacemaker activity. J Physiol. 1998;510:309–20.
31. Horisawa M, Watanabe Y, Torihashi S. Distribution of c-Kit immunopositive cells in normal human colon and in Hirschsprung's disease. J Pediatr Surg. 1998;33:1209–14.
32. Nemeth L, Yoneda A, Kader M, Devaney D, Puri P. Three-dimensional morphology of gut innervation in total intestinal aganglionosis using whole-mount preparation. J Pediatr Surg. 2001;36:291–5.
33. Hagger R, Finlayson C, Kahn F, De Oliveira R, Chimelli L, Kumar D. A deficiency of interstitial cells of Cajal in Chagasic megacolon. J Auton Nerv Syst. 2000;80:108–11.
34. Park HJ, Kamm MA, Abbasi AM, Talbot IC. Immunohistochemical study of the colonic muscle and innervation in idiopathic chronic constipation. Dis Colon Rectum. 1995;38:509–13.
35. Yamataka A, Fujiwara T, Nishiye H, Sunagawa M, Miyano T. Localization of intestinal pacemaker cells and synapses in the muscle layers of a patient with colonic hypoganglionosis. J Pediatr Surg. 1996;31:584–7.
36. Young HM, Ciampoli D, Southwell BR, Newgreen DF. Origin of interstitial cells of Cajal in the mouse intestine. Dev Biol. 1996;180:97–107.
37. Wu JJ, Rothman TP, Gershon MD. Development of the interstitial cell of Cajal: origin, kit dependence and neuronal and nonneuronal sources of kit ligand. J Neurosci Res. 2000; 59:384–401.
38. Young HM, Torihashi S, Ciampoli D, Sanders KM. Identification of neurons that express stem cell factor in the mouse small intestine. Gastroenterology. 1998;115:898–908.
39. Torihashi S, Ward SM, Sanders KM. Development of c-Kit-positive cells and the onset of electrical rhythmicity in murine small intestine. Gastroenterology. 1997;112:144–55.
40. Epperson A, Hatton WJ, Callaghan B *et al.* Molecular markers expressed in cultured and freshly isolated interstitial cells of Cajal. Am J Physiol Cell Physiol. 2000;279:C529–39.
41. Lecoin L, Gabella G, Le Douarin N. Origin of the c-kit-positive interstitial cells in the avian bowel. Development. 1996;122:725–33.

Section V
Nerve function modulating gut inflammation

17
Sensory nerve function in gut inflammation

G. F. GEBHART, K. BIELEFELDT, Y.-M. KANG and N. OZAKI

INTRODUCTION

Conceptually, altered sensations from the gut such as those associated with functional disorders can arise and be sustained wholly by either peripheral or central mechanisms. Given the innocuous stimuli that typically give rise to discomfort and pain in functional dyspepsia and irritable bowel syndrome, it is clear that peripheral mechanisms are important. In established functional disorders central mechanisms also certainly contribute significantly.

Although the discomfort and pain that characterize functional gut disorders arise in the absence of obvious cause, numerous reports in the clinical literature establish that conscious sensations from the gut are increased in functional gut disorders and the normal psychophysical function is shifted significantly leftward when the stomach (e.g. ref. 1) or distal colon[2] is distended.

Because hypersensitivity from the gut represents nervous system plasticity, both in the peripheral and central nervous systems, peripheral contributions to gut hypersensitivity would be reflected by an increased excitability of sensory receptors and a change in the functional characteristics of those receptors produced by peripheral mediators.

Experimentally, acute or chronic irritation or inflammation of the gut significantly alters the sensitivity and excitability of the extrinsic primary afferent (sensory) nerves that innervate it. Mechanoreceptors, chemoreceptors and/or thermoreceptors on these sensory nerve endings are affected when the gut is insulted and their axons or cell bodies can be studied electrophysiologically to assess changes in sensitivity and excitability. Most investigations have studied mechanosensitive visceral nociceptors, which sensitize after an experimental insult, suggesting that previously innocuous stimuli can lead to discomfort and pain.

In this summary we will review the characteristics of visceral afferent (sensory) fibres that innervate the gut, the process of sensitization and change in excitability, and consider some mediators that contribute to hypersensitivity.

CHARACTERISTICS OF VISCERAL AFFERENTS

The receptors that innervate the gut are associated with axons that are thinly myelinated or unmyelinated[3,4]; that is, information from the gut is conveyed by slowly and/or very slowly conducting axons. There are a limited number of more rapidly conducting axons (Aβ-fibres), but they are associated with Pacinian corpuscles associated with the mesentery[3]. Unlike the innervation of somatic structures, visceral afferent (sensory) fibres traverse both prevertebral and paravertebral ganglia *en route* to the spinal cord. These visceral sensory axons give off collaterals in prevertebral ganglia where they can influence secretory and motor function of the gut.

At the level of the spinal cord, visceral afferent fibres terminate in the superficial spinal dorsal horn (lamina I and II), in lamina V where they influence sympathetic and parasympathetic efferent outflow to viscera, and dorsal to the central canal in an area termed lamina X. The number of visceral afferent fibres is very low relative to somatic input to the spinal cord, but visceral afferent fibre terminals extensively arborize and spread within the spinal cord[5].

Relative to sensations from the gut, mechanoreceptors have been most extensively studied. Mechanoreceptor terminals are located in the muscle layers of the gut and respond to tension as hollow organs are filled and distended[3]. Because balloon distension in humans reproduces their symptoms and pattern of referred sensations[6], hollow organ distension in non-human animals has been widely used to study gut mechanoreceptors. For example, mechanoreceptors associated with pelvic nerve fibres that innervate the distal colon in the rat have been documented to have either low thresholds for response or high thresholds for response[7]. Receptors with low thresholds respond in the physiological range when the colon is distended, whereas those with high thresholds respond to mechanical distension in excess of the physiological range (e.g. > 30 mmHg). As previously reviewed[8], it has been documented for several hollow organs in different species that approximately 75% of the mechanoreceptors associated with hollow organs have low thresholds for response and approximately 25% have high thresholds for response. Similarly, low- and high-threshold mechanosensitive fibres in the splanchnic innervation of the rat stomach have recently been described[9]. Because of their high thresholds for response, it is likely that high-threshold mechanoreceptors function as nociceptors and signal acute pain associated with hollow organ distension. For reasons given below, we propose that low-threshold mechanoreceptors along the gut also contribute to acute sensations and that both low- *and* high-threshold receptors are important to the altered sensations associated with functional gut disorders.

When examined for responses to increasing intensities of organ distension, high-threshold mechanoreceptors, as one would expect of a nociceptor, encode the distending stimulus with increased responses to increasing intensities of organ distension (Fig. 1). Unexpectedly, it was found that low-threshold mechanoreceptors innervating hollow organs similarly encode distending pressures well into the noxious range (Fig. 1), exhibiting the ability to respond across a wide dynamic range of distending pressures. Unlike low-threshold cutaneous mechanoreceptors, which respond only to innocuous mechanical stimuli applied to the skin, these low-threshold mechanoreceptors innervating the gut

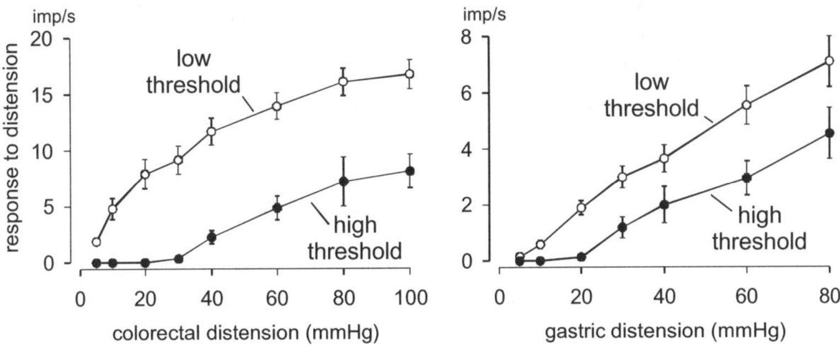

Fig. 1   Summary of responses of pelvic nerve (left) and splanchnic nerve (right) afferent fibres in the rat to graded intensities of distension of the colon and stomach, respectively. Two populations of mechanosensitive afferent fibres, low-threshold and high-threshold, innervate the gut. Low-threshold fibres typically have response thresholds $\leq$ 5 mmHg; high-threshold fibres typically have response thresholds $\geq$ 30 mmHg. Note that both low- and high-threshold fibres encode distending pressures in the noxious range (> 30 mmHg). See refs 7 and 9 for additional information

have the ability to contribute to discomfort and pain arising from over-distension of hollow organs. Moreover, as illustrated in Fig. 1, low-threshold mechano-receptors, on average, give greater magnitude responses to the same intensities of colon or gastric distension than high-threshold mechanoreceptors.

Another important characteristic of visceral afferent fibres is their ability to sensitize. By sensitization is meant an increase in response magnitude after tissue insult, often associated with a reduction in response threshold. In addition, spon-taneous activity is frequently increased after tissue insult and the receptive field area at the receptor terminal in the tissue often increases in size[10]. Cutaneous nociceptors are characterized by their unique ability to exhibit sensitization when tissue is injured. Similarly, high-threshold mechanoreceptors that innervate the gut sensitize in the presence of experimental inflammation. Unexpectedly, and different from the somatic realm, low-threshold mechanoreceptors that innervate the viscera also sensitize. The example shown in Fig. 2 illustrates an increase in response magnitude and in spontaneous activity for a low-threshold mechanoreceptor innervating the rat colon. A different, high-threshold mechanoreceptor is also shown to increase response magnitude after colon inflammation, and there is also a clear reduction in response threshold from 30 to 10 mmHg.

The significance of findings that low-threshold mechanoreceptors innervating the gut encode into the noxious range and can sensitize in the presence of an experimental inflammation reinforces the notion that both low-threshold and high-threshold mechanoreceptors innervating the gut can contribute significantly to discomfort and pain. It should be obvious from the example in Fig. 2 that a reduction in response threshold from the noxious range (30 mmHg) to the physio-logical range (10 mmHg) can lead to increased sensations associated with other-wise normal gut function. The ability of low-threshold mechanoreceptors to sensitize reveals that even distending pressures in the physiological range can lead to significantly increased input to the spinal cord and thus to greater input from the viscera to higher centres in the central nervous system.

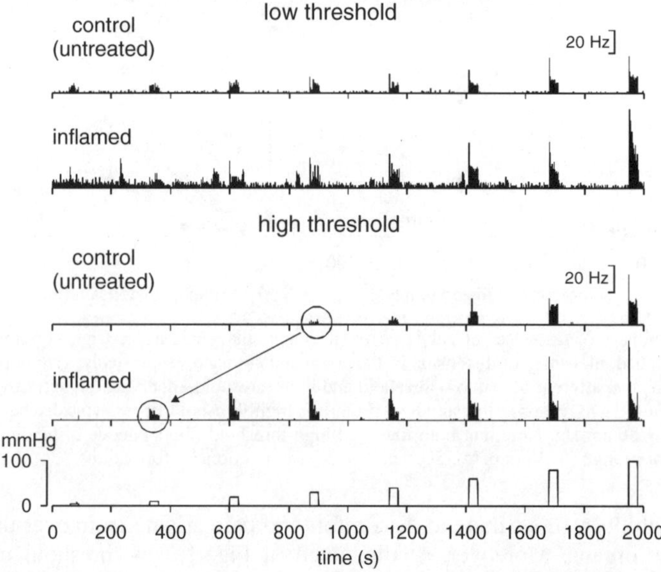

Fig. 2 Examples of sensitization of pelvic nerve afferent fibres in the rat after instillation of 2.5% acetic acid. Colorectal distending pressures are given bottom-most and responses are presented as peristimulus time histograms (1 s bin width) for a low-threshold and high-threshold fibre. Both spontaneous activity and response magnitude of the low-threshold fibre increase after colon inflammation; response threshold decreases and response magnitude increases for the high-threshold fibre after colon inflammation

A final characteristic of the visceral afferent innervation is that mechanoreceptors also exhibit sensitivity to chemical and/or thermal stimuli. In the somatic realm, C-polymodal nociceptors respond to noxious thermal, noxious chemical and noxious mechanical stimulation. Similarly, visceral mechanoreceptors respond to chemical and thermal stimulation, but this polymodal character is not restricted to the high-threshold mechanoreceptor population and includes also the low-threshold mechanoreceptor population. This is yet another distinguishing characteristic of the visceral innervation. In recent studies (Kang, Bielefeldt and Gebhart, unpublished), it has been found that gastric vagal mechanoreceptors are also chemosensitive and thermosensitive and, importantly, that innocuous thermal and chemical stimulation can sensitize gastric vagal mechanoreceptors. Accordingly, these data suggest that normal gut content can contribute to altered responses to activation of mechanoreceptors and probably other receptors in the gut.

The consequence of sensitization of the afferent innervation of the gut is that the stimulus–response function is shifted leftward. The early work of Ritchie[2], and others following, has clearly shown, in patients with functional gut disorders, increased sensitivity to distending stimuli. That is, their psychophysical function – the relationship between stimulus intensity and pain report – is shifted leftward. Figure 3 illustrates the leftward shift in the stimulus–response function of high-threshold mechanoreceptors that innervate the rat colon. At a low but

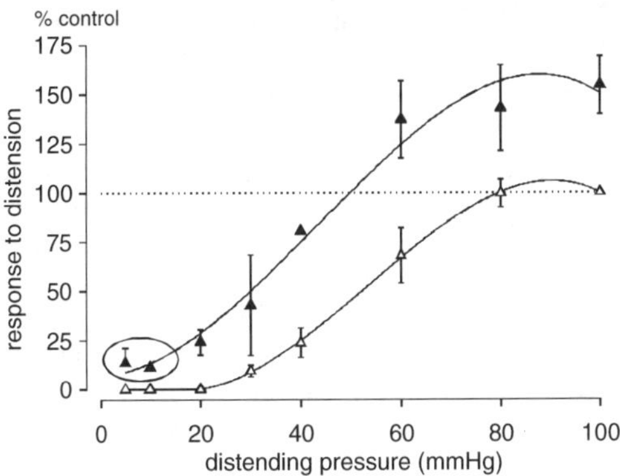

Fig. 3 Summary of responses of high-threshold pelvic nerve afferent fibres to graded intensities of colon distension before (unfilled symbols) and after (filled symbols) colon inflammation. The stimulus–response function is shifted significantly to the left; response magnitude is increased and the extrapolated response threshold is decreased after colon inflammation. Note that distending pressures in the physiological range (5 and 10 mmHg) activate high-threshold colon mechanoreceptors after colon inflammation (circled)

noxious intensity of distension (between 30 and 40 mmHg), response magnitude is approximately 20% of the maximum response to distension (defined as 100% at 100 mmHg distension). After the colon is experimentally inflamed, the stimulus–response function is shifted leftward and that same intensity of distension now produces a response that is approximately 60% of the maximum response in the absence of inflammation. Note also that, at low intensities of stimulation in the physiological range (e.g. 5–10 mmHg), response magnitude after inflammation is equivalent to higher intensity stimulation prior to colon inflammation. This illustration provides the operational definition of hypersensitivity, namely a leftward shift in the psychophysical or stimulus–response function associated with an increase in response magnitude and generally a reduction in the extrapolated response threshold.

ROLE OF SODIUM CHANNEL FUNCTION IN VISCERAL HYPERSENSITIVITY

Because voltage-gated sodium channels (Na_V) are important determinants of neuron excitability, it might be expected that their function is altered in the presence of tissue insult. There are nine known sodium channels that have been identified in mammals based on structure[11]. Most of these sodium channels are sensitive to tetrodotoxin (TTX), but two neuronal TTX-resistant sodium channels are of interest because they are predominantly associated with small-diameter sensory neurons in dorsal root ganglia, including visceral sensory neurons. Evidence has been accumulating for a role of these TTX-resistant sodium channels (Na_V 1.8 and Na_V 1.9) as contributing to increased excitability of sensory neurons following tissue insult. Recently we examined the behaviour of sodium channels in nodose and dorsal root ganglia after experimental ulceration[12] or irritation[13] of the stomach. In these experiments the stomach was ulcerated by injection of acetic acid into the wall of the stomach or irritated by ingestion of iodoacetamide in drinking water for 7 days. The cell bodies of vagal and splanchnic afferent fibres contained in the nodose and dorsal root ganglia, respectively, were identified by content of a fluorescent dye retrogradely transported from the stomach to the cell body. Changes in sodium channel function were found following both insults, but stomach ulceration, as might be expected, produced greater effects. When sodium currents in nodose or dorsal root ganglia cell bodies were examined 7 days following gastric ulceration with acetic acid, it was found that the peak sodium current was increased and that this was contributed almost exclusively by an increase in the TTX-resistant current (Fig. 4). It was also found that the time-course for recovery from inactivation was accelerated in these same neurons from the ulcerated stomach (see ref. 12). These outcomes suggest an increase in the excitability of gastric mechanoreceptors produced by gastric insult, although in these whole-cell patch clamp experiments it is not known whether the cell bodies studied are associated with mechanoreceptors at their terminals in the stomach. It would appear likely to be so, however, because, when examined 1 week following stomach ulceration, responses to gastric distension in the unanaesthetized animal were significantly enhanced, giving evidence of gastric hypersensitivity[14]. Given that gastric mechanoreceptors are polymodal in character, this outcome further suggests that chemical, thermal or mechanical stimulation would be affected, expressed as a lower threshold for action potential generation and a higher spike frequency. That is, analogous to recordings from the afferent fibres in response to mechanical distension, these experiments studying sodium channel function suggest a means by which excitability is increased and sensitization occurs.

It is, of course, necessary that some mediator or mediators in the viscera change in response to insult and thus contribute to modification of sodium channel (and other ion channel or receptor) function. The list of candidates is long, and includes amines, cytokines, products of arachidonic acid, neuropeptides, neurotrophins, etc. The roles of many mediators have been studied in different

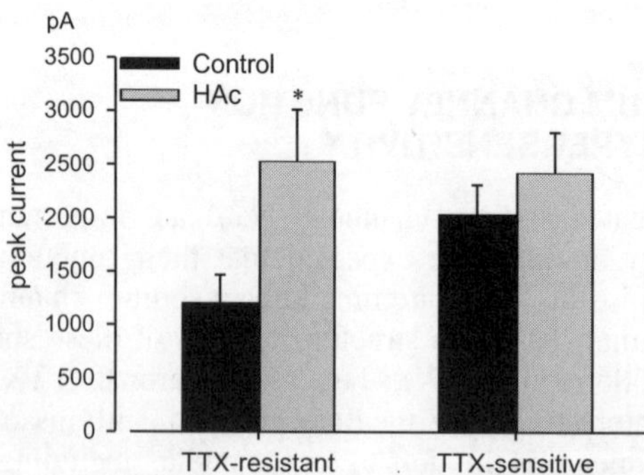

Fig. 4 Ulceration of the rat stomach (see ref. 14 for details) increases the peak sodium current in gastric nodose ganglion neurons (see ref. 12 for details). The increase in peak sodium current is contributed by the tetrodotoxin (TTX)-resistant component of the current; the TTX-sensitive component of the current is unaffected after gastric ulceration

experimental settings. For example, it is known that a mixture of mediators including bradykinin, serotonin, histamine, PGE_2 and protons (pH 6.0) sensitizes nociceptors innervating the skin better than do either one of the mediators applied alone and independent of the presence of other mediators[15]. Similar studies have not been done for visceral receptors, but the principle probably holds that no single mediator is responsible for sensitization of visceral mechanoreceptors, chemoreceptors or thermoreceptors. Rather, it is likely that multiple mediators contribute and perhaps that different mediators contribute differently in different parts of the gut. The neurotrophin nerve growth factor (NGF) has been studied and shown to produce hyperalgesia when injected into the rat skin[16] and also to sensitize visceral afferents[17]. Similarly, we[18] have examined the role of NGF on responses to gastric distension in the rat and on sodium currents in nodose ganglion cell bodies. Intragastric instillation of NGF produced an increase in response to gastric distension, providing evidence for sensitization, and this was supported by the effects of NGF on sodium currents recorded in nodose ganglion neurons. Similar to what was found following ulceration of the stomach wall, exposure of nodose ganglion neurons to NGF led to an increase in peak sodium current that was contributed almost exclusively by the TTX-R resistant component of the current.

EVIDENCE THAT INNOCUOUS STIMULI CAN ALTER MECHANOSENSATION

In a recent series of experiments, we (Kang, Bielefeldt and Gebhart, unpublished) have initiated experiments to examine the effect of normally innocuous stimuli on responses of vagal mechanoreceptors to gastric distension. The preliminary data suggest that instillation of warm saline into the stomach increases the spontaneous, resting activity of gastric mechanoreceptors and typically increases subsequent responses to gastric distension. Figure 5 shows the responses of a gastric vagal afferent fibre to increasing intensities of gastric distension before and following instillation of 46°C saline into the stomach. The instillation of saline increases spontaneous activity and also subsequent responses to gastric distension. The instillation of 37°C saline does not reproduce these effects. We have also examined concentration-dependent effects of instillation of hydrochloric acid (0.025–0.1 N) and glycocholic acid (2.5–10.0 mM) on resting activity of gastric vagal afferent fibres and responses to gastric distension. Hydrochloric acid has been found to sensitize some and desensitize other gastric mechanoreceptors, and glycocholic acid appears to desensitize responses to gastric distension. These intragastric treatments also certainly have effects on the intrinsic primary afferent neuron population and also produce changes in gastric compliance and motor activity. Accordingly, it is likely that through either direct action of chemical or thermal stimuli on polymodal vagal receptors or indirect influence by changes in motor function, mechanosensitivity of gastric vagal afferent fibres can be altered. Although it is generally held that the vagus nerve contributes no significant role to the discomfort and pain associated with functional gut disorders, it appears likely that the behaviour of mechanosensitive vagal afferents innervating the stomach does contribute in ways not yet understood.

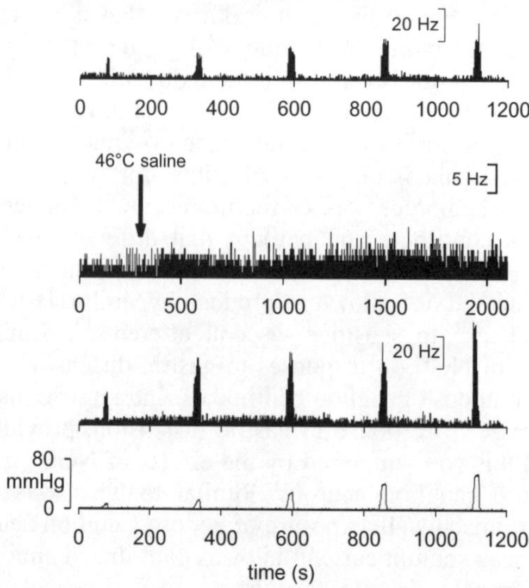

Fig. 5 Gastric vagal afferent fibre responses are sensitized by intragastric instillation of 46°C saline. Gastric distending pressures are given bottom-most and responses are presented as peristimulus time histograms (1 s bin width). Spontaneous activity (middle record) is significantly increased by 46 °C saline and response magnitude to gastric distension is significantly increased 30 min after saline instillation

Acknowledgements

We gratefully acknowledge Susan Birely for secretarial assistance and Michael Burcham for preparation of the graphics. The work was supported by NS19912 and NS 35790.

References

1. Mertz H, Fullerton S, Naliboff B, Mayer E. Symptoms and visceral perception in severe functional and organic dyspepsia. Gut. 1998;42:814–22.
2. Ritchie J. Pain from distension of the pelvic colon by inflating a balloon in the irritable colon syndrome. Gut. 1973;14:125–32.
3. Sengupta JN, Gebhart GF. Gastrointestinal afferent fibres and sensation. In: Jacobsen ED, Johnson LR, Christensen J, Alpers DA, Walsh JH, editors. Physiology of the Gastrointestinal Tract. New York: Raven Press, 1994:483–519.
4. Cervero F. Sensory innervation of the viscera: peripheral basis of visceral pain. Physiol Rev. 1994;74:95–138.
5. Sugiura Y, Tonosaki Y. Spinal organization of unmyelinated visceral afferent fibres in comparison with somatic afferent fibres. In: Gebhart GF, editor. Visceral Pain. Progress in Pain Research and Management, vol. 5. Seattle: IASP Press, 1995:41–59.
6. Ness TJ, Gebhart GF. Visceral pain: a review of experimental studies. Pain. 1990;41:167–234.
7. Sengupta JN, Gebhart GF. Characterization of mechanosensitive pelvic nerve afferent fibres innervating the colon of the rat. J Neurophysiol. 1994;71:2046–60.
8. Sengupta JN, Gebhart GF. Mechanosensitive afferent fibres in the gastrointestinal and lower urinary tracts. In: Gebhart GF, editor. Visceral Pain. Progress in Pain Research and Management, vol. 5. Seattle: IASP Press, 1995:75–98.

9. Ozaki N, Gebhart GF. Characterization of mechanosensitive splanchnic nerve afferent fibres innervating the rat stomach. Am J Physiol. 2001;281:G1449–59.
10. Pogatzki E, Gebhart GF, Brennan TJ. Activation and sensitization of cutaneous afferents and recruitment of MIAs one day after a plantar incision. J Neurophysiol. 2002;87:721–31.
11. Goldin AL. Resurgence of sodium channel research. Annu Rev Physiol. 2001;63:871–94.
12. Bielefeldt K, Ozaki N, Gebhart GF. Experimental ulcers alter voltage-sensitive sodium currents in rat gastric sensory neurons. Gastroenterology. 2002;122:394–405.
13. Bielefeldt K, Ozaki N, Gebhart GF. Mild gastritis alters voltage-sensitive sodium currents in gastric sensory neurons. Gastroenterology. 2002;122:752–61.
14. Ozaki N, Bielefeldt K, Sengupta J, Gebhart GF. Models of gastric hyperalgesia in the rat. Am J Physiol. 2002;283:G666–76.
15. Kress M, Reeh PW. Chemical excitation and sensitization in nociceptors. In: Belmont C, Cervero F, editors. Neurobiology of Nociceptors. Oxford: Oxford University Press, 1996;258–97.
16. Shu XQ, Mendell LM. Neurotrophins and hyperalgesia. Proc Natl Acad Sci. 1999;96:7693–6.
17. Dmitrieva N, McMahon SB. Sensitisation of visceral afferents by nerve growth factor in the adult rat. Pain. 1996;66:87–97.
18. Bielefeldt K, Ozaki N, Gebhart GF. Role of nerve growth factor in modulation of gastric afferent neurons in the rat. Am J Physiol. 2003;284:G499–G507.

18
Neuroimmunology and the gastrointestinal tract

K. BIELEFELDT

NEUROGENIC INFLAMMATION AND THE GASTROINTESTINAL TRACT

Clinical studies and animal experiments suggest that stress can modulate intestinal inflammation. These observations triggered interest in the potential interactions between the nervous system and inflammatory cells, a crosstalk that may take place at various levels. In this brief overview I will focus on the peripheral nerves and their role in the modulation of immune responses.

Early morphological investigations showed a close proximity between mast cells and nerves within the intestinal mucosa[1]. Is this proximity indeed functionally relevant? In the skin, injury-induced activation of sensory nerve terminals may contribute to the inflammatory response. As shown in Fig. 1, action potentials propagate past branch points into other terminations where they trigger the release of transmitters at the sensory terminals. This initiates a cascade of local reactions, leading to erythema and oedema – a phenomenon often referred to as axon reflex or neurogenic inflammation[2].

Is neurogenic inflammation also involved in the pathogenesis of gastrointestinal disease? In a model of acute enteritis, induced by administration of toxin A, treatment with capsazepine significantly blunted the severity of inflammation[3]. Capsazepine blocks the VR-1 receptor, a temperature-sensitive ion channel expressed in a subset of sensory neurons. Capsazepine also decreased the immunohistochemically determined endocytosis of substance P receptors in neurons within the myenteric plexus. Thus, these results point to a role of neurons in the pathogenesis of intestinal inflammation. Moreover, they provide some information about the involvement of an important signalling molecule, substance P, as endocytosis described above requires prior activation of a receptor. Substance P can be found in intrinsic and extrinsic neurons within the gastrointestinal tract. In spinal afferents it is primarily expressed in unmyelinated fibres that project to the outer layers of the dorsal horn, an area that plays a central role in the transmission of nociceptive information. Interestingly, the expression of substance P

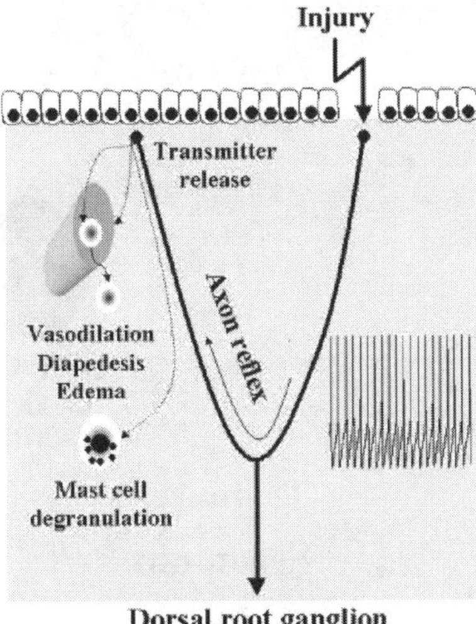

Fig. 1 Mechanism of neurogenic inflammation. Localized injury triggers action potentials, which invade other sensory terminals of the same axon and elicit transmitter release from these terminals. Transmitter molecules, in turn, interact with various targets, causing vasodilation, oedema due to capillary leak, chemotaxis and activation of immunocytes

as well as its receptor, the NK-1 receptor, increases in idiopathic inflammatory bowel disease[4,5]. Several lines of evidence suggest that substance P functions as a link between the nervous and immune system and contributes to the regulation of inflammation. Lamina propria lymphocytes and other immune competent cells express the NK-1 receptor[6]. This receptor is physiologically relevant as activation enhances chemotaxis of lymphocytes and monocytes[7] and increases tumour necrosis factor alpha (TNF-α) production in monocytes[8]. In the intestine substance P triggers histamine release, which can be inhibited by the neurotoxin tetrodotoxin or blockers of mast cell degranulation[9]. Comparable inhibitory effects of a compound on neurons and mast cells point to another important link between the nervous and immune systems.

NERVES, MAST CELLS AND INFLAMMATION

Recent studies in humans demonstrated that cold stress enhances the release of mast cell mediators into the jejunum in humans[10]. This raises questions concerning the role of these cells in inflammation and the interactions between the peripheral nervous system and immunocytes. Mast cells are part of the inflammatory infiltrate and increase after experimental injury and in chronic inflammatory diseases[11]. This change in number of mast cells is associated with elevation of tryptase release as a sign of mast cell activation[12]. Activated mast cells can produce a variety of signalling molecules that modulate the local immune response, such as leukotrienes, prostaglandins, TNF-α and various interleukins. In addition, mast cell granula contain histamine, serotonin and tryptase, which

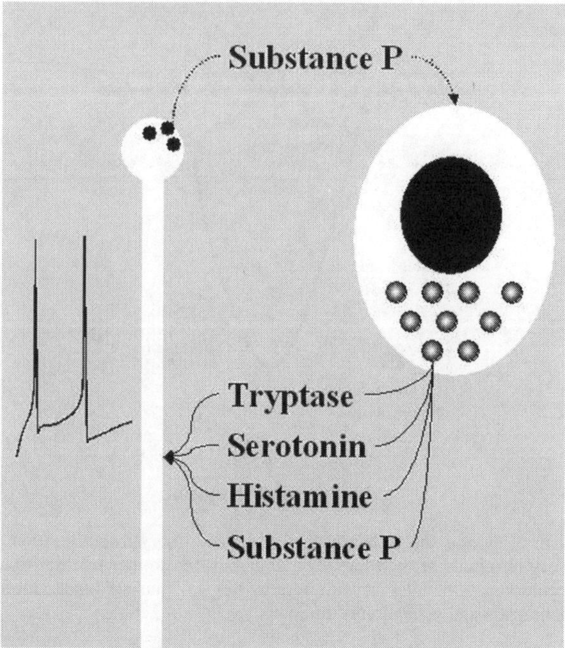

Fig. 2 Nerve–mast cell interactions. Activation of sensory neurons triggers substance P release, which functions as a chemoattractant for mast cells and may cause mast cell degranulation. Secretory granules contain serotonin, histamine and tryptase, which can activate receptors on sensory neurons, thereby augmenting the initial signal

may interact with many targets, including neurons. Tryptase cleaves the N-terminal of the type 2 proteinase-activated receptor (PAR-2), thereby triggering a cascade of intracellular signals, leading to an increase in cytosolic calcium and release of transmitters, such as substance P[13,14]. As this receptor is expressed on enteric and primary afferent neurons, tryptase release can initiate an interaction between mast cells and nerves. Mast cells, in turn, express receptors for neurotransmitters, such as serotonin, vasoactive intestinal peptide (VIP), somatostatin and substance P. This profile of signalling molecules and receptors and the observed proximity of nerves and mast cells provide a basis for a crosstalk where mast cells may cause nerve activation and vice-versa. The expression of PAR-2 receptors on neurons and of substance P receptors on mast cells may lead to an augmentation of the primary signal due to substance P release and consecutive mast cell activation (Fig. 2).

NERVE GROWTH FACTOR, INFLAMMATION AND HYPERALGESIA

We have recently demonstrated that experimental-induced inflammation is associated with an increase in nerve growth factor (NGF) and immunoreactivity

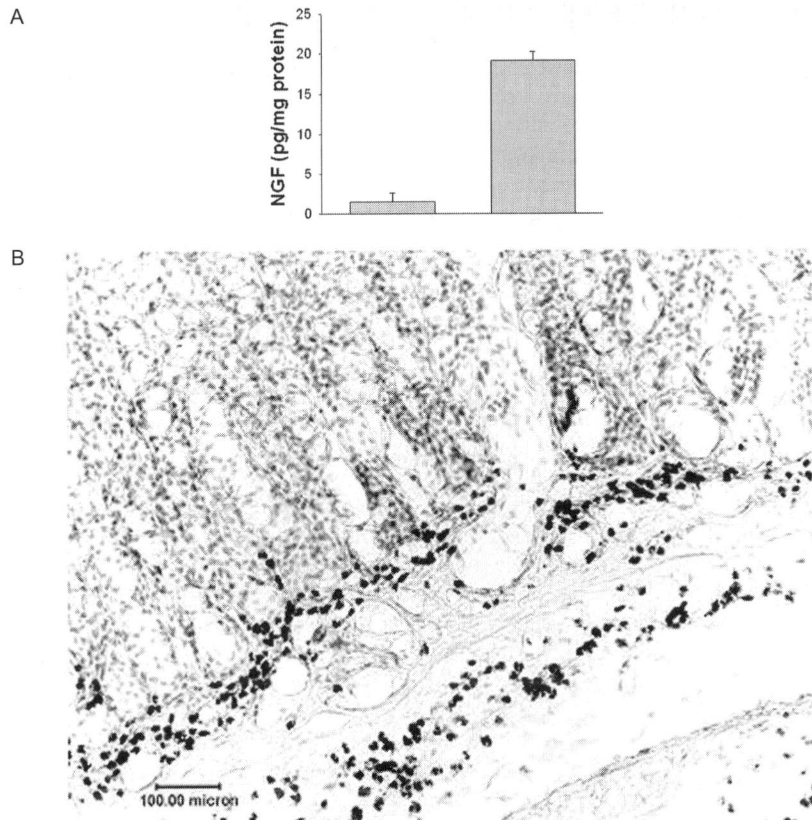

Fig. 3 Nerve growth factor and gastric injury. Experimentally induced gastric ulcers are associated with an increase in NGF within the gastric wall measured by ELISA (A). In parallel, a higher number of cells expressing the high-affinity NGF receptor can be found in the submucosa (B)

for its receptor within the gastric wall (Fig. 3). Similar changes have been described in idiopathic inflammatory bowel disease[15]. Exposure of primary afferent neurons to NGF alters the properties of voltage-sensitive sodium currents, consistent with the development of hyperalgesia[16]. At the level of the spinal cord, NGF changes the expression of transmitters at the synapse between first- and second-order neurons[17–19]. However, the effects of this neurotrophin go beyond the nervous system. Mast cells also express the high-affinity receptor for NGF[20]. Nerve growth factor functions as a chemoattractant for mast cells[8]. Mast cells are not only a potential target for NGF, they also produce this neurotrophin and may release it upon stimulation[21]. Therefore, NGF may directly enhance neuron excitability and indirectly contribute to the development of hyperalgesia by attracting and stimulating mast cells which then, in turn, may further increase NGF levels in the tissue.

TODAY'S CANDIDATES FOR TOMORROW'S TREATMENT?

Considering the role of mast cells and mediators, such as substance P or NGF, pharmacological agents have been developed and tested *in vitro* and *in vivo* to identify novel treatment options for patients with inflammatory diseases. Inhibitors of mast cell activation, such as cromolyn sodium or corticosteroids, blunt, but do not abolish the release of mediators *in vitro*[22]. Consistent with these findings, treatment before antigen challenge only partly inhibited changes in intestinal permeability triggered in animal models of allergic enteritis[23]. Strategies that rely on inhibition of mast cell mediators are the basis for the treatment of allergic rhinitis with histamine-1 receptor antagonists. While these agents do not play a role in the treatment of gastrointestinal inflammation, block of mast cell tryptase-induced changes could open up new therapeutic venues. Currently, no selective antagonists of the PAR-2 receptors exist. However, a recent study showed that inhibition of tryptase significantly improved the response of asthmatics to antigen challenge[24].

Experiments with other selective and potent inhibitors of signalling pathways described above are also encouraging. Substance P antagonists decrease the severity of colitis and pancreatitis in animal models of human diseases[25,26]. Similarly, these agents decrease hyperalgesia; however, such effects require administration of substance P antagonists before the initiating insult, raising questions concerning their effectiveness in the clinical context[27].

As discussed previously, gastrointestinal inflammation is associated with an increase in NGF, which in turn may contribute to the development of hyperalgesia. Tyrosine kinase inhibitors block the signal transduction of the high-affinity NGF receptor and blunt the development of hyperalgesia[28]. Unfortunately, interference with this important signalling pathway comes at a cost, as illustrated by an exacerbation of inflammation in an animal model of colitis[29]. This may at least in part be due to the involvement of NGF as a trophic factor in repair processes of neuronal and non-neuronal tissues[30,31]. In view of this role as trophic factor, the potential of NGF in post-traumatic or degenerative disorders of the nervous system has been tested. While initial results in animal experiments were encouraging, adverse effects with development of hyperalgesia[32–34] or worsening of nerve injury[35] limit the potential clinical utility of these approaches.

As discussed in this short overview, neurons and many immune competent cells share many signalling molecules and receptors. The translation of this information from the bench to the bedside is still in an early phase. Nonetheless, this overlap opens exciting opportunities for the development of new therapeutic approaches that simultaneously target sensory abnormalities and inflammation.

References

1. Stead RH, Tomioka M, Quinonez G, Simon GT, Felten SY, Bienenstock J. Intestinal mucosal mast cells in normal and nematode-infected rat intestines are in intimate contact with peptidergic nerves. Proc Natl Acad Sci USA. 1987;84:2975–9.
2. Willis WD. Dorsal root potentials and dorsal root reflexes: a double-edged sword. Exp Brain Res. 1999;124:395–421.
3. McVey DC, Vigna SR. The capsaicin VR1 receptor mediates substance P release in toxin A-induced enteritis in rats. Peptides. 2001;22:1439–46.

4. Vento P, Kiviluoto T, Keranen U, Jarvinen HJ, Kivilaakso E, Soinila S. Quantitative comparison of growth-associated protein-43 and substance P in ulcerative colitis. J Histochem Cytochem. 2001;49:749–58.

5. Renzi D, Pellegrini B, Tonelli F, Surrenti C, Calabrò A. Substance P (neurokinin-1) and neurokinin A (neurokinin-2) receptor gene and protein expression in the healthy and inflamed human intestine. Am J Pathol. 2000;157:1511–22.

6. Goode T, O'Connell J, Sternini C et al. Substance P (neurokinin-1) receptor is a marker of human mucosal but not peripheral mononulear cells: molecular quantitation and localization. J Immunol. 1998;161:2232–40.

7. Hood VC, Cruwys SC, Urban L, Kidd BL. Differential role of neurokinin receptors in human lymphocyte and monocyte chemotaxis. Regul Peptides. 2000;96:17–21.

8. Ho W-Z, Stavropoulos G, Lai J-P et al. Substance P C-terminal octapeptide analogues augment tumor necrosis factor-α release by human blood monocytes and macrophages. J Neuroimmunol. 1998;82:126–32.

9. Riegler M, Castagliuolo I, So PTC et al. Effects of substance P on human colonic mucosa in vitro. Am J Physiol. 1999;276:G1473–83.

10. Santos J, Saperas E, Nogueiras C et al. Release of mast cell mediators into the jejunum by cold pain stress in humans. Gastroenterology. 1998;114:640–8.

11. Nakajima S, Krishnan B, Ota H et al. Mast cell involvement in gastritis with or without Helicobacter pylori infection. Gastroenterology. 1997;113:746–54.

12. Raithel M, Winterkamp S, Pacurar A, Ulrich P, Hochberger J, Hahn EG. Release of mast cell tryptase from human colorectal mucosa in inflammatory bowel disease. Scand J Gastroenterol. 2001;36:174–9.

13. Coelho A-M, Vergnolle N, Guiard B, Fioramonti J, Bueno L. Proteinases and proteinase-activated receptor 2: a possible role to promote visceral hyperalgesia in rats. Gastroenterology. 2002; 122:1035–47.

14. Vergnolle N, Bunnett NW, Sharkey KA et al. Proteinase-activated receptor-2 and hyperalgesia: a novel pain pathway. Nature Med. 2001;7:821–6.

15. di Mola FF, Friess H, Zhu ZW et al. Nerve growth factor and Trk high affinity receptor (TrkA) gene expression in inflammatory bowel disease. Gut. 2000;46:670–9.

16. Bielefeldt K, Ozaki N, Gebhart GF. Nerve growth factor and sensitization of gastric afferent neurons. Digestion. 2001;63:267.

17. Bennett DLH, Dmietrieva N, Priestley JV, Clary D, McMahon SB. trkA, CGRP and IB4 expression in retrogradely labelled cutaneous and visceral primary sensory neurones in the rat. Neurosci Lett. 1996;206:33–6.

18. Huang FL, Zhuo H, Sinclair C, Goldstein ME, McCabe JT, Helke CJ. Peripheral deafferentation alters calcitonin gene-related peptide mRNA expression in visceral sensory neurons of the nodose and petrosal ganglia. Brain Res Mol Brain Res. 1994;22:290–8.

19. Tonra JR, Mendell LM. Effects of postnatal anti-NGF on the development of CGRP-IR neurons in the dorsal root ganglion. J Comp Neurol. 1998;392:489–98.

20. Nilsson G, Forsberg-Nilsson K, Xiang Z, Hallbook F, Nilsson K, Metcalfe DD. Human mast cells express functional TrkA and are a source of nerve growth factor. Eur J Immunol. 1997;27:2295–301.

21. Xiang Z, Nilsson G. IgE receptor-mediated release of nerve growth factor by mast cells. Clin Exp Allergy. 2000;30:1379–86.

22. Heiman AS, Newton L. Effect of hydrocortisone and disodium cromoglycate on mast cell-mediator release induced by substance P. Pharmacology. 1995;50:218–28.

23. Turner MW, Boulton P, Strobel S. Experimental intestinal hypersensitivity. Effect of four anti-allergic drugs on protein uptake, permeability to sugars and mucosal mast-cell activation. Clin Exp Allergy. 1995;25:448–55.

24. Krishna MT, Chauhan A, Little L et al. Inhibition of mast cell tryptase by inhaled APC 366 attenuates allergen-induced late-phase airway obstruction in asthma. J Allergy Clin Immunol. 2001;107:1039–45.

25. Di Sebastiano P, Grossi L, Di Mola FF et al. SR140333, a substance P receptor antagonist, influences morphological and motor changes in rat experimental colitis. Dig Dis Sci. 1999;44:439–44.

26. Grady EF, Yoshimi SK, Maa J et al. Substance P mediates inflammatory oedema in acute pancreatitis via activation of the neurokinin-1 receptor in rats and mice. Br J Pharmacol. 2000;130:505–12.

27. Traub RJ. The spinal contribution of substance P to the generation and maintenance of inflammatory hyperalgesia in the rat. Pain. 1996;67:151–61.
28. Owolabi JB, Rizkalla G, Tehim A *et al.* Characterization of antiallodynic actions of ALE-0540, a novel nerve growth factor receptor antagonist, in the rat. J Pharmacol Exp Ther. 1999;289:1271–6.
29. Reinshagen M, Rohm H, Steinkamp M *et al.* Protective role of neurotrophins in experimental inflammation of the rat gut. Gastroenterology. 2000;119:368–76.
30. Micera A, Vigneti E, Pickholtz D *et al.* Nerve growth factor displays stimulatory effects on human skin and lung fibroblasts, demonstrating a direct role for this factor in tissue repair. Proc Natl Acad Sci USA. 2001;98:6162–7.
31. Matsuda H, Koyama H, Sato H *et al.* Role of nerve growth factor in cutaneous wound healing: accelerating effects in normal and healing-impaired diabetic mice. J Exp Med. 1998;187:297–306.
32. Bergmann I, Reiter R, Toyka KV, Koltzenburg M. Nerve growth factor evokes hyperalgesia in mice lacking the low-affinity neurotrophin receptor p75. Neurosci Lett. 1998;255:87–90.
33. Koltzenburg M, Bennett DL, Shelton DL, McMahon SB. Neutralization of endogenous NGF prevents the sensitization of nociceptors supplying inflamed skin. Eur J Neurosci. 1999;11:1698–704.
34. Lewin GR, Ritter AM, Mendell LM. Nerve growth factor-induced hyperalgesia in the neonatal and adult rat. J Neurosci. 1993;13:2136–48.
35. Chen X, Levine JD. Hyper-responsivity in a subset of C-fiber nociceptors in a model of painful diabetic neuropathy in the rat. Neuroscience. 2001;102:185–92.

Section VI
What function is disturbed in functional gastrointestinal disorders and why?

19
Visceral hypersensitivity in functional gastrointestinal disorders

J. TACK

INTRODUCTION

Functional gastrointestinal disorders are characterized by episodes of gastrointestinal symptoms, in the absence of organic disease that readily explains them. The pathophysiology of functional gastrointestinal disorders is not established. Functional symptoms have been suggested to originate from abnormalities in gastrointestinal motor control or from abnormalities at the level of the central nervous system. More recently, visceral hypersensivity was put forward as a mechanism underlying functional bowel disorders[1]. Studies have demonstrated the presence of exaggerated sensitivity to balloon distension in patients with non-cardiac chest pain, functional dyspepsia and irritable bowel syndrome.

VISCERAL HYPERSENSITIVITY IN NON-CARDIAC CHEST PAIN

Patients with non-cardiac chest pain have significantly higher pain sensation scores during intra-oesophageal balloon distension than healthy control sujects[2]. This abnormal sensory perception appears to be independent of oesophageal contractions or oesophageal wall tone. Studies by de Caestecker *et al.* suggest that a stretch receptor, linked to the longitudinal muscle of the oesophageal wall, is mediating the sensory response, as edrophonium is increasing and atropine is reducing the sensitivity to balloon distension[3].

Drugs which interfere with pain perception may well be indicated in these patients. Tricyclic antidepressants were shown to decrease oesophageal sensitivity in humans[4,5]. Imipramine, a tricyclic antidepressant helpful in the management of patients with chronic pain syndromes, was evaluated in the treatment of patients with chest pain and normal coronary angiograms[6]. Imipramine reduced by approximately 50% the number of chest pain episodes, and it also reduced the sensitivity to cardiac pain during electrical stimulation. Oesophageal motility testing did not identify patients who were likely to respond to imipramine.

VISCERAL HYPERSENSITIVITY IN FUNCTIONAL DYSPEPSIA

Gastric barostat studies have confirmed that, as a group, patients with functional dyspepsia (FD) have lower thresholds for first perception and for discomfort or pain during balloon distension of the proximal stomach[7,8]. Hypersensitivity to gastric distension, defined as perception or discomfort thresholds outside the normal range, is found in a subset of patients with FD, but not in patients with organic causes of dyspepsia[9]. Furthermore, it does not exclusively exist in patients with FD, but also exists in dyspeptic subjects who are not health-care seekers, implying that the visceral hyperalgesia is not solely an expression of referral bias or personality factors[10]. However, different studies used different approaches to calculate sensitivity to distension and to determine the range of normality[7-10]. In a large study comparing sensitivity to gastric distension in healthy controls and in FD patients, we established that the increase of intra-balloon pressure over intra-abdominal pressure needed to induce discomfort or pain is the most appropriate expression of sensitivity to gastric distension as it yields a meaningful lower range of normal and it is independent from age and body mass index[11].

Using the mean $- 2\,\text{SD}$ from healthy control studies to define the range of normality, we found hypersensitivity to gastric distension in 34% of the patients, who did not differ from the other patients in demographic or other pathophysiological characteristics. In a study in 160 patients, hypersensitivity to distension was associated with a higher prevalence of postprandial pain, belching and weight loss[11]. Other groups, studying smaller groups of patients, found no association between the presence of hypersensitivity and symptom pattern in FD (Table 1)[9,13,14].

The use of intragastric barostat balloons has limited the number of studies investigating visceral sensitivity in FD. Attempts have been made to replace balloon distension with distension during a rapid or slow drinking test. Although patients with FD had impaired drinking capacity compared to controls, no correlation with thresholds to balloon distension was found[15,16].

Whether hypersensitivity to balloon distension in FD is limited to the stomach has been a matter of debate. While some groups observed hypersensitivity to duodenal distension[17], others failed to make the same observation[18].

Table 1 Association between hypersensitivity and symptom pattern in FD

Study	No.	Correlation
Tack et al., 2001[12]	160	Associated with pain, belching, weight loss
Mertz et al., 1998[9]	24	No correlation
Rehe et al., 2001	64	No correlation
Boeckxstaens et al., 2002[13]	44	No correlation

The contribution of enhanced chemosensitivity is also unclear. Recently, hypersensitivity of the duodenal bulb to acid infusion was suggested to play a role, as this induced nausea in a subset of FD patients[19]. A more recent study, however, which assessed spontaneous duodenal acid exposure in FD, failed to confirm this concept[20]. A high proportion of patients with FD demonstrate increased gastroduodenal sensitivity to meals of high energy or lipid content, not clearly associated with an altered gastric emptying[21]. In addition, duodenal infusion of lipids, but not glucose, sensitizes the stomach to distension in patients with FD in contrast to controls[22,23]. The response was shown to involve lipid digestion and activation of CCK-A receptors and 5-HT$_3$ receptors[24-26]. If confirmed with orally ingested meals, duodenal hypersensitivity to acid could play an important role in postprandial aggravation of symptoms in FD.

Perception of gastric distension requires the activation of mechanoreceptors, and studies in healthy volunteers have suggested involvement of in-series mechanoreceptors that respond to increases in tension within the stomach wall[27,28]. It has not been shown that perception or symptoms in patients with hypersensitivity to gastric distension are related to activation of tension-sensitive mechanoreceptors. Animal studies have shown that activation of in-series mechanoreceptors occurs during distension and during contraction against a resistance; they are inactivated during relaxation[29].

Using subthreshold isovolumetric distension of the proximal stomach, and using a symptom perception marker, we were able to establish that FD patients with visceral hypersensitivity perceive isovolumetric phasic contractions of the proximal stomach. These findings provide evidence that tension receptors in the proximal stomach mediate dyspeptic symptoms in hypersensitive FD[30].

The mechanism behind the gastric hypersensitivity in FD is not altogether clear, but an abnormal afferent sensory pathway has been proposed[18]. There are also contradictory results regarding the role of *Helicobacter pylori* for gastric sensitivity to distension[31,32], but large-scale studies failed to establish a role for *H. pylori* infection in gastric hypersensitivity[12,33]. As visceral hypersensitivity is also a feature of the irritable bowel syndrome (IBS), we investigated whether overlap between IBS and FD was explaining gastric hypersensitivity. Although patients with FD and coexisting IBS had a slightly higher prevalence of visceral hypersensitivity, IBS co-morbidity did not determine the presence of gastric hypersensitivity[34]. It is often suggested that post-infectious functional bowel disorders depend on post-inflammatory visceral hypersensitivity. However, in a subgroup with post-infectious FD, we did not find an increased prevalence of hypersensitivity to gastric distension[35].

A factor analysis revealed that hypersenstiivtiy to gastric distension was associated with a high prevalence of psychosocial disturbances, such as somatization, neuroticism, childhood abuse and low quality of life[36]. This was mainly the case for patients with symptoms of postprandial pain.

We used positron emission tomography (PET) to investigate cerebral patterns of activation during proximal gastric distension in healthy volunteers. Progressive distension of the stomach induced activation of the right gyrus frontalis inferior, and of both the lateral (left gyrus postcentralis or primary somatosensory cortex) and the medial pain system (left gyrus cingularis anterior, ACG). The same study was also performed in age- and sex-matched FD patients with established gastric hypersensitivity. In this group gastric distension induced a similar activation of the lateral pain system, but at significantly lower distending pressures. We did not find any activation of the left ACG in these patients[37]. The similar activation of the somatosensory cortex at lower distension levels seems to confirm the hypersensitivity status of these patients. The findings are compatible with central mechanisms of hypersensitivity (increased activation during normal afferent input) or with a failing antinociceptive system.

In order to obtain a better understanding of the neurophysiology of gastric hypersensitivity, we analysed the intensity of painful and non-painful symptoms during progressive gastric balloon distensions in FD patients with and without hypersensitivity. The results suggested that hypersensitivity in FD was not characterized by an up-regulation of specific 'high-threshold' pathways mediating the perception of pain, but rather by an up-regulation of non-specific 'low-threshold' pathways, which also generate non-painful symptoms such as nausea or fullness[38].

Drugs specifically aimed at improving hypersensitivity to gastric distension are lacking. There is some evidence that tricyclic antidepressants are effective in FD[39,40], and the mechanism behind the positive effect has been proposed to be due to an effect on gastric sensitivity. However, this could not be confirmed in a small-scale study by Mertz and co-workers[40]. The kappa opioid agonist, fedotozine, decreases gastric sensitivity to distensions[41] and in a placebo-controlled study in functional dyspeptics it showed superiority over placebo[42]. However, development of this drug has not continued. Psychological treatments have been reported to provide benefit in FD[43–46]. Given the association of hypersensitivity with psychosocial disturbances, it is conceivable that this subgroup is most likely to respond, but studies evaluating this hypothesis are still lacking.

If tension-sensitive mechanoreceptors are involved in symptom generation in dyspeptic patients with hypersensitivity to gastric distension, then inducing gastric relaxation might provide an approach to relieve symptoms. Preliminary studies with sumatriptan and clonidine in patients with visceral hypersensitivity seem to support this concept[30].

VISCERAL HYPERSENSITIVITY IN IBS

Several studies have now established that a variable subset of IBS patients have hypersensitivity to rectal or colonic balloon distension[47–52]. Recent studies suggested that hypersensitivity to rectal balloon distension is a marker for IBS, with good sensitivity and specificity[51,52]. However, across studies the prevalence of rectal hypersensitivity in IBS varies from 20% to 80%. Furthermore, hypersensitivity may be demonstrable only in response to repetitive stimuli rather than single stimuli[53]. The correlation between rectal sensory thresholds and symptoms is poor in most studies. One study reported a correlation with urge to defaecate[54].

The mechanoreceptors involved in hypersensitivity to distension in IBS have not been determined, but in healthy volunteers tension receptors mediate sensitivity to colonic distension[55].

Sensitivity testing is based on balloon distension, inducing conscious perception and reporting for stimulus intensity. Both perception of the stimulus (true hypersensitivity) as the reporting phase (attentional bias) may lead to hypersensitivity reporting. The pathogenic mechanism underlying hypersensitivity in IBS has not been determined, but evidence in favour of both peripheral or central mechanisms can be found in the literature. In favour of a peripheral mechanism are the presence of normal somatic pain thresholds[56] and the absence of correlation with anxiety, depression or sexual trauma[57]. In favour of central mechanisms are the observation that hypersensitivity patients rate sham distension higher, and that thresholds are correlated with attention to gastrointestinal sensations. A factor analysis confirmed the involvement of both types of mechanism[58].

The implications for treatment are unclear. In IBS, symptomatic responses to amitryptiline, but not to psychotherapeutic treatment, were associated with increased thresholds for pain during rectal distension[59].

References

1. Mayer EA, Gebhart FG. Basic and clinical aspects of visceral hyperalgesia. Gastroenterology. 1994;107:271–93.
2. Richter JE, Barish CF, Castell DO. Abnormal sensory perception in patients with esophageal chest pain. Gastroenterology. 1986;91:845–52.
3. De Caestecker JS *et al*. Site and mechanism of pain perception with esophageal balloon distension and intravenous edrophonium in patients with esophageal chest pain. Gut. 1992;33:580.
4. Pegini PL, Katz PO, Castell DO. Imipramine decreases oesophageal pain perception in human male volunteers. Gut. 1998;42:807–13.
5. Clouse RE, Lustman PJ, Eckert TC, Ferney DM, Griffith LS. Low dose trazodone for symptomatic patients with esophageal contraction abnormalities. Gastroenterology. 1987;92:1027–36.
6. Cannon RO, Quyyumi AA, Mincemoyer R *et al*. Imipramine in patients with chest pain despite normal coronary angiograms. N Engl J Med. 1994;19:1411–17.
7. Bradette M, Pare P, Douville P, Morin A. Visceral perception in health and functional dyspepsia. Crossover study of gastric distensions with placebo and domperidone. Dig Dis Sci. 1991;36:52–8.
8. Mearin F, Cucala M, Azpiroz F, Malagelada JR. The origin of symptoms on the brain–gut axis in functional dyspepsia. Gastroenterology. 1991;101:999–1006.
9. Mertz H, Fullerton S, Naliboff B, Mayer EA. Symptoms and visceral perception in severe functional and organic dyspepsia. Gut. 1998;42:814–22.
10. Holtmann G, Gschossmann J, Neufang-Huber J, Gerken G, Talley NJ. Differences in gastric mechanosensory function after repeated ramp distensions in non-consulters with dyspepsia and healthy controls. Gut. 2000;47:332–6.
11. Tack J, Coulie B, Wilmer A, Andrioli A, Janssens J. Influence of sumatriptan on gastric fundus tone and on the perception of gastric distension in man. Gut. 2000;46:468–73.
12. Tack J, Caenepeel P, Fischler B, Piessevaux H, Janssens J. Symptoms associated with hypersensitivity to gastric distention in functional dyspepsia. Gastroenterology. 2001;121:526–35.
13. Boeckxstaens GE, Hirsch DP, Kuiken SD, Heisterkamp SH, Tytgat GN. The proximal stomach and postprandial symptoms in functional dyspeptics. Am J Gastroenterol. 2002;97:40–8.
14. Rhee PL, Kim YH, Sung IK *et al*. Evaluation of individual symptoms cannot predict presence of gastric hypersensitivity in functional dyspepsia. Dig Dis Sci. 2000;45:1680–4.
15. Tack J, Caenepeel P, Piessevaux H, Cuomo R, Janssens J. Assessment of meal-induced gastric accommodation by a satiety drinking test in health and in severe functional dyspepsia. Gut. 2003 (In press).
16. Boeckxstaens GE, Hirsch DP, Van Den Elzen BD, Heisterkamp SH, Tytgat GN. Impaired drinking capacity in patients with functional dyspepsia: relationship with proximal stomach function. Gastroenterology. 2001;121:1054–63.
17. Holtmann G, Goebell H, Jockenhoevel F, Talley NJ. Altered vagal and intestinal mechanosensory function in chronic unexplained dyspepsia. Gut. 1998;42:501–6.
18. Mearin F, Cucala M, Azpiroz F, Malagelada JR. The origin of symptoms on the brain–gut axis in functional dyspepsia. Gastroenterology. 1991;101:999–1006.

19. Samsom M, Verhagen MA, vanBerge Henegouwen GP, Smout AJ. Abnormal clearance of exogenous acid and increased acid sensitivity of the proximal duodenum in dyspeptic patients. Gastroenterology. 1999;116:515–20.

20. Lee KJ, Demarchi B, Vos R, Demedts I, Janssens J, Tack J. Comparison of duodenal acid exposure in functional dyspepsia patients and healthy controls using 24-hour ambulatory duodenal pH monitoring. Gastroenterology. 2002;122:A102.

21. Houghton LA, Mangall YF, Dwivedi A, Read NW. Sensitivity to nutrients in patients with non-ulcer dyspepsia. Eur J Gastroenterol Hepatol. 1993;5:109–113.

22. Barbera R, Feinle C, Read NW. Nutrient-specific modulation of gastric mechanosensitivity in patients with functional dyspepsia. Dig Dis Sci. 1995;40:1636–41.

23. Barbera R, Feinle C, Read NW. Abnormal sensitivity to duodenal lipid infusion in patients with functional dyspepsia. Eur J Gastroenterol Hepatol. 1995;7:1051–7.

24. Feinle C, Read NW. Ondansetron reduces nausea induced by gastroduodenal stimulation without changing gastric motility. Am J Physiol. 1996;271:G591–7.

25. Feinle C, Meier O, Otto B, D'Amato M, Fried M. Role of duodenal lipid and cholecystokinin A receptors in the pathophysiology of functional dyspepsia. Gut. 2001;48:347–55.

26. Feinle C, Rades T, Otto B, Fried M. Fat digestion modulates gastrointestinal sensations induced by gastric distention and duodenal lipid in humans. Gastroenterology. 2001;120:1100–7.

27. Distrutti E, Azpiroz F, Soldevilla A, Malagelada JR. Gastric wall tension determines perception of gastric distention. Gastroenterology. 1999;116:1035–42.

28. Piessevaux H, Tack J, Wilmer A, Coulie B, Geubel A, Janssens J. Perception of changes in wall tension of the proximal stomach in humans. Gut. 2001;49:203–8.

29. Blackshaw LA, Grundy D, Scratcherd T. Vagal afferent discharge from gastric mechanoreceptors during contraction and relaxation of the ferret corpus. J Auton Nerv Syst. 1987;18:19–24.

30. Tack J, Vos R, Caenepeel P, Degreef T, Piessevaux H, Janssens J. Fundic tension receptors mediate perception in functional dyspepsia patients with hypersensitivity to gastric distensions. Gastroenterology. 2001;120:A1244.

31. Holtmann G, Talley NJ, Goebell H. Association between *H. pylori*, duodenal mechanosensory thresholds, and small intestinal motility in chronic unexplained dyspepsia. Dig Dis Sci. 1996;41: 1285–91.

32. Thumshirn M, Camilleri M, Saslow SB, Williams DE, Burton DD, Hanson RB. Gastric accommodation in non-ulcer dyspepsia and the roles of *Helicobacter pylori* infection and vagal function. Gut. 1999;44:55–64.

33. Mearin F, de Ribot X, Balboa A *et al*. Does *Helicobacter pylori* infection increase gastric sensitivity in functional dyspepsia? Gut. 1995;37:47–51.

34. Corsetti M, Caenepeel P, Fischler B, Janssens J, Tack J. Impact of co-existing irritable bowel syndrome on symptoms and pathophysiological mechanisms in functional dyspepsia. (Submitted for publication.)

35. Tack J, Demedts I, Dehondt G *et al*. Clinical and pathophysiological characteristics of acute-onset functional dyspepsia. Gastroenterology. 2002;122:1738–47.

36. Fischler B, Tack J, De Gucht V *et al*. Heterogeneity of symptom pattern, psychosocial and pathophysiological mechanisms in severe functional dyspepsia. Gastroenterology. 2003;124:903–10.

37. Vandenberghe J, Vos R, Janssens J, Tack J. Visceral hyperalgesia in functional dyspepsia: pain-specific or multimodal afferent pathways? Gastroenterology. 2002;122:302 (abstract).

38. Vandenberghe J, Tack J, Dupont P *et al*. The cortical processing of distention of the proximal stomach in man: a PET study. Gastroenterology. 2002;122: M1485 (abstract).

39. Clouse RE. Antidepressants for functional gastrointestinal syndromes. Dig Dis Sci. 1994; 39:2352–63.

40. Mertz H, Fass R, Kodner A, Yan-Go F, Fullerton S, Mayer EA. Effect of amitriptyline on symptoms, sleep, and visceral perception in patients with functional dyspepsia. Am J Gastroenterol. 1998;93:160–5.

41. Coffin B, Bouhassira D, Chollet R *et al*. Effect of the kappa agonist fedotozine on perception of gastric distension in healthy humans. Aliment Pharmacol Ther. 1996;10:919–25.

42. Read NW, Abitbol JL, Bardhan KD, Whorwell PJ, Fraitag B. Efficacy and safety of the peripheral kappa agonist fedotozine versus placebo in the treatment of functional dyspepsia. Gut. 1997;41:664–8.

43. Calvert EL, Houghton LA, Cooper P, Whorwell P. Hypnotherapy is effective in the long-term treatment of functional dyspepsia. Gastroenterology. 2001;120:618.

44. Gonsalkorale WM, Houghton LA, Whorwell PJ. Hypnotherapy in irritable bowel syndrome: a large-scale audit of a clinical service with examination of factors influencing responsiveness. Am J Gastroenterol. 2002;97:954–61.
45. Hamilton J, Guthrie E, Creed F *et al*. A randomized controlled trial of psychotherapy in patients with chronic functional dyspepsia. Gastroenterology. 2000;119:661–9.
46. Haug TT, Wilhelmsen I, Svebak S, Berstad A, Ursin H. Psychotherapy in functional dyspepsia. J Psychosom Res. 1994;38:735–44.
47. Ritchie J. Pain from distension of the pelvic colon by inflating a balloon in the irritable colon syndrome. Gut. 1973;14:125–32.
48. Prior A, Maxton DG, Whorwell PJ. Anorectal manometry in irritable bowel syndrome: differences between diarrhoea and constipation predominant subjects. Gut. 1990;31:458–62.
49. Bradette M, Delvaux M, Staumont G, Fioramonti J, Bueno L, Frexinos J. Evaluation of colonic sensory thresholds in IBS patients using a barostat. Dig Dis Sci. 1994;39:449–57.
50. Whitehead WE, Holtkotter B, Enck P *et al*. Tolerance for rectosigmoid distention in irritable bowel syndrome. Gastroenterology. 1990;98:1187–92.
51. Mertz H, Naliboff B, Munakata J, Niazi N, Mayer EA. Altered rectal perception is a biological marker of patients with irritable bowel syndrome. Gastroenterology. 1995;109:40–52.
52. Bouin M, Plourde V, Boivin M *et al*. Rectal distention testing in patients with irritable bowel syndrome: sensitivity, specificity and predictive values of pain sensory thresholds. Gastroenterology. 2002;122:1771–7.
53. Munakata J, Naliboff B, Harraf F *et al*. Repetitive sigmoid stimulation induces rectal hyperalgesia in patients with irritable bowel syndrome. Gastroenterology. 1997;112:55–63.
54. Steens J, Van Der Schaar PJ, Penning C, Brussee J, Masclee AA. Compliance, tone and sensitivity of the rectum in different subtypes of irritable bowel syndrome. Neurogastroenterol Motil. 2002;14:241–7.
55. Corsetti M, Gevers AM, Caenepeel P, Tack J. The role of tension receptors in colonic mechanosensitivity. (Submitted for publication.)
56. Accarino AM, Azpiroz F, Malagelada JR. Selective dysfunction of mechanosensitive intestinal afferents in irritable bowel syndrome. Gastroenterology. 1995;108:636–43.
57. Whitehead WE, Palsson OS. Is rectal pain sensitivity a biological marker for irritable bowel syndrome? Psychological influences on pain perception. Gastroenterology. 1998;115:1263–71.
58. Naliboff BD, Munakata J, Fullerton S *et al*. Evidence for two distinct perceptual alterations in irritable bowel syndrome. Gut. 1997;41:505–12.
59. Poitras P, Riberdy Poitras M, Plourde V, Boivin M, Verrier P. Evolution of visceral sensitivity in patients with irritable bowel syndrome. Dig Dis Sci. 2001;46:2542–8.

20
Motor function and dysfunction in functional dyspepsia and irritable bowel syndrome

V. STANGHELLINI, R. COGLIANDRO, G. BARBARA,
R. de GIORGIO, L. COGLIANDRO and R. CORINALDESI

INTRODUCTION

Gastrointestinal motility is a complex function characterized by myoelectrical smooth muscle activity, gut wall movements, intraluminal phasic and tonic pressure changes, and movement of intraluminal contents. No single technique is available to simultaneously measure all the above-mentioned motor events and we still have only limited information both in health and disease.

Functional digestive syndromes are characterized by multifactorial pathogenetic mechanisms. Among these abnormal motor patterns of the alimentary canal have long been considered with variable success. After a decade in oblivion their potential pathogenetic role is currently regaining momentum. More specifically, the complex interplay among smooth muscle cells, mechanoreceptors, neural reflexes and afferent pathways is currently attracting the interest of investigators.

Gastrointestinal motor abnormalities found in functional dyspepsia are rather aspecific and restricted to subsets of patients with different symptom manifestations. Delayed gastric emptying and over-distended gastric antrum are found in patients primarily complaining of fullness, nausea and vomiting, while inability of the gastric fundus to adapt to meal ingestion is more frequently found in patients complaining of early satiety. Meta-analysis studies confirm the efficacy of prokinetic drugs in dyspeptic patients, but the studies involved were often of questionable quality and difficult to interpret.

In irritable bowel syndrome (IBS) patients, altered motor patterns have been detected throughout the gastrointestinal tract, including the oesophagus, stomach, and biliary tract, but interest has traditionally been focused on colonic and small intestinal motility. It has been reported that the colon of patients with diarrhoea-predominant and constipation-predominant IBS shows respectively more and less propagated contractions, as well as accelerated and delayed intestinal transit time. In the small bowel of IBS patients characteristic, although aspecific, motor abnormalities have been detected, some of which are coincident to perception of abdominal pain. Consistent evidence also suggests that IBS patients display exaggerated intestinal motor responses to environmental or intraluminal stimuli. Mild inflammation as well as intraluminal contents may interfere with neuromuscular functions in the gut and contribute to symptom perception.

The clinical relevance of gastrointestinal motor abnormalities remains to be established, but it is likely that abnormalities of neuro–muscle interactions will be recognized as being of pivotal relevance in the determination of digestive functional syndromes.

MOTOR FUNCTION AND DYSFUNCTION IN FUNCTIONAL DYSPEPSIA

Gastrointestinal manometric abnormalities are invariably found in patients with very severe functional digestive syndromes such as chronic idiopathic intestinal pseudo-obstruction[1]. In less severe syndromes such as functional dyspepsia, interdigestive and/or postprandial antral hypomotility has been reported in up to 50% of dyspeptic patients[2–5]. Sporadic abnormalities have also been observed in the proximal small bowel, but usually only in patients with secondary dyspepsia[2] or in patients with overlapping IBS[3]. No correlation has been found between symptoms and manometric findings in functional dyspepsia[3,6].

The majority of studies investigating motility disorders in dyspepsia have focused on gastric emptying and this parameter has been found to be on average abnormal whenever appropriate inclusion criteria and techniques were adopted. Specifically, delayed gastric emptying of digestible solids has been found in 30–80% of these patients, while lower frequencies have generally been reported of delayed liquid emptying[7]. Technical differences, and different inclusion criteria, may account for the wide range of results obtained, and may make comparisons difficult. Delayed gastric emptying has been observed using radiographic[8], ultrasonographic[9], electrogastrographic[10] and breath test[11] techniques. Nevertheless, the majority of studies have applied scintigraphy, which is considered the gold standard technique for indirectly measuring this motor pattern. Interpretation of studies evaluating the relationship between dyspeptic symptoms and gastric emptying times is made difficult not only by the small numbers of patients included[12–17], but also by the different inclusion criteria adopted. Studies carried out on patients presenting with pain (with or without other associated dyspeptic symptoms) showed no difference, compared to healthy controls when either the whole group of patients[16], or only male patients were considered[13]. In contrast, studies including patients with symptoms of gastroparesis consistently found a delayed gastric emptying[15,17–20]. In the largest studies carried out so far, including appropriate control groups, gastric emptying of digestible solids resulted delayed in 24–34% of patients[18–20].

Table 1 summarizes the main results and characteristics of the studies which have investigated the relationship between gastric emptying of solids and dyspeptic symptoms in functional dyspepsia. The studies which failed to identify a relationship have a number of potential pitfalls: limited number of patients

Table 1 Studies investigating correlations between gastric emptying of solids and symptoms in functional dyspepsia

References	Percentage delayed gastric emptying[*]	Related symptoms
Jain *et al.*, 1989[12]	30 (28)	Prolonged digestion higher in gastroparesis
Talley *et al.*, 1989[13]	Only females[†] (32)	No relationship
Waldron *et al.*, 1991[14]	42 (50)	No relationship
Tucci *et al.*, 1992[15]	40 (45)	Postprandial fullness higher in gastroparesis
Scott *et al.*, 1993[16]	11 (75)	No relationship
Caballero-Plasencia *et al.*, 1995[17]	78 (50)	No relationship
Stanghellini *et al.*, 1996[18]	34 (348)	Relevant fullness, vomiting
Stanghellini *et al.*, 1999[19]	32 (483)	Predominant discomfort
Talley *et al.*, 2001[20]	24 (551)	No relationship

* Figures in parentheses indicate no. of patients.
† Percentage unknown.

evaluated (with the consequent risk of type 2 errors); inclusion of patients with secondary dyspepsia, definitions of dyspepsia focused on the presence of pain or, on the contrary, inclusion restricted to patients with symptoms suggestive of gastroparesis; inadequate gastric emptying techniques, and absence of quantitative analysis of symptoms[18]. A relationship between delayed gastric emptying and symptoms could not be demonstrated in the studies evaluating only subpopulations of patients characterized by dominant epigastric pain, probably because in these patients gastric emptying is similar to that of asymptomatic control subjects[15]. Such a relationship could also not be detected when individual symptoms were neglected and analysis was carried out on global symptom scores including different, and perhaps opposite, symptoms. Similarly, studies simply analysing the presence/absence of symptoms, or of clusters of symptoms, are inadequate, since the mere perception of digestive symptoms is extremely frequent in the general population and probably of limited value. Finally, the negative results of these studies could be influenced by the use of a low-calorie test meal, and/or inclusion of secondary forms of dyspepsia, or of symptoms suggestive of digestive syndromes other than dyspepsia. Among all the large studies carried out so far only Talley and colleagues failed to identify a correlation between delayed gastric emptying of solids and non-painful symptoms[20]. However, this was a multinational therapeutic trial which involved many centres without a specific interest in the field and symptom evaluation may require some training[21].

Nevertheless, measurement of gastric emptying only provides a broad and indirect indication of the complex series of motor events necessary to empty the stomach of its contents. An abnormal distribution of intragastric contents seems to occur in some patients with functional dyspepsia, characterized by rapid emptying from the proximal stomach and a sudden yet prolonged distension of the antrum[22,23]. Another study carried out in patients with dysmotility-like symptoms supported the existence of an abnormally elevated proximal gastric tone after meal ingestion, similar to what has been described after truncal vagotomy[24]. Impaired postprandial gastric relaxation is specifically associated with moderate/severe early satiety and weight loss[25] and it is likely that disorders of gastric wall tension could contribute to the pathogenesis of some dyspeptic symptoms when no gross motor abnormality is detected.

The relationship between gastrointestinal motor disorders and dyspeptic symptoms remains controversial. Dyspeptic patients often have normal gastrointestinal motility and, vice-versa, occasionally digestive motor abnormalities occur in asymptomatic individuals[26]. However, it is well known that even major pathological conditions such as myocardial infarction can be asymptomatic, but nobody would argue that ischaemia of heart muscle cells contributes to perception of chest pain. If altered motility *per se* were the direct cause of dyspepsia, a temporal relationship would be expected with perception of symptoms. Data on this aspect remain scanty, but some studies suggest that such a relationship might exist: (a) a close relationship was observed between the onset of tachygastria and of dyspeptic symptoms in 15 healthy subjects exposed to a nauseating stimulus (illusory self-motion)[27]; (b) the progressive delay in gastric emptying induced by infusion of increasing doses of carbohydrates in the terminal ileum of healthy subjects was accompanied by the onset of increasingly more frequent dyspeptic symptoms, such as nausea and vomiting[28]; (c) in healthy controls, postprandial fullness was found to be directly related to gastric emptying times of the aqueous phase (more full when gastric emptying was slower) and postprandial hunger was inversely related to gastric emptying rates of oil (less hungry when more oil was emptied into the small bowel)[29]; (d) although marked inflation of an intragastric rubber balloon induces pain at lower pressure levels, it promptly generates a rather monotonous and reproducible response characterized by sensations that are suggestive of gastric motor derangement such as epigastric fullness and pressure[30].

A number of reasons explain the apparent inability of investigators to clarify this important aspect of the genesis of dyspeptic symptoms: (a) symptoms are difficult to investigate in appropriate studies due to their high daily variability[31]; (b) evaluation of simulated cases of dyspepsia by 27 general practitioners from the UK showed an overall agreement for each of the symptom complexes evaluated, but the accuracy and consistency of assessment varied considerably among doctors for individual symptoms[33]; (c) training is needed to improve the reproducibility of symptom evaluation by doctors[21]; (d) techniques available for measuring gastrointestinal motility are sub-optimal and none of them can simultaneously measure all motor patterns potentially associated with perception of symptoms; (e) wall movements of the small intestine or colon may give rise to the same symptoms as distension of the stomach[33,34]; (f) some symptoms in IBS, such as upper abdominal pain related to meals, are similar to those occurring in dyspepsia[35]; (g) there is a considerable overlap between nerve projections from organs of the upper and lower gut.

MOTOR FUNCTION AND DYSFUNCTION IN IBS

IBS is a functional gastrointestinal disease characterized by symptoms that are strongly suggestive of an underlying digestive motor disorder such as disturbed defaecation, abdominal pain or abdominal distension[36]. Despite the benign nature of the syndrome it causes significant distress in affected individuals, with relevant deterioration of their quality of life. It is the most common disease seen by gastroenterologists, although only 10–30% of affected individuals actually seek medical help[36]. Women are four times as likely as men to present to their doctors in industrialized countries[37], but not in other areas of the world[38]. Both severity of symptoms and psychosocial aspects probably determine health-care utilization.

The pathophysiology of IBS is extremely complex and yet largely unknown. Beyond gut dysmotility, altered visceral perception and psychological disturbances are probably involved. Evidence suggests that there is a critical interplay among these mechanisms, each one affecting the outcome of the others. Part of the most recent research focuses on the identification of putative factors implicated in the altered sensory and motor function observed in IBS. Studies are now evaluating the role of enteric flora, gastrointestinal infections, offending foods and mucosal inflammation in the pathophysiology of IBS. These fields of investigation hopefully will improve our understanding of the mechanisms underlying symptom generation and, ultimately, the management of affected individuals. Compared to functional dyspepsia, understanding of motor disturbances and their potential role in the pathophysiology of IBS is even poorer. This probably reflects our poor understanding of intestinal functions and of their great variability both in health and disease. Many studies have investigated intestinal motility in IBS, but they were generally carried out on small numbers of patients, using a variety of protocols and methodologies. Furthermore, only a few descriptive studies evaluated the potential correlation between motor abnormalities and symptom perception.

Although altered motor patterns have been detected throughout the gastrointestinal tract, including the oesophagus, stomach, and biliary tract, interest has traditionally been focused on colonic and small intestinal motility. Identification of palpable bowel loops at physical examination, as well as endoscopic visualization of painful contractions in the sigmoid colon, have driven attention of investigators to the large bowel. Despite 'three cycles per minute' colonic myoelectric activity being reported as a typical hallmark of IBS patients[39,40] in the 1970s, this finding has not been confirmed in more recent studies[41,42]. Several studies failed to detect any motor abnormality in IBS patients in terms of rectal compliance[43] or colonic tone[44]. Table 2 summarizes the main colonic motor abnormalities described so far in IBS. It has been reported that the colon of patients with diarrhoea-predominant and constipation-predominant IBS shows respectively more[43] and less[45] propagated contractions than that of healthy individuals. In keeping with these observations the intestinal transit time is accelerated in diarrhoea-predominant IBS and delayed in constipation-predominant IBS[46]. Analysis of frequency and amplitude of colonic contractions in different subgroups of IBS patients provides conflicting results. Connell originally described frequency of colonic contractions as being decreased in IBS patients with diarrhoea and increased in those with constipation[47]. More recently Bazzocchi and colleagues described decreased frequency of high-amplitude contractions in patients with constipation-predominant IBS[48], and increased frequency of both high-amplitude contractions[45] and of postprandial contractions in general[49] in those with diarrhoea-predominant IBS. Recent evidence has confirmed the relatively high frequency of high-amplitude propagated contractions in diarrhoea-predominant IBS, possibly associated with episodes of abdominal pain[50].

Probably due to the many difficulties encountered in exploring and understanding colonic motor patterns, or to the emerging evidence of IBS as a diffuse digestive disorder, the focus of motility studies has moved to the small intestine (Table 3)[51]. In the small bowel of IBS patients short bursts of rhythmic contractions, termed discrete clustered contractions[52], bursts of uncoordinated contractions[53], and high-pressure contractions[54] have been reported in the small bowel of affected individuals, coincident to perception of abdominal pain. However, the results of these studies have never been confirmed and their consistency remains to be established. In general, the most consistent finding is represented by an increased contractile activity that can be expressed as a long sequence of regularly spaced clustered contractions[54–57] or by more irregular activities such as irregular bursts[53], ileal high-pressure contractions[54], increased frequency of diurnal migrating motor complexes[55] or of contractions[56] in diarrhoea-predominant IBS. Other motor disorders include: increased frequencies of phase III-like activity[57], and increased contractile response to feeding with increased contraction amplitude in constipated IBS patients[58]. Orocaecal transit time has been found to be accelerated in patients with diarrhoea[59], while more recently a correlation has been found between IBS symptoms and intestinal contractions retrogradely propagated during phase II[60].

Table 2 Colonic dysmotility in IBS

Frequency contractions ↑ in C-IBS ↓ in D-IBS (Connel, 1962[47])
↑ frequency of 3 c/m slow waves (Snape *et al.*, 1976[40])
transit time ↑ in C-IBS ↓ in D-IBS (Cann *et al.*, 1983[46])
↓ frequency high-amplitude contractions in C-IBS (Bazzocchi *et al.*, 1998[48])
↑ frequency high-amplitude contractions in D-IBS (Bazzocchi *et al.*, 1990[45])
↑ postprandial colonic contractions in D-IBS (Bazzocchi *et al.*, 1991[49])
Abdominal pain = 90% of HAPCs in D IBS (Chey *et al.*, 2001[50])

C-IBS: constipation-IBS; D-IBS: diarrhoea-IBS; HAPCs: high-amplitude propagated contractions.

Table 3 IBS and small bowel motility

DCC associated with abdominal pain (Horowitz and Farrar, 1962[52])
Stress: no MMC, ↑ bursts in IBS vs HC (Kumar and Wingate, 1985[53])
Jejunal DCC and ileal HPC temporally linked to pain (Kellow and Phillips, 1987[54])
↓ feeding, ↑ frequency of diurnal MMC in D-IBS vs C-IBS, ↑ DCC (Kellow *et al.*, 1990[55])
↓ orocaecal TT in D-IBS (Godard *et al.*, 1994[59])
↑duration DCC, ↑ contractility in D-IBS vs HC (Schmidt *et al.*, 1996[56])
↑ MI, DCC, phase III-like activity (in hypersensitivity) (Evans *et al.*, 1996[57])
↑ postprandial contraction frequency vs HC; ↓ contraction amplitude in C-IBS vs HC (Small *et al.*, 1997[58])
Correlation between retrograde phase II contractions and symptoms (Simren *et al.*, 2000[60])

MMC: migrating motor complexes; DCC: discrete clustered contractions; TT: transit time; MI: motility index

As previously mentioned for dyspepsia, there is an emerging body of literature considering a possible inflammatory basis for symptom generation in a subgroup of patients with IBS. A particular interest has been directed to the identification of mast cells in intestinal mucosal biopsies of IBS patients[61,62]. These cells have been shown to degranulate in response to neuropeptides, and this event is associated with changes in muscle contraction[63], and excitability of enteric nerves[64]. In IBS patients mast cells may be increased not only in the intestinal mucosa but also in the muscularis propria, as reported by Hiatt and Katz as long ago as 1962[65]. Other studies have shown that other inflammatory cells may be increased in both the small intestine and colon of IBS patients, particularly in those with predominant diarrhoea[61,66]. Studies in animal models provide a solid background to explain changes in bowel physiology in the presence of mucosal inflammation even when the inflammatory infiltrate is mild and limited to the lamina propria[67]. Recent studies support the original observation of Chaudhary and Truelove[68] that acute episodes of infectious gastroenteritis may lead to IBS in some 7–31% of previously healthy subjects[69–73]. Gwee *et al.* described post-infectious changes in gut physiology including faster whole-gut transit times[71] and decreased rectal sensitivity compared to healthy subjects[69, 71]. Post-infectious changes in gut transit times were observed both in patients who developed IBS and in those who did not. Therefore, abnormal gut transit times were not sufficient *per se* to determine IBS symptoms; thus the authors postulated that psychological factors were required to perceive such changes as symptoms[71]. This hypothesis is supported by the finding that subjects who develop IBS after an acute gastrointestinal infection display higher scores for psychological difficulties than the asymptomatic group[70, 71].

The mechanisms underlying post-infectious IBS are yet to be understood; however, the persistence of a mild inflammatory infiltrate in the colonic mucosa of patients with persistent IBS symptoms may play a critical role[71]. Studies in animal models have certainly demonstrated that mucosal inflammation may alter both motor and sensory gut functions[67]. In many instances these changes occur in the absence of any discernible inflammatory involvement of the neuromuscular layers. Recent studies also indicate that gut sensory and motor changes may persist long after the resolution of an acute inflammatory insult of the mucosa[72]. Accordingly, research has focused on local (neuromuscular) sources of mediator, and recent studies indicate that smooth muscle cells represent both the source of and the target for cytokines such as interleukins IL1-β and IL-6[73].

CONCLUSIONS

Various abnormalities in the motor functions of the alimentary canal can be detected in subgroups of patients with functional dyspepsia and IBS, but the relationship of these abnormalities and digestive symptoms is certainly a very complex one and has not been fully clarified. A variety of methodological and conceptual shortcomings characterize many of the studies investigating the relationship between gastrointestinal motility disorders and dyspeptic symptoms, and this obviously contributes to a higher level of uncertainty in the field. Advances in this field will require application of comprehensive and accurate quantitative techniques for measuring both gastrointestinal motility and symptoms. For instance, techniques are needed to simultaneously measure gastrointestinal wall tension, pressure events and transit. Symptoms are even more difficult to measure since investigators can rely upon nothing but the words used by patients to describe their sensations, so that cultural factors inevitably play a pivotal role. Instruments for measuring individual complains of patients and their severity need to be created and validated in different cultural settings. Studies with appropriate inclusion criteria, sample size, methods and analysis will help to clarify the relationship between gastrointestinal motor events and digestive symptoms. The causes of abnormal motor activities are unclear. They could represent a primary abnormality of gastrointestinal neural or muscular cells, or a normal motor response to abnormal intraluminal contents, or the result of disturbed central or autonomic neural control mechanisms, or the immune-mediated response to different kinds of pathogens. Whatever the cause, gastrointestinal motility cannot be enucleated from neural events and motor–sensory abnormal interactions must represent the target of future research in this area.

References

1. Stanghellini V, Camilleri M, Malagelada JR. Chronic idiopathic intestinal pseudoobstruction: clinical and intestinal manometric findings. Gut. 1987;28:5–12.
2. Malagelada JR, Stanghellini V. Manometric evaluation of functional upper gut symptoms. Gastroenterology. 1985;88:1223–31.
3. Stanghellini V, Ghidini C, Ricci Maccarini M *et al.* Fasting and postprandial gastrointestinal motility in ulcer and non-ulcer dyspepsia. Gut. 1992;33:184–90.
4. Jebbink HJ, van Berge-Henegouwen GP, Akkermans LM, Smout AJ. Small intestinal motor abnormalities in patients with functional dyspepsia demonstrated by ambulatory manometry. Gut. 1996;38:694–700.
5. Kusano M, Sekiguchi T, Kawamura O *et al.* Further classification of dysmotility-like dyspepsia by interdigestive gastroduodenal manometry and plasma motilin level. Am J Gastroenterol. 1997;92:481–4.
6. Wilmer A, Van Cutsem E, Andrioli A *et al.* Ambulatory gastrojejunal manometry in severe motility like dyspepsia. Lack of correlation between dysmotility, symptoms, and gastric emptying. Gut. 1998;42:235–42.
7. Malagelada JR. Gastrointestinal motor disturbance in functional dyspepsia. Scand J Gastroenterol. 1991;30:745–51.
8. Bekhti A, Rutgeers L. Domperidone in the treatment of functional dyspepsia in patients with delayed gastric emptying. Postgrad Med J. 1979;55(Suppl. 1):30–2.
9. Bolondi L, Bortolotti M, Santi V *et al.* Measurement of gastric emptying time by real-time ultrasonography. Gastroenterology. 1985;89:752–9.
10. Geldof H, Van Der Schee EJ, Van Blankenstein M, Grashuis JL. Electrogastrographic study of gastric myoelectrical activity in patients with unexplained nausea and vomiting. Gut. 1986;27:799–808.
11. Maes BD, Ghoos YF, Hiele MI, Rutgeers PJ. Gastric emptying rate of solids in patients with nonulcer dyspepsia. Dig Dis Sci. 1997;42:1158–62.
12. Jian R, Ducrot F, Ruskone A *et al.* Symptomatic, radionuclide and therapeutic assessment of chronic idiopathic dyspepsia. A double-blind placebo-controlled evaluation of cisapride. Dig Dis Sci. 1989;34:657–64.
13. Talley NJ, Shuter B, McGrudden G *et al.* Lack of association between gastric emptying of solids and symptoms in nonulcer dyspepsia. J Clin Gastroenterol. 1989;11:625–30.
14. Waldron B, Cullen PT, Kumar R *et al.* Evidence for hypomotility in non-ulcer dyspepsia: a prospective multifactorial study. Gut. 1991;32:246–51.
15. Tucci A, Corinaldesi R, Stanghellini V *et al. Helicobacter pylori* infection and gastric function in patients with chronic idiopathic dyspepsia. Gastroenterology. 1992;103:768–74.

16. Scott AM, Kellow JE, Shuter B *et al.* Intragastric distribution and gastric emptying of solids and liquids in functional dyspepsia. Lack of influence of symptom subgroups and *H. pylori*-associated gastritis. Dig Dis Sci. 1993;38:2247–54.
17. Caballero-Plasencia AM, Muros Navarro MC, Martin-Ruiz JL *et al.* Dyspeptic symptoms and gastric emptying of solids in patients with functional dyspepsia. Role of *Helicobacter pylori* infection. Scand J Gastroenterol. 1995;30:745–51.
18. Stanghellini V, Tosetti C, Paternicò A *et al.* Risk indicators of delayed gastric emptying of solids in 343 patients with functional dyspepsia. Gastroenterology. 1996;110:1036–42.
19. Stanghellini V, Tosetti C, Paternico A *et al.* Predominant symptoms identify different subgroups in functional dyspepsia. Am J Gastroenterol. 1999;94:2080–5.
20. Talley NJ, Verlinden M, Jones M. Can symptoms discriminate among those with delayed or normal gastric emptying in dysmotility-like dyspepsia? Am J Gastroenterol. 2001;96:1422–8.
21. Stanghellini V, Vaira D, Morselli Labate AM *et al.* Training improves the reliability of a questionnaire for functional dyspepsia (FD) in a multicenter setting. Gastroenterology. 1999;112: A831p(abstract).
22. Troncon LEA, Bennett RJM, Ahluwalia NK, Thompson DG. Abnormal intragastric distribution of food during gastric emptying in functional dyspepsia patients. Gut. 1994;35:327–32.
23. Ahluwalia NK, Thompson DG, Mamtora H, Hindle J. Evaluation of gastric antral motor performance in patients with dysmotility-like dyspepsia using real-time high-resolution ultrasound. Neurogastroenterol Motil. 1996;8:333–8.
24. Troncon LEA, Thompson DG, Ahluwalia NK *et al.* Relations between upper abdominal symptoms and gastric distension abnormalities in dysmotility-like functional dyspepsia and after vagotomy. Gut. 1995;37:17–22.
25. Tack J, Piessevaux H, Coulie B *et al.* In functional dyspepsia, impaired gastric accommodation is associated with early satiety and weight loss. Neurogastroenterol Mot. 1998;10:102(abstract).
26. Loo FD, Palmer DW, Soergel KH *et al.* Gastric emptying in patients with diabetes mellitus. Gastroenterology. 1994;86:485–94.
27. Stern RM, Koch KL, Stewart WR, Lindblad IM. Spectral analysis of tachygastria recorded during motion sickness. Gastroenterology. 1987;92:92–7.
28. Jain NK, Boivin M, Zinsmeister AR *et al.* Effect of ileal perfusion of carbohydrates and amylase inhibitor on gastrointestinal hormones and emptying. Gastroenterology. 1989;96:377–87.
29. Jones VA, McLaughlan P, Shorthouse M, Workman E, Hunter JO. Food intolerance: a major factor in the pathogenesis of irritable bowel syndrome. Lancet. 1982;2:1115–17.
30. Rouillon JM, Azpiroz F, Malagelada JR. Reflex changes in intestinal tone: relationship to perception. Am J Physiol. 1991;261:G280–6.
31. Johannessen T, Petersen H, Kristensen P *et al.* The intensity and variability of symptoms in dyspepsia. Scand J Primary Health Care. 1993;11:50–5.
32. Heading RC, Wagner E, Tooley PJ. Reliability of symptom assessment in dyspepsia. Eur J Gastroenterol Hepatol. 1997;9:779–81.
33. Azpiroz F, Malagelada JR. Perception and reflex relaxation of the stomach in response to gut distension. Gastroenterology. 1990;98:1193–8.
34. Ritchie J. Pain from the distension of the pelvic colon by inflating a balloon in the irritable colon syndrome. Gut. 1973;14:125–32.
35. Talley NJ, Phillips SF. Non-ulcer dyspepsia: potential causes and pathophysiology. Ann Intern Med. 1988;108:865–79.
36. Camilleri M, Heading RC, Thompson WG. Consensus report: clinical perspective, mechanisms, diagnosis and management of irritable bowel syndrome. Aliment Pharmacol Ther. 2002;16: 1407–10.
37. Everhart JE, Renault PF. Irritable bowel syndrome in office-based practice in the United States. Gastroenterology. 1991;100:998–1005.
38. Jain AP, Gupta OP, Jajoo UN, Sidhwa HK. Clinical profile of irritable bowel syndrome at a rural based teaching hospital in central India. J Assoc Phys India. 1991;39:385–6.
39. Taylor I, Duthie DL, Smallwood R. The effect of stimulation on the myoelecrtrical activity of the rectosigmoid of man. Gut. 1974;15:599–607.
40. Snape WJ, Carlson GM, Cohen S. Colonic myoelectric activity in the irritable bowel syndrome. Gastroenterology. 1976;70:326–30.
41. Welgan P, Meshkinpour H, Hoehler F. The effect of stress on colon motor and electrical activity in irritable bowel syndrome. Psychosom Med. 1985;47:139–49.

42. Latimer PR, Sarna SK, Campbell D, Latimer MR, Waterfall WE, Daniel EE. Colonic motor and myoelectrical activity: a comparative study of normal patients, psychoneurotic patients and patients with irritable bowel syndrome. Gastroenterology. 1981;80:893–901.
43. Whitehead WE, Engel BT, Schuster MM. Irritable bowel syndrome. Physiological and psychological differences between diarrhoea-predominant and constipation-predominant patients. Dig Dis Sci. 1980;25:404–13.
44. Vassallo M, Camilleri M, Phillips SF, Brown ML, Chapman NJ, Thomforde GM. Transit through the proximal colon influences stool weight in the irritable bowel syndrome. Gastroenterology. 1992;102:102–8.
45. Bazzocchi G, Ellis J, Villaneuva-Meyer J et al. Postprandial colonic transit and motor activity in chronic constipation. Gastroenterology. 1990;98:686–93.
46. Cann PA, Read NW, Brown C, Hobson N, Holdsworth CG. Irritable bowel syndrome: relationship of disorders in the transit of a single solid meal to symptom patterns. Gut. 1983;24:405–11.
47. Connell AM. The motility of the pelvic colon. Part II. Paradoxical motility in diarrhea and constipation. Gut. 1962;3:342–8.
48. Bazzocchi G, Ellis J, Meyer J. Colonic scintigraphy and manometry in constipation, diarrhea and inflammatory bowel disease. Gastroenterology. 1988;94:A29(abstract).
49. Bazzocchi G, Ellis J, Villanueva-Meyer J, Reddy SN, Mena I, Snape WJ Jr. Effect of eating on colonic motility and transit in patients with functional diarrhea. Simultaneous scintigraphic and manometric evaluations. Gastroenterology. 1991;101:1298–306.
50. Chey WY, Jin HO, Lee MH, Sun SW, Lee KY. Colonic motility abnormality in patients with irritable bowel syndrome exibiting abdominal pain and diarrhea. Am J Gastroenterol. 2001;96:1499–506.
51. Quigley EMM. Disturbances in small bowel motility. Bailliere's Clin Gastroenterol. 1999; 13:385–95.
52. Horowitz L, Farrar JT. Intraluminal small intestinal pressure in normal patients and in patients with functional gastrointestinal disorders. Gastroenterology. 1962;42:455–64.
53. Kumar D, Wingate DL. The irritable bowel syndrome: a paroxysmal motor disorder. Lancet. 1985;2:973–7.
54. Kellow JE, Phillips SF. Altered small bowel motility in irritable small bowel syndrome is correlated with symptoms. Gastroenterology. 1987;92:1885–93.
55. Kellow JE, Gill RC, Wingate DL. Prolonged ambulant recordings of small bowel motility demonstrate abnormalities in the irritable bowel syndrome. Gastroenterology. 1990;98:1208–18.
56. Schmidt T, Hackelsberger N, Widmer R, Meisel C, Pfeiffer A, Kaess H. Ambulatory 24-hour jejunal motility in diarrhea-predominant irritable bowel syndrome. Scand J Gastroenterol. 1996;31;581–9.
57. Evans PR, Bennett EJ, Bak YT, Tennant CC, Kellow JE. Jejunal sensorimotor dysfunction in irritable bowel syndrome: clinical and psychosocial features. Gastroenterology. 1996;110:393–404.
58. Small PK, Loudon MA, Hau CM, Noor N, Campbell FC. Large-scale ambulatory study of postprandial jejunal motility in irritable bowel. Scand J Gastroenterol. 1997;32:39–47.
59. Godard DA, Libby GW, Farthing MJG. Ambulatory small intestinal motility in 'diarrhoea' predominant irritable bowel syndrome. Gut. 1994;35:203–10.
60. Simren M, Castedal M, Svelund J, Abrahamsson H, Bjornsson E. Abnormal propagation patterns of duodenal pressure waves in the irritable bowel syndrome. Dig Dis Sci. 2000;45:2151–61.
61. Weston AP, Biddle WL, Bhatia PS, Miner PB Jr. Terminal ileal mucosal mast cells in irritable bowel syndrome. Dig Dis Sci. 1993;38:1590–5.
62. Read NW. Irritable bowel syndrome (IBS) – definition and pathophysiology. Scand J Gastroenterol (Suppl). 1987;130:7–13.
63. Vermillion DL, Ernest PB, Scicchitano R, Collins SM. Antigen-induced contraction of jejunal smooth muscle in the sensitized rat. Am J Physiol. 1988;255:G701–8.
64. Palmer JM. Immunomodulation of electrical and synaptic behaviour of myenteric neurons of guinea pig small intestine during infection with *Trichinella spiralis*. In: Snape J, Collins SM, editors. Effect of Immune Cells and Inflammation on Smooth Muscle and Enteric Nerve. Boca Raton, FL: CRC Press, 1991:181–95.
65. Hiatt RB, Katz L. Mast cells in inflammatory conditions of the gastrointestinal tract. Am J Gastroenterol. 1962;37:541–5.

66. Salzmann JL, Peltier-Koch F, Bloch F, Petite JP, Camilleri JP. Methods in laboratory investigation: morphometric study of colonic biopsies: a new method of estimating inflammatory diseases. Lab Invest. 1992;60:847–51.
67. Collins SM. The immunomodulation of enteric neuromuscular function: implications for motility and inflammatory disorders. Gastroenterology. 1996;111:1683–99.
68. Chaudhary NA, Truelove SC. The irritable colon syndrome. A study of the clinical features, predisposing causes, and prognosis in 130 cases. Q J Med. 1962;31:307–22.
69. Bergin AJ, Donnelly TC, McKendrick MW, Read NW. Changes in anorectal function in persistent bowel disturbance following *Salmonella* gastroenteritis. Eur J Gastroenterol Hepatol. 1993; 5:617–20.
70. Gwee KA, Graham JC, McKendrick MW *et al*. Psychometric scores and persistence of irritable bowel after infectious diarrhoea. Lancet. 1996;347:150–3.
71. Gwee KA, Leong Y-L, Graham C *et al*. The role of psychological and biological factors in postinfective gut dysfunction. Gut. 1999;44:400–6.
72. Neal KR, Hebden J, Spiller R. Prevalence of gastrointestinal symptoms six months after bacterial gastroenteritis and risk factors for development of the irritable bowel syndrome: postal survey of patients. Br Med J. 1997;314:779–82.
73. Garcia Rodriguez LA, Ruigomez A. Increased risk of irritable bowel syndrome after bacterial gastroenteritis: cohort study. Br Med J. 1999;318:565–6.

21
A rational approach to *Helicobacter pylori* eradication in patients with functional dyspepsia

A. QASIM, M. BUCKLEY, H. O'CONNOR and C. A. O'MORAIN

INTRODUCTION

The prevalence of dyspepsia has been estimated to be 40% or more over a 6-month period in most communities, and accounts for 2–3% of general practice consultations[1]. There is an increased tendency for self-medication, substantial loss of workdays, and overall reduction in quality of life in patients with dyspepsia[2]. Consensus on a clear definition of the disorder has been difficult. The Rome II criteria are postprandial upper abdominal pain or discomfort, early satiety, nausea, vomiting, abdominal bloating and anorexia in the absence of known organic disease, and which have been present for 3 of the past 12 months[3]. The underlying pathophysiological mechanisms may include gastrointestinal motor abnormalities, altered visceral sensation, and psychosocial factors. Almost 50% of dyspeptic patients show evidence of motor disorders including impaired fundic relaxation, antral muscular dysfunction, gastroparesis, or impaired gastroduodenal reflexes. Attempts have been made to define various symptom complexes on the presence of predominant pathophysiological abnormalities such as impaired gastric accommodation resulting in early satiety and gastric hypersensitivity correlating with pain and belching. However, gastric motility studies in general have not shown significant differences between dyspeptic and control populations[4].

ROLE OF *HELICOBACTER PYLORI* INFECTION IN FUNCTIONAL DYSPEPSIA

Epidemiological studies have shown that *H. pylori* infection occurs more frequently in functional dyspepsia compared to matched control populations[5]. The contribution or association of *H. pylori* in the pathophysiology and clinical symptoms of functional dyspepsia is not completely understood, and remains a matter of debate. Increased postprandial epigastric sensation is a more frequent complaint in *H. pylori*-positive patients as compared with controls[6]. Fasting and meal-induced gastrin secretion at baseline and 6 months post-eradication were significantly different in those cured of infection; possibly an effect of resolution of antral gastritis[7]. Attempts to associate infection with a subgroup of these patients based on predominant symptom type have been unsuccessful. Conflicting results of systemic reviews add further confusion on account of their inability to synthesize a definitive role of eradication therapy[8,9]. Several factors may explain the conflicting results, such as geographical variations, selection bias, endpoint differences, and study duration. Randomized trials on the role of *H. pylori* eradication in functional dyspepsia have yielded equivocal conclusions[10,11]. In this chapter we will analyse the factors which may be responsible for the conflicting results.

DYSPEPSIA SCORING IN EVALUATION OF TREATMENT SUCCESS

The current definition of functional dyspepsia includes various symptoms, and the response from different therapy approaches is evaluated using a variety of scoring systems[12–15]. Several individual studies and meta-analyses have demonstrated no or minimal symptomatic benefit from *H. pylori* eradication, advocating a non-eradication policy in functional dyspepsia[8,10,16]. In a placebo-controlled study involving dyspepsia patients Koskenpato *et al.* found no clear benefit of *H. pylori* eradication on symptom improvement[16]. Of the 136 patients completing 1-year follow-up the reduction in mean dyspepsia score was seen in 28.8% and 21.7% of patients in the eradication and control groups, respectively. A significant improvement of abdominal pain, vomiting, early satiety, bloating, and nausea was maintained more effectively in the eradication group at the 12-month follow-up. However, significant recurrence of the regurgitation and heartburn was seen in both study arms at the 12-month follow-up, and resulted in an overall negative outcome for the study. The possible existence of non-erosive oesophagitis among the included patients cannot be entirely ruled out. *H. pylori* has not been identified as an aetiological or disease-aggravating factor in reflux oesophagitis[17].

In another randomized trial Talley *et al.* demonstrated no significant improvement in dyspepsia at 1-year follow-up after *H. pylori* eradication[10]. However, certain aspects of this study need further consideration. Firstly, co-presence or inadvertent inclusion of patients with microscopic oesophagitis cannot be ruled out as patient exclusion was based on symptom evaluation or presence of erosive oesophagitis. Secondly, despite the fact that dyspepsia is a common disorder, the numbers of patients included from more than 20 participating centres were surprisingly low, at less than six. In addition, subgroups with motility-type dyspepsia were over-represented. Interpretation of symptom scoring has produced widely variable results even in homogeneous patient populations[10,11,18–21] (Fig. 1). These differences cannot be explained on the basis of the therapies or scoring systems employed, as exclusively selecting dyspepsia-free patients at follow-up also demonstrated significant variability of the results[10,18–20] (Table 1). This was also true for other studies conducted by the same investigators.

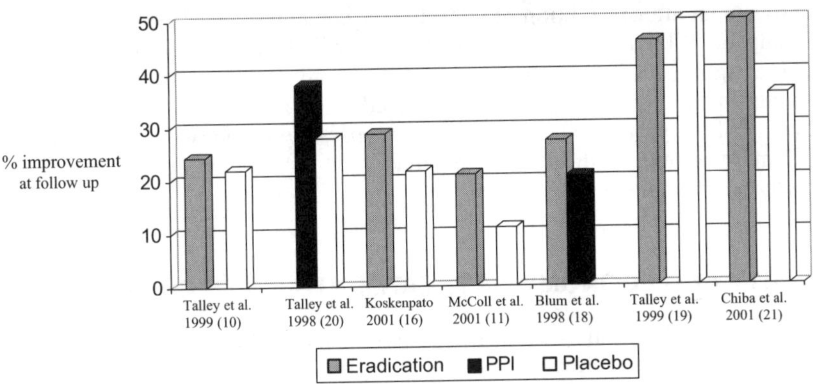

Fig. 1 Follow-up evaluation demonstrating huge variation in symptoms scoring in well-designed clinical studies

Table 1 Complete relief of symptoms in functional dyspepsia patients during follow-up period

Reference	No. of patients	Treatment duration	Symptom-free patients at 1 month			Symptom-free patients at 12 months		
			Eradication	PPI	Placebo	Eradication	PPI	Placebo
Talley *et al.*, 1999[10]	278	1 week	15% or less		11% or less	15%		11%
Blum *et al.*, 1998[18]	245	1 week	13% or less	10% or less		13%	10%	
Talley *et al.*, 1999[19]	337	2 weeks	28% or less		23% or less	28%		23%
Talley *et al.*, 1998[20]	1262	4 weeks		38%*	28%			

PPI = proton pump inhibitor.
* Maximum improvement was evident at the end of first week of therapy.

Such unreliability of results must be considered when deciding against an eradication policy in functional dyspepsia.

INTERRELATION BETWEEN *H. PYLORI* GASTRITIS AND DYSPEPSIA SCORING

H. pylori infection is associated with variable degree and topography of gastritis. Improvement of gastritis following eradication appears to be a universal phenomenon. Koskenpato *et al.* demonstrated significant reduction ($p < 0.0001$) of chronic gastritis scores at 1-year follow-up after eradication therapy, which was not associated with symptomatic improvement[16]. In a recent study, however, the same investigators demonstrated a significant association of antral gastritis with dyspepsia symptoms after *H. pylori* eradication[22]. In a separate study, symptomatic improvement after resolution of inflammatory changes was also demonstrated in a group of 251 patients at 3-month follow-up[23]. In an earlier study by Talley *et al.* a significant improvement of gastritis score was demonstrated in 81% of patients in the eradication group compared with 13% in the placebo group[10]. Severity of the gastritis was not evaluated separately in the two groups, although 15% more patients with little or no persisting gastritis were symptom-free even on secondary analysis.

SAFETY AND ECONOMY OF TREATMENT APPROACHES

To achieve symptomatic benefit in one functional dyspeptic patient, 15 patients need treatment, an effect similar to therapy using proton-pump inhibitors (PPI)[24,25]. Trials involving *H. pylori* are, however, more robust as a significantly higher number of patients is included. *H. pylori* eradication involves 1 week of therapy compared to ongoing acid-suppression therapy. Health economic models suggest that the cost of *H. pylori* eradication in functional dyspepsia is similar to that achieved by acid-suppression therapy in reflux disease[24]. These factors have led the Maastricht 2-2000 Consensus Report to suggest that *H. pylori* eradication is advisable in functional dyspepsia[15].

The strongest argument in favour of eradicating *H. pylori* is the finding that PPI therapy, in some *H. pylori*-positive patients, may promote progressive corpus atrophic gastritis, a potentially precancerous process. The *H. pylori*-negative stomach appears relatively immune to PPI therapy-related changes in the topography and severity of chronic gastritis. A prolonged inflammatory process in the gastric mucosa is associated with destruction of glandular units. Loss of parietal and chief cells without glandular destruction is also described, which ultimately leads to gastric atrophy and intestinal metaplasia[26,27]. Kuipers *et al.* found that atrophic corpus gastritis developed in 18 of 59 *H. pylori*-positive patients (31%) treated with PPI, compared with only two of 46 (4%) *H. pylori*-negative patients[28]. Accelerated atrophic corpus gastritis, following long-term PPI treatment, has also been described by other investigators[29]. Solcia *et al.* have shown that corpus gastritis regresses quickly once PPI therapy is withdrawn[30]. In a recent prospective study Moayyedi *et al.* randomized 41 *H. pylori*-positive patients to either 1-week eradication therapy or placebo, and continued antisecretory therapy[31]. At 1 year none of eight patients cured of *H. pylori* had corpus atrophy compared with six of 11 *H. pylori*-positive patients. Harbouring *H. pylori* infection over long periods of time, and particularly when treated with PPI therapy, changes the pattern of gastritis from the duodenal ulcer phenotype to the gastric cancer phenotype[32–34].

Similarly, in a prospective study involving 100 patients treated with daily PPI for 1 year, Schenk *et al.* randomized *H. pylori*-positive patients to double-blind treatment with 1-week eradication therapy or placebo and assessed gastritis parameters at 1 year[35]. In patients with persistent *H. pylori* infection the severity of corpus gastritis increased. There was a significant decrease in corpus inflammation in patients cured of *H. pylori*. In a recent study, a consecutive series of patients undergoing treatment with PPI ($n = 113$) or histamine$_2$-receptor antagonists (H$_2$-RAs) ($n = 37$), and 76 non-treated dyspeptic controls were investigated[36].

Gastric mucosal *H. pylori* and non-*H. pylori* bacteria, histological gastritis, *H. pylori* serology, and circulating interleukins (IL)-1β, IL-6, and IL-8 were examined. *H. pylori*-positive patients on long-term acid inhibition displayed non-*H. pylori* bacterial growth, increased cytokine levels, and a higher risk of atrophic gastritis. It was suggested that double infection with *H. pylori* and non-*H. pylori* bacteria could be a major factor in the development of atrophic gastritis during gastric acid inhibition. Current evidence suggests that long-term PPI-induced acid suppression in *H. pylori*-infected individuals, particularly in young patients, may increase the risk of severe corpus gastritis and atrophy[37]. Such an approach should therefore be avoided in these patients.

FUNCTIONAL DYSPEPSIA: 'TEST AND TREAT'

Potential factors influencing the eradication decision in functional dyspepsia include cost of eradication, prevalence and emergence of antibiotic resistance, and therapy-related complications including the long-term effects of eradication on the gastric and oesophageal environment. The 'test-and-treat' paradigm has been validated in many studies. There is overwhelming evidence not only in favour of symptom relief in dyspepsia from *H. pylori* eradication but also the possible beneficial effect in gastric cancer prevention. Chiba *et al.* demonstrated 14% clinical gain by adopting a 'test-and-treat' eradication policy in a dyspeptic population. The treat to success ratio was 7[21]. This approach reduced mean annual cost by 53 Canadian dollars per patient.

It is interesting to note that eradication rates are generally inferior in patients suffering with non-ulcer dyspepsia[38]. Meta-analysis reveal that one patient in 15 will become completely asymptomatic[24]. Although the effect is modest it is similar to what can be achieved with other therapies such as PPI or motility drugs. The cost-effectiveness and safety of 'test-and-treat' *H. pylori* eradication is also supported by results of a recent meta-analysis conducted by Moayyedi *et al.* in which a significant peptic ulcer risk reduction was demonstrated among 2541 patients from nine included studies (Table 2). There was a 9% relative risk reduction in the eradication group and no significant heterogeneity between the nine included studies. The future risk of developing complications, including peptic ulceration, is evident from the results of study by Blum *et al.* who demonstrated a 5% 1-year incidence of peptic ulcer in *H. pylori*-positive functional dyspepsia. However, this study is mainly quoted for its negative results in dyspepsia improvement[18]. The substantial risk of peptic ulcer among the functional dyspepsia population is also evident from the results of a study by Talley *et al.*[20]. Out of 180 patients with persistent *H. pylori* infection in treatment and control groups, 10 patients (5.5%) developed peptic ulcer at 1-year follow-up (peptic ulcer prevention in one out of 18 eradicated patients), confirming the importance of eradication in functional dyspepsia. Maastricht 2000-2 Guidelines recommend non-invasive testing of all those patients under the age of 45 years without alarm symptoms at first presentation, and treating all those positive for infection[15]. Both Canadian and American guidelines have been published, and generally suggest a test-and-treat strategy, although on a case-by-case basis[39,40].

Table 2 Meta-analysis of nine trials on *H. pylori* eradication in non-ulcer dyspepsia by Moayyedi *et al.*[24]

Reference	Functional dyspepsia patients (treatment vs. placebo)	Risk ratio (95% CI)
Blum *et al.*	119 vs. 130	0.92 (0.81–1.03)
Koelz *et al.*	67 vs. 73	0.95 (0.81–111)
McColl *et al.*	121 vs. 143	0.85 90.77–0.93)
Talley *et al.*	101 vs. 111	0.97 (0.86–1.34)
Talley *et al.*	81 vs. 72	1.07 (0.86–1.34)
Miwa *et al.*	33 vs. 28	0.91 (0.70–1.18)
Malferthiener *et al.*	269 vs. 143	0.88 (0.77–0.990)
Bruley des Varannes *et al.*	74 vs. 86	0.83 (0.68–1.00)
Froehlich *et al.*	31 vs. 34	0.86 (0.60–1.24)
Total	*896 vs. 820*	*0.91 (0.86–0.96)*

NNT = 15

H. PYLORI ERADICATION 'SEARCH AND TREAT'

H. pylori is acquired during infancy or childhood and persists unless efforts are made to eradicate it. In spite of an apparent asymptomatic course in the majority of the infected population, occurrences of chronic gastritis, subsequent atrophic gastritis, metaplasia, and cancer risk have all been well documented[41]. Patients with functional dyspepsia are shown to have a relatively higher risk of developing gastric cancer compared to asymptomatic controls. Relatives of patients with gastric cancer also have a higher incidence of *H. pylori* infection, and increased prevalence of precancerous changes can be reversed by *H. pylori* eradication[42].

Intestinal metaplasia is associated with a wide range of genetic changes including telomere reduction; microsatellite instability; and mutations in p53, APC, and k-ras even before the onset of dysplasia[43]. The increased risk of malignant transformation is relatively more common with type III intestinal metaplasia, whereas such a risk is minimal with type I and type II[44]. *H. pylori* eradication may be related to healing and improvement of advanced atrophic gastritis and intestinal metaplasia in an elderly population[45]. Resolution of inflammation subsequent to *H. pylori* eradication also leads to reversal of gastric atrophy and intestinal metaplasia[46]. *H. pylori*-associated atrophic gastritis in patients with truncating APC gene mutation is related to development of gastric adenoma in familial adenomatous polyposis[47]. El-Nujumi *et al.* have shown that eradicating *H. pylori* reduces the rise in gastrin seen during subsequent long-term acid-inhibition therapy[48]. *H. pylori* eradication before the development of such changes seems the most logical approach. Infection with certain *H. pylori* genotypes prevalent in high-risk gastric cancer areas may change the balance between gastric mucosal proliferation and apoptosis. Such an association has recently been demonstrated with higher gastric proliferation rates in those harbouring babA2+ strains[49]. Considering these factors the new paradigm may be 'search and treat'.

CONCLUSIONS

Symptomatic as well as long-term benefits of eradication far outweigh the risk of developing drug resistance, and are cost-effective in treating functional dyspepsia. Symptom evaluation in functional dyspepsia is subject to variability and may, with other factors, explain the conflicting results of treatment trials. The future development of a *H. pylori* vaccine, a global 'search-and-treat' eradication policy, and possible identification of high-risk *H. pylori* strains will show a way forward in gastric cancer prevention.

References

1. Jones R, Lydeard S. Prevalence of symptoms of dyspepsia in the community. Br Med J. 1989;289:30–2.
2. Knill-Jones RP. Geographical differences in the prevalence of dyspepsia. Scand J Gastroenterol. 1991;26(Suppl. 182):17–24.
3. Talley NJ, Stanghellini V, Heading RC *et al.* Functional gastroduodenal disorder. Gut. 1999; 45(Suppl. 2):II37–42.
4. Goh KL, Paramsothy M, Azian M *et al.* Does *Helicobacter pylori* infection affect gastric emptying in patients with functional dyspepsia? J Gastroenterol Hepatol. 1997;12:790–4.
5. Buckley M, O'Morain CA. Prevalence of *Helicobacter pylori* in non-ulcer-dyspepsia. Aliment Pharmacol Ther. 1995;9(Suppl. 2):53–8.
6. Thumshrin M, Camilleri M, Saslow SB *et al.* Gastric accommodation in non-ulcer dyspepsia and the roles of *Helicobacter pylori* infection and vagal function. Gut. 1999;44:55–64.
7. Parente F, Imbesi V, Maconi G *et al.* Effects of *Helicobacter pylori* eradication on gastric function indices in functional dyspepsia. A prospective controlled study. Scand J Gastroenterol. 1998;33:461–7.
8. Laine L, Schoenfeld P, Fennerty B. Therapy for *Helicobacter pylori* in patients with nonulcer dyspepsia. Ann Intern Med. 2001;134:361–9.
9. Moayyedi P, Soo S, Deeks J *et al.* Eradication of *Helicobacter pylori* for non-ulcer dyspepsia. Cochrane Database Syst Rev. 2001;CD002096.
10. Talley NJ, Janssens J, Lauritsen K *et al.* Eradication of *Helicobacter pylori* in functional dyspepsia: randomised double blind placebo controlled trial with 12 month's follow up. The Optimal Regimen Cures Helicobacter Induced Dyspepsia (ORCHID) Study Group. Br Med J. 1999;318:833–7.
11. McColl K, Murray L, El-Omer *et al.* Symptomatic benefit from eradicating *H. pylori* infection in patients with nonulcer dyspepsia. N Engl J Med. 1998;339:1869–74.
12. Rosenstoch S, Kay L, Rosenstock C *et al.* Relation between *H. pylori* infection and gastrointestinal symptoms and syndromes. Gut. 1997;41:169–76.
13. Parsonnet J, Blaser MJ, Perez-Perez I *et al.* Symptoms and risk factors of *Helicobacter* infection in a cohort of epidemiologists. Gastroenterology. 1992;102:41–6.
14. Pilotto A, Franceschi M, Leandro G *et al.* Efficacy of 7 day lansoprazole-based triple therapy for *Helicobacter pylori* infection in elderly patients. J Gastroenterol Hepatol. 1999;14:464–71.
15. Malfertheiner P, Megraud F, O'Morain C *et al.* Current concept in the management of *Helicobacter pylori* infection – the Maastricht 2-2000 Consensus Report. Aliment Pharmacol Ther. 2002;16:167–80.
16. Kostenpato J, Farkkila M, Sipponen P. *Helicobacter pylori* eradication and standardized 3-month omeprazole therapy in functional dyspepsia. Am J Gastroenterol. 2001;96:2866–72.
17. O'Connor HJ, O'Morain CA. *Helicobacter pylori* and gastroesophageal reflux disease: to treat or not to treat? Scand J Gastroenterol. 2001;7:677–82.
18. Blum AL, Talley NJ, O'Morain C *et al.* Lack of effect of treating *Helicobacter pylori* infection in patients with nonulcer dyspepsia. Omeprazole plus Clarithromycin and Amoxicillin Effect One Year after Treatment (OCAY) Study Group. N Engl J Med. 1998;339:1875–81.
19. Talley NJ, Vakil N, Ballard ED 2nd, *et al.* Absence of benefit of eradicating *Helicobacter pylori* in patients with nonulcer dyspepsia. N Engl J Med. 1999;341:1106–11.

20. Talley NJ, Meineche-Schmidt P, Duckworth P *et al.* Efficacy of omeprazole in functional dyspepsia: double-blind, randomised, placebo-controlled trials (the Bond and Opera studies). Aliment Pharmacol Ther. 1998;12:1055–65.
21. Chiba N, Vedhuyzen van Zanten SJO, Sinclair P *et al.* Treating *Helicobacter pylori* infection in primary care patients with uninvestigated dyspepsia: the Canadian adult dyspepsia empiric treatment – *Helicobacter pylori* positive (CADET-Hp) randomised controlled trial. Br Med J. 2002; 324:1012.
22. Koskenpato J, Farkkila M, Sipponen P. *Helicobacter pylori* and different topographic types of gastritis: treatment response after successful eradication therapy in functional dyspepsia. Scand J Gastroenterol. 2002;37:778–84.
23. Kyzekove J, Arlt J, Arltova M. Is there any relationship between functional dyspepsia and chronic gastritis associated with *Helicobacter pylori* infection? Hepatogastroenterology. 2001;48:594–602.
24. Moayyedi P, Soo S, Deeks J *et al.* Systematic review and economic evaluation of *Helicobacter pylori* eradication treatment for non-ulcer dyspepsia. Dyspepsia Review Group. Br Med J. 2000; 321:659.
25. Soo S, Moayyedi P, Deeks J *et al.* Pharmacological interventions for non-ulcer dyspepsia (Cochrane Review). In: The Cochrane Library. Issue 2. Oxford: Update Software, 2002.
26. Asaka M, Kato M, Kudo M *et al.* Atrophic changes of gastric mucosa are caused by *Helicobacter pylori* infection rather than ageing: studies in asymptomatic Japanese adults. Helicobacter. 1996;1:52–6.
27. DeLuca VA, West AB, Haque S *et al.* Long-term symptom patterns, endoscopic findings, and gastric histology in *Helicobacter pylori*-infected and uninfected patients. J Clin Gastroenterol. 1998;26:106–12.
28. Kuipers EJ, Uyterlinde AM, Pena AS *et al.* Increase of *Helicobacter pylori*-associated corpus gastritis during acid suppressive therapy: implications for long-term safety. Am J Gastroenterol. 1995;90:1401–6.
29. Eissele R, Brunner G, Simon B, Solcia E, Arnold R. Gastric mucosa during treatment with lansoprazole: *Helicobacter pylori* is a risk factor for argyrophil cell hyperplasia. Gastroenterology. 1997;112:707–17.
30. Solcia E, Fiocca R, Villani L *et al.* Effects of permanent eradication or transient clearance of *Helicobacter pylori* on histology of gastric mucosa using omeprazole with or without antibiotics. Scand J Gastroenterol. 1996;31(Suppl. 215):105–10.
31. Moayyedi P, Morrow S, Peacock R *et al.* Changing patterns of *H. pylori* gastritis in long-standing acid suppression. Gut. 1999;44(Suppl. 1):A117.
32. Logan RPH, Walker MM, Misiewicz JJ *et al.* Changes in the intragastric distribution of *Helicobacter pylori* during treatment with omeprazole. Gut. 1995;36:12–16.
33. Meining A, Bosseckert H, Caspary WF *et al.* H2-receptor antagonists and antacids have an aggravating effect on *Helicobacter pylori* gastritis in duodenal ulcer patients. Aliment Pharmacol Ther. 1997;11:729–34.
34. Stolte M, Meining A, Schmitz JM *et al.* Changes in *Helicobacter pylori*-induced gastritis in the antrum and corpus during 12 months of treatment with omeprazole and lansoprazole in patients with gastro-oesophageal reflux disease. Aliment Pharmacol Ther. 1998;432:311–14.
35. Schenk BE, Kuipers EJ, Nelis GF *et al. H. pylori* eradication for chronic gastritis during omeprazole treatment for GERD. Gastroenterology. 1998;114(Suppl.):A279.
36. Sanduleanu S, Jonkers D, De Bruïne A, Hameeteman W, Stockbrügger RW. Double gastric infection with *Helicobacter pylori* and non-*Helicobacter pylori* bacteria during acid-suppressive therapy: increase of pro-inflammatory cytokines and development of atrophic gastritis. Aliment Pharmacol Ther. 2001;15:1163–75.
37. Labenz J. Does *Helicobacter pylori* affect the management of gastroesophageal reflux disease? Am J Gastroenterol. 1999;94:867–9.
38. Spliller RC. Is there any difference in *Helicobacter pylori* eradication rates in patients with active peptic ulcer, inactive peptic ulcer and functional dyspepsia? Eur J Gastroenterol Hepatol. 1999;11(Suppl. 2);discussion S4305.
39. American Gastroenterological Association. American Gastroenterological Association medical position statement. Evaluation of dyspepsia. Gastroenterology. 1998;114:549–58.
40. Hunt R, Thompson ABR. Canadian *Helicobacter* consensus conference. Can J Gastroenterol. 1998;12:31–41.
41. Vaira D *et al.* Prevalence of peptic ulcer in *H. pylori* positive blood donors. Gut. 1994;35: 309–12.

42. El-Omer EM, Oien K, Murray LS *et al*. Increased prevalence of precancerous changes in relatives of gastric cancer patients: critical role of *H. pylori*. Gastroenterology. 2000;118:22–30.

43. Tahara E. Molecular biology of gastric cancer. World J Surg. 1995;19:484–8.

44. Rokkas T, Filepe MI, Sladen GE. Detection of an increased incidence of early gastric cancer in patients with intestinal metaplasia type III who are closely followed up. Gut. 1991;32:1110–13.

45. Kokkola A, Sipponen P, Rautelin H *et al*. The effect of *Helicobacter pylori* eradication on the natural course of atrophic gastritis with dysplasia. Aliment Pharmacol Ther. 2002;16:515–20.

46. El-Omer EM, Oien K, El-Nujumi *et al*. *Helicobacter pylori* infection and chronic gastric acid hyposecretion. Gastroenterology. 1997;113:15–24.

47. Nakamura S, Matsumoto T, Kobori Y *et al*. Impact of *Helicobacter pylori* infection and mucosal atrophy on gastric lesions in patients with familial adenomatous polyposis. Gut. 2002;51:485–9.

48. El-Nujumi A, Williams C, Ardill JE, Oien K, McColl KEL. Eradicating *Helicobacter pylori* reduces hypergastrinaemia during long-term omeprazole treatment. Gut. 1998;42:159–65.

49. Yu J, Leung WK, Go MYY *et al*. Relationship between *Helicobacter pylori* babA2 status with gastric epithelial cell turnover and premalignant gastric lesions. Gut. 2002;51:480–4.

22
Con: *Helicobacter pylori* eradication – a rational approach for the treatment of patients with functional dyspepsia?

N.B. VAKIL

DEFINITIONS

Dyspepsia (also called uninvestigated dyspepsia) is defined as pain or discomfort centred in the upper abdomen[1]. Non-ulcer dyspepsia or functional dyspepsia refers to a group of patients who have been investigated to rule out organic causes of dyspepsia. These patients should be distinguished from those who have symptoms of dyspepsia but have not undergone investigation (uninvestigated dyspepsia). To meet the criteria for the definition of this condition, patients must have a chronic course and have no abnormalities at endoscopy that could explain the symptoms. Non-ulcer dyspepsia is therefore defined as: at least 12 weeks, which need not be consecutive, within the preceding 12 months of:

1. persistent or recurrent dyspepsia (as defined above);
2. no evidence of organic disease (including upper endoscopy) that is likely to explain the symptoms;
3. no evidence that the dyspepsia is exclusively relieved by defaecation or associated with the onset of a change in stool frequency or stool form (i.e. not irritable bowel syndrome)[1].

The minimum work-up for a diagnosis of functional dyspepsia is a careful history, physical examination and upper endoscopy during a symptomatic period off antisecretory therapy.

ENDOSCOPIC FINDINGS IN UNSELECTED DYSPEPTIC PATIENTS IN PRIMARY CARE

When unselected, consecutive patients with dyspepsia in primary care are investigated, 10–20% of them have peptic ulcer disease, 5–15% have oesophagitis,

10–12% have abnormalities that are less specific (gastritis, duodenitis) and approximately 50% have no visible abnormalities at endoscopy. Kagevi *et al.*[2] studied 172 patients with dyspepsia who were evaluated in a primary-care centre. After history taking, physical examination, laboratory tests, upper endoscopy and flexible sigmoidoscopy a final diagnosis was established. Six per cent of patients had oesophagitis, 13% had peptic ulcer disease, and 64% had non-ulcer dyspepsia. In another study, Gear *et al.*[3] studied 346 patients and found that a gastric ulcer was present in 6% of cases and a duodenal ulcer in 12% of cases presenting with dyspepsia in primary care. Sixty per cent of patients in that study did not have specific findings at endoscopy. Given the large numbers of patients with dyspepsia in primary care, and the large numbers of patients who have no specific findings at endoscopy, several empirical treatment strategies have been proposed, among which *Helicobacter pylori* eradication has aroused considerable interest. Non-ulcer dyspepsia is a difficult area for investigation. Placebo response rates are high and there is no symptom complex that predicts response to any single form of therapy. *H. pylori* infection is known to cause gastritis and peptic ulcer disease, and trials of eradication therapy are based on the premise that resolution of the inflammation might improve symptoms. The role of *H. pylori* infection in non-ulcer dyspepsia may be evaluated by assessing the prevalence of the infection and by trials of eradication therapy. These are discussed in more detail below.

Prevalence of *H. pylori* infection in patients with non-ulcer dyspepsia

A number of population-based studies have been performed to determine the prevalence of *H. pylori* infection in non-ulcer dyspepsia. A population-based study in Norway suggested that there may be a higher prevalence of *H. pylori* infection in non-ulcer dyspepsia, but another Scandinavian study found no increase in *H. pylori* infection in non-ulcer dyspepsia[4]. A study in Dutch workers found no association between *H. pylori* infection and dyspeptic symptoms[5]. Conflicting results in population-based studies are often due to confounding factors such as socioeconomic status and childhood living conditions. Low socioeconomic status and crowding in childhood have been shown to be important risk factors for the early acquisition of *H. pylori* infection. There are therefore no conclusive data to suggest that *H. pylori* infection is more prevalent in subjects with non-ulcer dyspepsia.

Randomized controlled trials of *H. pylori* eradication in non-ulcer dyspepsia

There are now several large, double-blind, randomized, placebo-controlled trials that evaluate the efficacy of *H. pylori* eradication in non-ulcer dyspepsia. While the overall design of the studies is excellent, the results are not uniform. As a result there is a debate on the usefulness of eradicating *H. pylori* in non-ulcer dyspepsia. These studies will be considered individually in more detail.

Blum *et al.*[6] randomly assigned 438 patients to proton-pump inhibitor triple therapy or omeprazole alone for 1 week, and followed patients for 1 year.

The study was carefully designed with appropriate controls and blinding, Treatment success was reported in 27% of patients in the triple-therapy group and 21% of patients in the placebo group (not significant). Talley *et al.*[7] randomly treated 278 patients with triple therapy for 1 week or placebo for 1 week. Relief of dyspepsia at 1 year was similar in the two groups (24% in active treatment and 22% in placebo). Data from another well-designed, large US multi-centre trial also show no benefit for eradication therapy in non-ulcer dyspepsia[8]. Of 337 patients randomized to either *H. pylori* eradication therapy or placebo, and followed for 1 year, 46% of patients in the active treatment group and 50% in the placebo group had a successful response to therapy ($p = 0.55$). If a more stringent endpoint of no dyspepsia was considered, 28% of patients on triple therapy compared with 23% on placebo had no symptoms at 12 months by intent-to-treat analysis. No significant association was found between the symptom type (ulcer-like, reflux-like or dysmotility-like) and the outcome, and there was no correlation with improvement in chronic gastritis at 12 months. An important element of the design of this study was that endoscopy was performed at the end of the trial and showed a low prevalence of ulcer disease in the placebo group (4% duodenal ulcer and 2% gastric ulcer). This is an important finding because it suggests that the number of patients with occult ulcer disease in this population was quite small. In contrast, in a single-centre study from Scotland, a significant benefit was reported with eradication therapy. McColl *et al.*[9] reported that symptoms resolved in a significantly greater proportion of patients (21%) with *H. pylori* triple therapy compared to 7% in the placebo group. There are several possibilities for the results of this study. The first is that the inclusion criteria permitted the inclusion of patients with gastro-oesophageal reflux disease into the trial. Patients with symptoms of reflux disease were excluded from the other studies. Excluding these patients is important because there is little likelihood of success with eradication therapy in patients with reflux disease. Another possibility is that the baseline prevalence of *H. pylori*-related ulcer disease is very high in Scotland and eradication therapy may cure a larger pool of occult ulcer disease than in other countries. In an earlier study of dyspeptic patients in Scotland the same authors found ulcer disease in 40% of 182 *H. pylori*-infected dyspeptic patients in their population. When the prevalence of *H. pylori*-related ulcer disease in a population is high, there is an increased likelihood of including patients with healed peptic ulcer disease in a trial of non-ulcer dyspepsia. These patients are more likely to demonstrate a long-term response to eradication therapy. Finally, the placebo response rate in the Scottish study is much lower than in other trials, suggesting that the population studied may differ from the patients seen in other countries in Western Europe and in the United States. The patients were not subjected to endoscopy at the end of the trial, as in the US study, but the low placebo response rate suggests that many of these patients may have had ulcer disease and relapsed over the course of the year. In another US study, 100 patients were randomized to therapy with omeprazole and clarithromycin or placebo. At 1 year the reduction in dyspepsia scores was similar in the two groups[10]. The study, however, had significant limitations: it did not use a validated symptom scale, was not powered to detect small differences and used a two-drug treatment regimen (omeprazole and clarithromycin) that is obsolete. The FROSCH trial from Germany and Switzerland randomized

180 patients to omeprazole and amoxycillin or omeprazole for 14 days and followed them for 6 months[11]. The primary outcome was defined as no need for further therapy or investigations in the last 3 months of the trial, and there was no significant difference between the study groups. A small study from Japan randomized patients to omeprazole, amoxycillin and clarithromycin therapy ($n = 50$) and 40 patients to omeprazole twice daily with placebos in lieu of the antibiotics[12]. Gastritis improved with eradication therapy but dyspeptic symptoms did not change. The final results from the ELAN study, a large European study of 860 patients randomized to lansoprazole or lansoprazole triple therapy, will be of great interest. In an abstract 2 years ago the authors reported preliminary data from this study[13]. The primary objective of the study, response in the intent-to-treat groups, is not yet available; however, if patients were classified as responders (dyspepsia score less than or equal to 1) or non-responders, there was a higher proportion of responders (44%) in patients with successful eradication compared to patients without eradication (36%). These data can only be considered preliminary at this time. The final results are awaited with interest.

Meta-analyses of *H. pylori* eradication in non-ulcer dyspepsia

A recent meta-analysis has suggested that eradication therapy may have modest benefit with one responder for every 15 patients treated[14]. Nine studies were included for analysis, including the ELAN study mentioned above which is still in abstract form. No significant heterogeneity was found. Another recent meta-analysis has reached the opposite conclusion, suggesting that there is no benefit for eradication therapy[15]. This study found seven trials that met their inclusion criteria, and the authors found significant heterogeneity and noted that this was caused by the Scottish randomized controlled trial described in detail above.

Problems with eradication therapy in non-ulcer dyspepsia

Cost and effectiveness

With the most optimistic estimates for eradication therapy suggesting that one patient will be cured for every 15 treated, the anticipated cost of an eradication strategy in functional dyspepsia is high. For example, if one were to consider 100 dyspeptic patients presenting in primary care, approximately half ($n = 50$) would have non-ulcer dyspepsia. In most developed countries the prevalence of *H. pylori* infection is 20–30% in this population. This would mean that 15–20 patients would have functional dyspepsia and *H. pylori* infection. With the most optimistic estimates of response suggesting a cure in one of 15 patients, it is easy to see that this strategy is unlikely to have a significant impact on dyspepsia with a cure in only one or two patients of 100 presenters with dyspepsia.

Antimicrobial resistance

Treatment for *H. pylori* infection fails in 25–30% of cases, and secondary resistance develops in a significant number of these patients. Clarithromycin resistance rates have been rising in many countries, and treatment of a large number of patients with functional dyspepsia will certainly add to the burden of resistance with *H. pylori*[16,17].

Unknown long-term side-effects of eradication therapy

Labenz *et al.*[18] studied 450 patients with duodenal ulcer disease without evidence of reflux oesophagitis at baseline. They reported data on 244 patients who had successful eradication of *H. pylori* and 216 with persistent infection. All patients underwent annual endoscopy. Using life-table analysis the authors estimated that the incidence of oesophagitis was 25.8% at 3 years in patients with eradication of *H. pylori* compared with 12.9% in patients with ongoing infection. While these results have been contested by other studies, the possibility that eradication of *H. pylori* may have potentially deleterious effects remains a matter of conjecture.

Alternative strategies: acid-suppressive therapy

There have been mixed results with the use of H_2 receptor antagonists in non-ulcer dyspepsia. A recent meta-analysis concluded that there was some benefit, but a large number of the studies had to be excluded from the analysis (only 18 of 150 studies met the inclusion criteria)[19]. This suggests that many studies have been poorly conducted. The overall results suggest that H_2 receptor antagonists have a modest effect. With cimetidine the therapeutic benefit above placebo was 14% (95% CI 3–24%) and with ranitidine the therapeutic benefit was 33% (95% CI 23–43%). A recent Cochrane review suggested that H_2 receptor antagonists were effective (eight trials generating 1125 patients; relative risk reduction 30%; 95% CI 4–48%)[20].

Three recent studies evaluated the effectiveness of proton-pump inhibitors in functional dyspepsia. A total of 1262 patients with functional dyspepsia were enrolled in two studies (BOND or OPERA studies) to omeprazole 20 mg or 10 mg a day or identical placebo for 4 weeks[21]. Complete symptom relief was seen on the last 3 days of therapy in 38% of patients receiving omeprazole 20 mg, 36% in patients receiving omeprazole 10 mg, and 28% on placebo ($p = 0.002$). Symptom relief was similar in patients who were *H. pylori*-positive or -negative. Similar data have been reported in preliminary form with lansoprazole in a US population. Peura *et al.*[22] reported complete symptom relief in 44% of patients given lansoprazole 30 mg for 8 weeks compared to 33% of controls given placebo in a trial lasting 8 weeks. The Cochrane review found four trials with 1248 patients and a relative risk reduction of 12% (95% CI 1–24%)[12].

CONCLUSIONS

The utility of *H. pylori* eradication in non-ulcer dyspepsia is controversial. The most optimistic estimates suggest that only a small number of patients benefit from eradication therapy and there is the risk of adverse effects from the widespread use of eradication therapy in these patients. For any approach to be considered rational in functional dyspepsia it should meet the requirements of efficacy, safety and cost-effectiveness. *H. pylori* eradication does not meet these criteria.

References

1. Talley NJ, Stanghellii V, Heading RC, Koch KL, Malagelada JR, Tytgat GNJ. Functional gastroduodenal disorders. Gut. 1999;45(Suppl. II):1137–42.

2. Kagevi I, Lofstedt S, Persson L-G. Endoscopic findings and diagnoses in unselected dyspeptic patients at a primary health care center. Scand J Gastroenterol. 1989;24:145–50.
3. Gear MWL, Barnes RJ. Endoscopic studies of dyspepsia in general practice. Br Med J. 1980;1: 1136–7.
4. Berensen B, Johnsen R, Bostad L *et al.* Is *Helicobacter pylori* the cause of dyspepsia. Br Med J. 1992;304:1276–9.
5. Schlemper RJ, van der Werf S, Vandenbroucke JP *et al.* Non-ulcer dyspepsia in a Dutch working population and *H. pylori.* Arch Intern Med. 1995;155:82–7.
6. Blum AL, Talley NJ, O'Morain C *et al.* Lack of effect of treating *Helicobacter pylori* infection in patients with nonulcer dyspepsia. N Engl J Med. 1998;339:1875–81.
7. Talley NJ, Jenssens J, Lauritsen K *et al.* Eradication of *Helicobacter pylori* in functional dyspepsia – randomized double blind placebo controlled trial with 12 months follow up. Br Med J. 1999;318: 833–7.
8. Talley NJ, Vakil N, Ballard ED, Fennerty B. Absence of benefit of eradicating *Helicobacter pylori* in patients with nonulcer dyspepsia. N Engl J Med. 1999;341:1106–11.
9. McColl K, Murray L, El-Omar E *et al.* Symptomatic benefit from eradicating *H. pylori* in patients with nonulcer dyspepsia. N Engl J Med. 1998;339:1869–74.
10. Greenberg P, Cello J. Lack of effect of treatment for *Helicobacter pylori* on symptoms of non-ulcer dyspepsia. Arch Intern Med. 1999;159:2283–8.
11. Koelz HR, Arnold R, Stolte M, Blum AL. Treatment of *Helicobacter pylori* does not improve symptoms of functional dyspepsia. Gastroenterology. 1998;114:A182.
12. Miwa H, Hirai S, Nagahara A *et al.* Cure of *H. pylori* infection does not improve symptoms in non-ulcer dyspepsia patients: a double-blind placebo controlled study. Aliment Pharacol Ther. 2000;14:317–24.
13. Malfertheiner P, Fischbach W, Layer P *et al.* ELAN study proves symptomatic benefit of *Helicobacter pylori* eradication in functional dyspepsia. Gastroenterology. 2000;118:A440.
14. Moayyedi P, Soo S, Deeks J *et al.* Systematic review and economic evaluation of *Helicobacter pylori* eradication treatment for non-ulcer dyspepsia. Br Med J. 2000;321:659–64.
15. Laine L. Schoenfeld P, Fennerty MB. *H. pylori* therapy is not effective for treatment of non-ulcer dyspepsia: meta-analysis of randomized controlled trials. Ann Intern Med. 2001;134:361–9.
16. Megraud F, Lehn N, Lind T *et al.* Antimicrobial susceptibility testing of *Helicobacter pylori* in a large multicenter trial: the MACH 2 study. Antimicrob Agents Chemother. 1999;43:2747–52.
17. Vakil N, McSorley D, Hahn B, Ciociola A, Webb D. Clarithromycin resistant *Helicobacter pylori* in the United States. Am J Gastroenterol. 1998;93:1432–5.
18. Labenz J, Blum AL, Bayerdorffer E, Meining A, Stolte M, Borsch G. Curing *Helicobacter pylori* infection in patients with duodenal ulcer may provoke reflux esophagitis. Gastroenterology. 1997;112:1442–7.
19. Finney JS, Kinnersley N, Hughes M, Bryan Tear C, Lothian J. Meta analysis of anti secretory and gastrokinetic compounds in functional dyspepsia. J Clin Gastroenterol. 1998;26:312–20.
20. Soo S. Pharmacological interventions for non-ulcer dyspepsia. Cochrane Database Syst Rev. 2000(2):CD001960.
21. Talley N, Meineche-Schmidt V, Pare P *et al.* Effect of omeprazole in functional dyspepsia: double-blind, randomized, placebo-controlled trials (the Bond and Opera studies). Aliment Pharmacol Ther. 1998;12:1055–65.
22. Peura D, Kovacs T, Metz D, Gudmundson J, Pilmer B. Low-dose lansoprazole: effective for non-ulcer dyspepsia (NUD). Gastroenterology. 2000:A439(abstract).

Section VII
Animal models on the role of inflammation in gastrointestinal function

23
Animal models for visceral sensitivity

T. LIEBREGTS, B. ADAM, J. M. GSCHOSSMANN,
G. GERKEN and G. HOLTMANN

INTRODUCTION

Disturbed gastrointestinal sensory function is believed to play a key role for the development of symptoms in patients with so-called functional gastrointestinal (GI) disorders. While the precise pathomechanisms that are linked to the development of these disturbances are mostly unknown, various factors such as inflammation, stressful life events or genetic differences are postulated to lead to altered sensory function. In clinical studies the incidence of irritable bowel syndrome (IBS) is increased following a *Salmonella* infection[1]. Animal studies have now been used to confirm the concept of postinflammatory alterations of sensory function and to address the precise mechanisms in detail.

Based on the observation that IBS tends to run in families[2], genetically engineered animal models have been examined to determine their influence on the development of visceral hypersensitivity. There is abundant information on the modulation of somatic pain and sensory function; in contrast, limited data are available on the modulation of visceral sensory function.

Currently established animal models differ with regard to two points: (1) the assessment of sensory function and (2) modalities of modulation of sensory thresholds. Key studies and the most important animal models will be reviewed in this chapter.

In general, a nociceptive stimulus can be applied by electrical, thermal, mechanical or chemical means. The response to a stimulus can be detected by measuring a behavioural response such as tail-flicking, paw withdrawal, hyperextension of the hindlimbs, concave arching of the back or licking and biting behaviour, or by measuring alterations of physiological functions such as heart rate or electromyographic (EMG) activity. Gebhart and Ness[3] introduced the frequently used measurement of the visceromotor reflex (VMR). A pseudo-affective response to a colorectal distension (CRD) by a balloon catheter is measured by EMG of the abdominal wall muscles.

STRESS

Neonatal maternal separation and water avoidance

Early life stressors such as physical or sexual abuse or deprivation during child-hood are associated with an increased risk for the development of IBS. Coutinho and co-workers[4] developed a rat model with an early adverse life event in the form of neonatal maternal separation (MS) and also studied the responsiveness of the MS rats to acute water avoidance (WA) stress by recording the VMR to CRD and the somatic sensitivity by measuring the tail-flick latency (TFL) exposing the dorsal surface of the tail to radiant heat and recording the time taken to withdraw the tail from the noxious thermal stimulus. Male Long Evans rat pups underwent MS 180 min daily on postnatal days 2–14 in the study group and were not handled in controls. At the age of 2 months the VMR to CRD and TFL were assessed at baseline and after 60 min acute WA stress. The VMR at baseline and after WA was significantly elevated in the MS rats compared to controls. The cutaneous analgesia, measured by TFL and caused by acute WA stress, was significantly lower in the MS rats compared to controls. These data suggest early life events as a predisposing factor for the development of visceral hyperalgesia and reduced somatic analgesia in adult male Long Evans rats.

The neonatal MS model proved to be a useful tool to further investigate the mechanisms of altered sensory function. The most striking advantage is the possibility to induce long-lasting alterations of perception thresholds at baseline and also to cause hyperresponsiveness to acute stress. Potential morpho-logical or functional changes concerning the enteric or central nervous system following stress in the vulnerable neonatal period need to be investigated further.

Soederholm et al.[5] reported that neonatal MS predisposes adult rats to colonic barrier dysfunction in response to mild stress via mechanisms involving peripher-ally located corticotropin-releasing hormone receptors, and that chronic stress itself induces bacterial adherence initiating mucosal inflammation, supporting the concept of an acute inflammation as a pathogenetic cofactor in the development of altered sensory function. The MS could be a model for at least a subgroup of patients with IBS, and allows us to further investigate stress-related symptoms.

CHEMICAL STIMULATION, INFECTION AND INFLAMMATION

Zymosan

The intracolonic administration of zymosan causes an acute inflammation with extensive crypt damage and an increasing epithelial infiltration with inflammatory cells such as neutrophils. Coutinho et al.[6] assessed the VMR to colorectal distension 1, 2, 3, 4 and 6 h after intracolonic treatment and found an elevated EMG response in zymosan-treated animals compared to saline-treated controls with a maximum at 3–4 h and persisting for up to 6 h. This enhancement of the VMR was produced by noxious visceral stimuli as well as by non-noxious stim-uli, and can be caused by a variety of different mechanisms, because zymosan is known to cause multiple proinflammatory activities such as histamine release, cytokine liberation or intestinal barrier dysfunction with bacterial translocation.

Because of the number of different systems activated by intracolonic administration of zymosan this model might be useful to characterize the interactions of the particular pathway involved. However, the effect on visceral sensitivity seems to be limited to the acute inflammatory phase with a maximum 6h after induction, because no long-term changes are reported to date.

Mustard oil

Mustard oil (MO), which is believed to activate C-fibre nociceptor selectively, and causes neurogenic inflammation, was topically applied in male Sprague-Dawley rat pups and adults (age from 2 days to adult) on the surface area of the left leg by Jiang and Gebhart[7]. The nociceptive response to electrical stimulation of the hind foot was measured by EMG in spinal transected rats at thoracic spinal level T4–T5, or by measuring the TFL in intact rats after MO treatment. The effect of MO on the EMG response to electrical stimulation was multiply recorded for 2h after topical application in EMG experiments and 50min following MO application in tail-flick experiments. These experiments showed age-dependent alterations of visceral sensitivity with an enhancement of EMG response in young rats only to the initial stimulus, which increases in duration with age. The thermal response in tail-flick experiments also decreased in all groups after MO application, but was weak and short-lived in younger rats compared to adults. A hypoalgesic period after initial hyperalgesia was seen in pups, which was not observed in adults. One of the authors' conclusions is that the maturation of MO-produced hyperalgesia might be linked to the conduction velocities of primary afferents which show a peripheral and central delay in young rats. These data interestingly show a long-term facilitation process of nociception from neonates to adults, and suggest a potential role of neuroplastic changes in the development of hyperalgesia.

Capsaicin

Based on the observation made by Giamberardino et al.[8], showing that visceral pain is associated with a referred hyperalgesia of superficial structures such as muscles or body wall parts, Laird et al.[9] invented a mouse model which allows measurement of visceral pain-related behaviours to intracolonic chemical irritation, and a referred hyperalgesia by testing the response to the application of von Frey hairs to the abdomen. Colonic irritation was performed by rectal instillation of saline, MO or capsaicin, and the behavioural response to this chemical stimulation, as well as the response to mechanical stimulation of the abdomen by von Frey hairs, was observed 20min after injection. Intracolonic saline evoked a small number of licking behaviours and was considered as pain-related behaviour, while MO and capsaicin caused significantly greater dose-dependent pain-related behavioural responses. The withdrawal response to mechanical stimulation was significantly enhanced by intracolonic instillation of MO and capsaicin, but not by saline. The inflammatory changes of the colon caused by chemical irritation were determined by plasma extravasation of prior intravenously administered Evans blue. Capsaicin caused a smaller inflammatory reaction than did MO, while saline showed no inflammation at all. With this study the authors offered a model which worked well for further testing acute effects of chemical irritants or pharmacological agents influencing visceral pain and referred hyperalgesia. Some of the potential mechanisms have already been investigated further in a genetically engineered model by Laird *et al.*[10,11], and will be discussed later in this chapter.

Acetic acid

Intracolonic instillation of acetic acid causes a colonic inflammation with typical inflammatory responses with mucosal infiltration by leucocytes. This has been well described in male Sprague-Dawley rats[12]. The colonic mucosa was observed for inflammatory signs at 4, 6, 12 and 24 h after application, and showed a significant increase in leucocytes only at 24 h, which was the last time-point of observation. To quantify the alterations of visceral sensitivity the visceromotor response to phasic noxious colorectal distension was measured 6 and 24 h after treatment as abdominal EMG activity. The resting EMG activity was recorded in untreated as well as in acetic acid- or saline-treated rats. These experiments showed that colonic irritation, either by saline or acetic acid instillation, produced an increase in resting EMG activity compared to untreated rats without any significant difference between saline and acetic acid. The EMG response to CRD was significantly greater after colorectal manipulation than in untreated controls, and was significantly enhanced in acetic acid-treated rats compared to saline-treated controls at both time-points. These data suggest that mechanical irritation causes altered visceral sensitivity, which can be further enhanced by acute inflammation. Because the inflammatory signs were apparent only 24 h after acetic acid treatment, but the changes in EMG response were also observed after 6 h, the presence of inflammation as established by leucocyte infiltration is not a sufficient explanation for the enhancement of the VMR to CRD which might be linked to an early local sensitization by inflammatory mediators before detectable leucocyte infiltration. These experiments nicely showed two different mechanisms (colonic irritation and inflammation) in the development of visceral hyperalgesia, but did not show potential long-term changes in nociception after acute sensitizing events.

Trinitrobenzene sulphonic acid

Treatment with trinitrobenzene sulphonic acid (TNB) after destruction of the mucosal barrier with ethanol causes a colitis with infiltration of inflammatory cells in all layers. CRD experiments in male Lewis rats after intracolonic instillation of TNB were performed by Gschossmann and co-workers[13,14] to assess alterations of visceral sensitivity by measuring the EMG activity of the abdominal wall musculature as a pseudoaffective reflex to a standardized visceral stimulus. The TNB was found to cause a transient colitis with a maximum of histological alterations 5 days after instillation and a complete histological healing at day 14. In two different experiments the effect of a TNB colitis on visceral sensitivity was observed during the acute inflammation with CRDs at days 3, 5 and 14 after instillation and in long-term experiments 2, 4 and 15 weeks after a single intracolonic TNB application. The VMR to CRD reached a transient significant increase compared to saline-treated controls with a maximum at day 5, correlating with the most severe histological tissue alterations, and returned to baseline levels at day 14. In long-term experiments the VMR was significantly enhanced with a maximum at 15 weeks after TNB instillation compared to saline controls. These data showed decreased sensory thresholds during an acute colorectal inflammation and chronic alterations of visceral sensitivity following a transient colitis, strongly supporting the thesis that a transient inflammatory process can trigger long-lasting changes in visceral nociception. This animal model can be used to further investigate the mechanisms potentially involved in long-term alterations of visceral sensory function.

COLORECTAL MANIPULATION

Colon irritation

Mechanical or chemical colon irritation was performed by Al-Chaer and co-workers[15] in postnatal male Sprague-Dawley rats between day 8 and 21 and periadolescent and adult rats starting at postnatal day 21 or 45 by repetitive CRD or intracolonic injection of MO or repetitive perianal touch in control animals. The altered visceral sensitivity was measured by behavioural testing and neuronal recordings from spinal cord neurons at the ages of 5, 6 and 7 weeks, and at 3 months. The abdominal withdrawal reflex showed a persisting significant increase in CRD- and MO-treated neonatal rats compared to controls, and to periadolescent and adult rats which did not differ from controls. The neuronal firing rate was also significantly higher in neonatal rats than in the other groups. These data indicate, similar to the MO experiments performed by Jiang and Gebhart 2 years previously[6], that the nervous system shows a specific vulnerability in the neonatal period.

GENETICALLY ENGINEERED MODELS

Nav 1.8 (SNS/PN3) knockout mice

In the development of visceral hypersensitivity the sensitization of nociceptors is an important pathogenetic factor. This sensitization is postulated to be mediated by voltage-gated sodium channels and has been further investigated by Laird et al.[10] utilizing tetrodotoxin (TTX)-resistant sodium channel α subunit Nav 1.8-deficient mice. The TTX-resistant sodium channel α subunit is known to be expressed exclusively in primary sensory neurons and has been previously described by Akopian et al.[16] Knockout mice (Nav 1.8 null, $-/-$) and littermate wild-type ($+/+$) mice were observed for their behavioural response to intraperitoneal injection of acetylcholine and to colonic stimulation by instillation of saline, capsaicin or MO. Nav 1.8 null mice showed no difference compared to wild-type mice in response to intracolonic saline instillation or intraperitoneal acetylcholine as an acute noxious visceral stimulus, but the behavioural response to capsaicin and to MO was reduced in $-/-$ mice. The authors concluded that the Nav 1.8 is not required for responses to acute noxious visceral stimuli such as intracolonic saline and intraperitoneal acetylcholine, which is known to excite nociceptors without sensitizing them[17], but plays an important role in mediating the activity in sensitized nociceptors because of the altered response to MO and capsaicin which are known to sensitize nociceptors.

Alpha 1b subunit calcium channel-deficient mice

Synaptic transmission at spinal dorsal horn neurons is mediated by calcium influx through N-type calcium channels. Kim *et al.*[18] generated knockout mice for the pore-forming α1B subunit of the calcium channel and measured the response to visceral inflammatory pain caused by subcutaneous injection of formalin into the dorsal surface of the left hindpaw. Writhing tests and paw-withdrawal latency tests were performed to quantify the response. The response to visceral pain was divided into an early phase 1 response (0–10 min) and a late phase 2 response (20–60 min). The formalin at a concentration of 0.2% induced only a first phase response, whereas at a concentration of 2% it induced both a first and second phase response in wild-type mice. The calcium subunit-deficient mice showed a significant decrease in withdrawal latency and writhing motions compared to wild-type mice in phase 2 response after 2% formalin injection without any difference in phase 1 response. However, the phase 2 onset time for α1B knockout mice was 40 min after formalin injection, whereas for wild-type mice onset occurred at 20 min. These data suggest an important role of N-type calcium channels in central processing of visceral nociceptive stimuli because of the difference in phase 2 response representing central sensitization while the early phase 1 response is linked to direct activation of C-fibres by formalin. This animal model characterizes a molecular defect responsible for altered visceral sensory function.

NK-1 knockout mice

Noxious stimuli such as intracolonic instillation of MO or capsaicin are known to excite and sensitize primary sensory nociceptive neurons which, in response, release tachykinins such as substance P, stimulating the neurokinin 1 receptor (NK-1). Partly adapting their above-described model of visceral pain and referred hyperalgesia, Laird *et al.*[11] focused on the role of NK-1 receptors in the nociceptive responses to mechanical and chemical stimulation of the viscera in NK-1 knockout compared to wild-type mice. In a comprehensive study protocol the most interesting part of this work was the altered behavioural response such as licking, stretching, squashing of the abdomen and abduction of the hindpaw caused by chemical stimulation of the colon by intracolonic instillation of MO or capsaicin, which was observed 20 min after manipulation. In wild-type mice (+/+) intracolonic MO and capsaicin evoked a significantly greater spontaneous behavioural response than did saline, without differences between MO and capsaicin. In NK-1 knockout mice (−/−) there was no difference in behavioural response between intracolonic capsaicin and saline. However, colonic instillation of MO in (+/+) mice showed the same effect as in (−/−) mice. The inflammatory changes caused by MO and capsaicin were determined by plasma extravasation of prior intravenously administered Evans blue. In contrast to MO, capsaicin was found to cause a pure neurogenic inflammation. Because of the missing altered behavioural response to intracolonic capsaicin in (−/−) mice the authors concluded that SP and NK-1 receptors play an essential role in mediating central nociceptive responses evoked by neurogenic inflammation, but that there seems to be another NK-1-independent hyperalgesic pathway in response to other inflammatory stimuli because of the enhanced behavioural response of $(-/-)$ mice to intracolonic MO instillation.

CONCLUSION

While clinical studies clearly point to the role of alterations of sensory function for the manifestation of symptoms in patients with functional GI disorders, animal studies have contributed greatly to our current understanding of the mechanisms of visceral sensitivity. While the enigma of functional GI disorder is currently a diagnosis of exclusion, the data from animal studies greatly support the concept that morphological or functional alterations on the level of the receptor, transmitter and the down- or up-regulation of specific genes leads to altered functions causing symptoms in GI disorders. Thus animal models will ultimately contribute to our understanding of the pathomechanisms and may allow us to develop the 'cure' for these disorders.

References

1. McKendrick MW, Read NW. Irritable bowel syndrome–post salmonella infection, J Infect. 1994;29:1–3.
2. Locke GR, Zinsmeister AR, Talley NJ, Fett SL, Melton LJ. Familial association in adults with functional gastrointestinal disorders. Mayo Clin Proc. 2000;75:907–12.
3. Ness TJ, Gebhart GF. Colorectal distension as a noxious visceral stimulus: physiologic and pharmacologic characterizationof pseudaffective reflexes in the rat. Brain Res. 1988;450:153–69.
4. Coutinho SV, Plotsky PM, Sablad M *et al.* Neonatal maternal separation alters stress-induced responses to viscerosomatic nociceptive stimuli in rat. Am J Physiol Gastrointest Liver Physiol. 2002;282:G307–16.
5. Soederholm JD, Yates DA, Gareau MG, Yang PC, McQueen G, Perdue M. Neonatal maternal separation predisposes adult rats to colonic barrier dysfunction in response to mild stress. Am J Physiol Gastrointest Liver Physiol. 2002;283:1257–63.
6. Coutinho SV, Meller ST, Gebhart GF. Intracolonic zymosan produces visceral hyperalgesia in the rat that is mediated by spinal NMDA and non-NMDA receptors. Brain Res. 1996;736:7–15.
7. Jiang MC, Gebhart GF. Development of mustard oil-induced hyperalgesia in rats. Pain. 1998;77:305–13.
8. Giamberardino MA, Valente R, De Bigontina P, Vecchiet L. Artificial ureteral calculosis in rats; behavioural characterization of visceral pain episodes and their relationship with referred lumbar muscle hyperalgesia. Pain. 1995;61:459–69.
9. Laird JMA, Souslova V, Wood JN, Cervero F. Deficits in visceral pain and referred hyperalgesia in Nav 1.8 (SNS/PN3)-null mice. J Neurosci. 2002;22:8352–6.
10. Laird JMA, Martinez-Caro L, Garcia-Nicas E, Cervero F. A new model of visceral pain and referred hyperalgesia in the mouse. Pain. 2001;92:335–42.
11. Laird JMA, Olivar T, Roza C, De Felipe C, Hunt SP, Cervero F. Deficits in visceral pain and hyperalgesia of mice with a disruption of the tachykinin NK1 receptor gene. Neuroscience. 2000;98:345–52.
12. Burton MB, Gebhart GF. Effects of intracolonic acetic acid on response to colorectal distension in the rat. Brain Res. 1995;672:77–82.
13. Gschossmann JM, Adam B, Liebregts T *et al.* Effect of transient chemically induced colitis on the visceromotor response to mechanical colorectal distension. Eur. J Gastroenterol Hepatol. 2002;14:1067–72.
14. Gschossmann JM, Liebregts T, Adam B *et al.* Long-term effects of a transient chemically induced colitis on the visceromotor response to mechanical colorectal distension. (In press.)

15. Al-Chaer ED, Kawasaki M, Pasricha P. A new model of chronic visceral hypersensitivity in adult rats induced by colon irritation during postnatal development. Gastroenterology. 2000;119:1276–85.

16. Akopian AN, Souslova V, England S *et al*. The tetrodotoxin-resistant sodium channel SNS has a specialized function in pain pathways. Nat Neurosci. 1999;2:541–8.

17. Steen KH, Reeh PW. Actions of cholinergic agonists and antagonists on sensory nerve endings in rat skin, *in vitro*. J Neurophysiol. 1993;70:397–405.

18. Kim C, Jun K, Lee T *et al*. Altered nociceptive response in mice deficient in the alpha 1b subunit of the voltage dependent calcium channel. Mol Cell Neurosci. 2001;18:235–45.

24
Descending modulation of visceral hyperalgesia

S. V. COUTINHO and G. F. GEBHART

INTRODUCTION

It is well known that spinal nociceptive transmission is modulated by descending pathways from supraspinal sites. One such site is the midbrain periaqueductal grey (PAG), which has been shown to play a pivotal role in descending modulation (see refs 1–3 for reviews). However, anatomical studies have demonstrated very few direct spinopetal fibres from the PAG to the spinal cord that could account for this modulation[4,5]. Instead, the major output from the PAG projects to the rostral ventromedial medulla (RVM) which contains several nuclei including the nucleus raphe magnus (RMg), reticularis gigantocellularis (Gi) and reticularis paragigantocellularis lateralis (LPGi)[4,6–8]. On the other hand, direct connections from the RVM to the spinal cord have been well documented[4], and numerous studies have demonstrated that the RVM serves as a medullary relay for descending modulation from the PAG. For example, electrical or chemical stimulation in the PAG produces an inhibition of behavioural and spinal dorsal horn neuronal responses, which can be attenuated or blocked by lesions in, or microinjections of local anesthetic into, the RVM[9–11]. Although initial studies focused on the inhibitory nature of descending systems, recent studies have demonstrated that facilitatory modulation can also occur[12–19]. Similar to its cutaneous counterpart, visceral nociceptive transmission is also subject to descending inhibitory and facilitatory modulation[20–23]. This is evident in the responses of dorsal horn neurons at the level of thoracic and lumbar spinal cord to noxious colorectal distension that were inhibited by electrical or chemical stimulation applied within the PAG or the RMg[21,23–27]. More recently the visceromotor response (contraction of abdominal and hind limb musculature), as well as spinal dorsal horn neuronal responses to colorectal distension, have been shown to be modulated in a biphasic manner by chemical stimulation in the brainstem RVM[28–30]. Whereas low doses of glutamate or neurotensin were facilitatory, higher doses were inhibitory. Tonic descending modulation of spinal viscerosensitive neurons has also been reported[23,31,32]. Tattersall et al.[31] observed that responses of neurons at the thoracic spinal level to distension of the biliary system could be attenuated or abolished by a reversible cold block of the cervical spinal cord. Ness and Gebhart[23,32] have demonstrated that responses of spinal dorsal horn neurons to noxious CRD could also be attenuated or enhanced by a reversible cold block (which prevents neurotransmission) of the cervical spinal cord.

Prolonged noxious stimulation or peripheral tissue injury can lead to an altered sensory state of increased sensitivity to pain, a phenomenon known as hyperalgesia. Although it is clear from the aforementioned account that descending systems from supraspinal sites significantly influence spinal nociceptive transmission, studies on mechanisms fundamental to hyperalgesia have focused mainly on peripheral afferent and spinal mechanisms. Investigations of the involvement of descending systems in modulating hyperalgesia are of relatively recent origin[33–38]. A clear involvement of the RVM was demonstrated by Urban et al.[35]. These investigators induced hyperalgesia (facilitation of the tail-flick reflex) by topical application of mustard oil to the hind leg, and this hypersensitivity was abolished by electrolytic lesions in the RVM. Similarly, paw or hind limb or knee joint inflammation-induced facilitation of the paw-withdrawal response was attenuated by chemical inactivation of the RVM[36].

A growing body of evidence suggests that the pain and discomfort accompanying inflammatory and functional bowel disorders represents the equivalent of hyperalgesia (see ref. 39 for review). For example, increased sensitivity to colorectal distension and expanded areas of viscerosomatic referral have been observed in patients with functional bowel disorders[39]. Despite the prevalence of these disorders, our knowledge of visceral hyperalgesia is not very extensive, and the available animal models are scarce. A few models of inflammatory and non-inflammatory visceral hyperalgesia have been developed in non-human animals, that utilize quantification of visceromotor, cardiovascular or behavioural responses to gastrointestinal or colonic inflammation (for example, refs 40–43). As in somatic hyperalgesia models, most studies in these models of visceral hyperalgesia have focused on peripheral (spinal and vagal afferent) mechanisms, and those intrinsic to the spinal cord. While a role for descending pain modulatory systems in modulating visceral hyperalgesia has been proposed[39], the hypothesis has not been extensively tested.

In the following account we will focus on two neurotransmitter systems that play a key role in the descending modulation of visceral hyperalgesia.

ROLE OF SUPRASPINAL EXCITATORY AMINO ACIDS (EAAs)

Numerous investigations have demonstrated a role for EAAs in nociception and hyperalgesia. Although the vast majority of these studies have focused on spinal EAAs, the possible involvement of peripheral EAAs has also received some attention (for example, refs 44–46). In contrast, evidence for the participation of supraspinal EAAs in modulating nociception and hyperalgesia is relatively sparse. EAA receptors have been found to be localized to relevant supraspinal sites including the PAG and RVM, and probably play a role in nociceptive processing[48–50]. Furthermore, glutamate serves as the neurotransmitter of the ascending projections of many dorsal horn nociceptive neurons[51,52] and descending projections from the PAG to the RVM (see ref. 53 for review). Supportive of a role for supraspinal EAAs in nociceptive processing, it has been shown that intracerebral administration of glutamate or N-methyl D-aspartic acid (NMDA) into the RVM results in spontaneous pain-like behaviours[54]. The idea that supraspinal EAA receptors, particularly those in the RVM, are involved in modulating spinal nociceptive transmission via descending projections is further bolstered by recent studies[28,29] in which microinjection of glutamate into the RVM resulted in biphasic effects; low doses were facilitatory whereas higher doses were inhibitory.

Since the RVM is involved in modulating the hyperalgesia following a peripheral cutaneous insult, and because activation of EAA receptors in the RVM modulates spinal nociceptive transmission, we examined the possible participation of EAA receptors in the RVM in a model of inflammatory visceral hyperalgesia. These data appear in a full report elsewhere[55]. Intracolonic instillation of zymosan produces a robust hyperalgesia at 3 h post-treatment, characterized by an increase in the magnitude of the visceromotor response to noxious colorectal distension in awake rats[41]. Microinjection of the selective NMDA receptor antagonist, DL-2-amino-5-phosphonovaleric acid (APV), into the RVM at the 3-h time point dose-dependently and significantly attenuated zymosan-produced visceral hyperalgesia. The onset of effect was within 3–6 min following drug administration and lasted about 30 min. The most effective dose of APV (100 fmol) was without effect in animals treated with intracolonic saline. These data strongly suggest that endogenous activation of NMDA receptors in the RVM following colonic inflammation exerts a descending facilitatory influence and thereby contributes to the visceral hyperalgesia. This conclusion is supported by the fact that administration of the agonist NMDA into the RVM of naïve, uninflamed rats produced a short-lived, receptor-mediated facilitation of the VMR to noxious CRD. It should be pointed out that, while APV attenuated visceral hyperalgesia, it did not completely abolish the response to distension in zymosan-inflamed animals. Furthermore, APV was without effect on the response to noxious CRD in normal, uninflamed animals (i.e. was not analgesic).

In contrast to the effect of APV, intra-RVM microinjection of the non-NMDA receptor antagonist, 6,7-dinitroquinoxaline-2,3-dione (DNQX), 3 h post-zymosan further enhanced the already-exaggerated responses to noxious CRD for about 30 min. The highest dose of DNQX tested (10 nmol) was without effect in uninflamed, saline-treated animals. These results imply that activation of non-NMDA receptors in the RVM mediates descending inhibition of visceral hyperalgesia, but is not involved in mediating normal responses to a noxious visceral stimulus. Altogether, these observations support a role for NMDA and non-NMDA receptors in the RVM in mediating descending facilitation and inhibition, respectively.

ROLE OF SUPRASPINAL NITRIC OXIDE (NO•)

In the spinal cord the ingress of calcium through the activated NMDA receptor channel, and the subsequent production of NO•, leads to a cascade of events that contribute to central sensitization and hyperalgesia (see ref. 56 for review).

Given that zymosan-produced visceral hyperalgesia is modulated by activation of NMDA receptors in the RVM, we also examined the involvement of supraspinal NO•. There is abundant evidence implicating supraspinal NO• in nociceptive modulation. The enzyme nitric oxide synthase (NOS) has been found to be widely distributed throughout the brain, including the RVM, and supraspinal NO• has been shown to promote nociception[57–61].

Three hours post-zymosan inflammation, intra-RVM administration of the NOS inhibitor, N-nitro-L-arginine methyl ester (L-NAME), but not its inactive stereoisomer, N-nitro-D-arginine methyl ester (D-NAME), significantly attenuated zymosan-produced visceral hyperalgesia in a reversible manner without completely abolishing the response to colorectal distension. The time-course of the effect of L-NAME was similar to that observed with APV (30 min duration). Additionally, the highest effective dose of L-NAME (600 nmol) was ineffective in uninflamed animals treated with intracolonic saline. Thus, while production of NO• as a post-NMDA receptor activation event mediates descending facilitation of visceral hyperalgesia, it does not modulate normal responses to colorectal distension.

We further investigated the involvement of NO• in the RVM with the aid of NADPH-diaphorase (NADPH-d) histochemistry and neuronal NOS (nNOS) immunocytochemistry. Consistent with an earlier report[58], we found large stained neurons in the midline RMg and bilaterally in the LPGi in saline-treated animals. Intracolonic instillation of zymosan resulted in a significant increase in NADPH-d-labelled cells in the RMg as well as in the LPGis at the 3-h time point. This increase in NADPH-d suggested either an increase in the enzyme activity of NOS or an induction of the enzyme protein. To address these possibilities we used immunocytochemical staining with an antibody specific for nNOS. The pattern of nNOS immunostaining in the RVMs of control animals was virtually identical to that seen with NADPH-d staining. Large nNOS immunoreactive (nNOS-ir) neurons, morphologically similar to NADPH-d-labelled neurons, were seen in the RMg and bilaterally in the LPGi. Three hours post-zymosan there was a significant increase in the number of nNOS-ir cells in the RMg as well as LPGi, similar in magnitude to the increase in NADPH-d labelling. The profile of stained cells suggested that the cells stained for NADPH-d or nNOS are probably the same. Thus, it appears that colonic inflammation causes the induction of nNOS protein in the RVM. Although nNOS is constitutively expressed, its induction under pathological conditions is not without precedent[62,63].

These observations document a role for supraspinal NO•, produced as a consequence of induction of nNOS and activation of NMDA receptors in the RVM in mediating descending facilitation.

SUMMARY

It appears that intracolonic instillation of zymosan produces colonic inflammation which engages two concurrent, but opposing, descending modulatory systems from the RVM: a facilitatory system mediated by activation of NMDA receptors and production of NO•, and an inhibitory component mediated by activation of non-NMDA receptors. These systems counter each other, and the balance between the two determines the magnitude of the hyperalgesia. We, as well as others, have examined the role of descending systems in models of cutaneous hyperalgesia and have obtained complementary results[19,35,36]. Although intra-colonic zymosan sensitizes colonic afferent fibres, they revert to control (pre-zymosan) at $3\,h^{64}$, a time at which the hyperalgesia is robust and descending systems are active. The counteraction between descending facilitation and inhibition results in a net facilitatory effect, which maintains the visceral hyperalgesia in this model. Such an imbalance in descending modulation may provide a plausible mechanistic basis to account for the visceral hyperalgesia accompanying functional and inflammatory bowel diseases.

References

1. Basbaum AI, Fields HL. Endogenous pain control systems: brainstem spinal pathways and endorphin circuitry. Annu Rev Neurosci. 1984;7:309–38.
2. Fields HL, Heinricher MM, Mason P. Neurotransmitters in nociceptive modulatory circuits. Annu Rev Neurosci. 1991;14:219–45.
3. Millan MJ. Descending control of pain. Prog Neurobiol. 2002;66:355–474.
4. Mantyh PW, Peschanski M. Spinal projections from the periaqueductal grey and dorsal raphe in the rat, cat and monkey. Neuroscience. 1982;7:2769–76.
5. Mantyh PW. The terminations of the spinothalamic tract in the cat. Neurosci Lett. 1983;38:119–24.
6. Abols IA, Basbaum AI. Afferent connections of the rostral medulla of the cat: a neural substrate for midbrain–medullary interactions in the modulation of pain. J Comp Neurol. 1981;201:285–97.
7. Beitz AJ. The nuclei of origin of brain stem enkephalin and substance P projections to the rodent nucleus raphe magnus. Neuroscience. 1982;7:2753–68.
8. Marchand JE, Hagino N. Afferents to the periaqueductal gray in the rat. A horseradish peroxidase study. Neuroscience. 1983;9:95–106.
9. Gebhart GF, Sandkuhler J, Thalhammer JG, Zimmermann M. Inhibition of spinal nociceptive information by stimulation in midbrain of the cat is blocked by lidocaine microinjected in nucleus raphe magnus and medullary reticular formation. J Neurophysiol. 1983;50:1446–59.
10. Sandkuhler J, Gebhart GF. Relative contributions of the nucleus raphe magnus and adjacent medullary reticular formation to the inhibition by stimulation in the periaqueductal gray of a spinal nociceptive reflex in the pentobarbital-anesthetized rat. Brain Res. 1984;305:77–87.
11. Prieto GJ, Cannon JT, Liebeskind JC. N. raphe magnus lesions disrupt stimulation-produced analgesia from ventral but not dorsal midbrain areas in the rat. Brain Res. 1983;261:53–7.
12. Haber LH, Martin RF, Chung IM, Willis WD. Inhibition and excitation of primate spinothalamic tract neurons by stimulation in region of nucleus reticularis gigantocellularis. J Neurophysiol. 1980;43:1578–93.
13. Light AR, Casale EJ, Menetrey DM. The effects of focal stimulation in nucleus raphe magnus and periaqueductal gray on intracellularly recorded neurons in spinal laminae I and II. J Neurophysiol. 1986;56:555–71.
14. Zhuo M, Gebhart GF. Biphasic modulation of spinal nociceptive transmission from the medullary raphe nuclei in the rat. J Neurophysiol. 1997;78:746–58.
15. Zhuo M, Gebhart GF. Characterization of descending facilitation and inhibition of spinal nociceptive transmission from the nuclei reticularis gigantocellularis and gigantocellularis pars alpha in the rat. J Neurophysiol. 1992;67:1599–614.
16. Urban MO, Gebhart GF. Characterization of biphasic modulation of spinal nociceptive transmission by neurotensin in the rat rostral ventromedial medulla. J Neurophysiol. 1997;78:1550–62.
17. Fields HL, Basbaum AI, Clanton CH, Anderson SD. Nucleus raphe magnus inhibition of spinal cord dorsal horn neurons. Brain Res. 1977;126:441–53.
18. McMahon SB, Wall PD. Descending excitation and inhibition of spinal cord lamina I projection neurons. J Neurophysiol. 1988;59:1204–19.
19. Porreca F, Ossipov MH, Gebhart GF. Chronic pain and medullary descending facilitation. Trends Neurosci. 2002;25:319–25.
20. Giesler GJ Jr, Liebeskind JC. Inhibition of visceral pain by electrical stimulation of the periaqueductal gray matter. Pain. 1976;2:43–8.

21. Cervero F, Lumb BM, Tattersall JE. Supraspinal loops that mediate visceral inputs to thoracic spinal cord neurones in the cat: involvement of descending pathways from raphe and reticular formation. Neurosci Lett. 1985;56:189–94.
22. Tattersall JE, Cervero F, Lumb BM. Viscerosomatic neurons in the lower thoracic spinal cord of the cat: excitations and inhibitions evoked by splanchnic and somatic nerve volleys and by stimulation of brain stem nuclei. J Neurophysiol. 1986;56:1411–23.
23. Ness TJ, Gebhart GF. Quantitative comparison of inhibition of visceral and cutaneous spinal nociceptive transmission from the midbrain and medulla in the rat. J Neurophysiol. 1987;58:850–65.
24. Ammons WS. Cardiopulmonary sympathetic afferent excitation of lower thoracic spinoreticular and spinothalamic neurons. J Neurophysiol. 1990;64:1907–16.
25. Ammons WS, Blair RW, Foreman RD. Raphe magnus inhibition of primate T1–T4 spinothalamic cells with cardiopulmonary visceral input. Pain. 1984;20:247–60.
26. Chandler MJ, Garrison DW, Brennan TJ, Foreman RD. Effects of chemical and electrical stimulation of the midbrain on feline T2–T6 spinoreticular and spinal cell activity evoked by cardiopulmonary afferent input. Brain Res. 1989;496:148–64.
27. Chapman CD, Ammons WS, Foreman RD. Raphe magnus inhibition of feline T1–T4 spinoreticular tract cell responses to visceral and somatic inputs. J Neurophysiol. 1985;53:773–85.
28. Zhuo M, Sengupta JN, Gebhart GF. Biphasic modulation of spinal visceral nociceptive transmission from the rostroventral medial medulla in the rat. J Neurophysiol. 2002;87:2225–36.
29. Zhuo M, Gebhart GF. Facilitation and attenuation of a visceral nociceptive reflex from the rostroventral medulla in the rat. Gastroenterology. 2002;122:1007–19.
30. Urban MO, Coutinho SV, Gebhart GF. Biphasic modulation of visceral nociception by neurotensin in rat rostral ventromedial medulla. J Pharmacol Exp Ther. 1999;290:207–13.
31. Tattersall JE, Cervero F, Lumb BM. Effects of reversible spinalization on the visceral input to viscerosomatic neurons in the lower thoracic spinal cord of the cat. J Neurophysiol. 1986;56:785–96.
32. Ness TJ, Gebhart GF. Characterization of neurons responsive to noxious colorectal distension in the T13–L2 spinal cord of the rat. J Neurophysiol. 1988;60:1419–38.
33. Wiertelak EP, Furness LE, Horan R, Martinez J, Maier SF, Watkins LR. Subcutaneous formalin produces centrifugal hyperalgesia at a non-injected site via the NMDA-nitric oxide cascade. Brain Res. 1994;649:19–26.
34. Ren K, Dubner R. Enhanced descending modulation of nociception in rats with persistent hindpaw inflammation. J Neurophysiol. 1996;76:3025–37.
35. Urban MO, Jiang MC, Gebhart GF. Participation of central descending nociceptive facilitatory systems in secondary hyperalgesia produced by mustard oil. Brain Res. 1996;737:83–91.
36. Urban MO, Zahn PK, Gebhart GF. Descending facilitatory influences from the rostral medial medulla mediate secondary, but not primary hyperalgesia in the rat. Neuroscience. 1999;90:349–52.
37. Ren K, Ruda MA. Descending modulation of Fos expression after persistent peripheral inflammation. NeuroReport. 1996;7:2186–90.
38. Pogatzki EM, Urban MO, Brennan TJ, Gebhart GF. Role of the rostral medial medulla in the development of primary and secondary hyperalgesia after incision in the rat. Anesthesiology. 2002;96:1153–60.
39. Mayer EA, Gebhart GF. Basic and clinical aspects of visceral hyperalgesia. Gastroenterology. 1994;107:271–93.
40. Coutinho SV, Plotsky PM, Sablad M et al. Neonatal maternal separation alters stress-induced responses to viscerosomatic nociceptive stimuli in rat. Am J Physiol Gastrointest Liver Physiol. 2002;282:G307–16.
41. Coutinho SV, Meller ST, Gebhart GF. Intracolonic zymosan produces visceral hyperalgesia in the rat that is mediated by spinal NMDA and non-NMDA receptors. Brain Res. 1996;736:7–15.
42. Al-Chaer ED, Kawasaki M, Pasricha PJ. A new model of chronic visceral hypersensitivity in adult rats induced by colon irritation during postnatal development. Gastroenterology. 2000;119:1276–85.
43. Laird JM, Martinez-Caro L, Garcia-Nicas E, Cervero F. A new model of visceral pain and referred hyperalgesia in the mouse. Pain. 2001;92:335–42.
44. Carlton SM, Hargett GL, Coggeshall RE. Localization and activation of glutamate receptors in unmyelinated axons of rat glabrous skin. Neurosci Lett. 1995;197:25–8.
45. Jackson DL, Graff CB, Richardson JD, Hargreaves KM. Glutamate participates in the peripheral modulation of thermal hyperalgesia in rats. Eur J Pharmacol. 1995;284:321–5.

46. Zhou S, Bonasera L, Carlton SM. Peripheral administration of NMDA, AMPA or KA results in pain behaviors in rats. NeuroReport. 1996;7:895–900.
47. Coderre TJ, Katz J, Vaccarino AL, Melzack R. Contribution of central neuroplasticity to pathological pain: review of clinical and experimental evidence. Pain. 1993;52:259–85.
48. Clements JR, Madl JE, Johnson RL, Larson AA, Beitz AJ. Localization of glutamate, glutaminase, aspartate and aspartate aminotransferase in the rat midbrain periaqueductal gray. Exp Brain Res. 1987;67:594–602.
49. Beitz AJ. Relationship of glutamate and aspartate to the periaqueductal gray-raphe magnus projection: analysis using immunocytochemistry and microdialysis. J Histochem Cytochem. 1990;38:1755–65.
50. Tolle TR, Berthele A, Zieglgansberger W, Seeburg PH, Wisden W. The differential expression of 16 NMDA and non-NMDA receptor subunits in the rat spinal cord and in periaqueductal gray. J Neurosci. 1993;13:5009–28.
51. De Biasi S, Amadeo A, Spreafico R, Rustioni A. Enrichment of glutamate immunoreactivity in lemniscal terminals in the ventropostero lateral thalamic nucleus of the rat: an immunogold and WGA-HRP study. Anat Rec. 1994;240:131–40.
52. Magnusson KR, Clements JR, Larson AA, Madl JE, Beitz AJ. Localization of glutamate in trigeminothalamic projection neurons: a combined retrograde transport-immunohistochemical study. Somatosens Res. 1987;4:177–90.
53. Gebhart GF. Descending inhibition of nociceptive transmission. In: Olesen J, Edvinsson L, editors. Basic Mechanisms of Headache. Amsterdam: Elsevier; 1988: 201–12.
54. Jensen TS, Yaksh TL. Brainstem excitatory amino acid receptors in nociception: microinjection mapping and pharmacological characterization of glutamate-sensitive sites in the brainstem associated with algogenic behavior. Neuroscience. 1992;46:535–47.
55. Coutinho SV, Urban MO, Gebhart GF. Role of glutamate receptors and nitric oxide in the rostral ventromedial medulla in visceral hyperalgesia. Pain. 1998;78:59–69.
56. Meller ST, Gebhart GF. Nitric oxide (NO) and nociceptive processing in the spinal cord. Pain. 1993;52:127–36.
57. Moore PK, Oluyomi AO, Babbedge RC, Wallace P, Hart SL. L-NG-nitro arginine methyl ester exhibits antinociceptive activity in the mouse. Br J Pharmacol. 1991;102:198–202.
58. Vincent SR, Kimura H. Histochemical mapping of nitric oxide synthase in the rat brain. Neuroscience. 1992;46:755–84.
59. Kawabata A, Umeda N, Takagi H. L-Arginine exerts a dual role in nociceptive processing in the brain: involvement of the kyotorphin–Met-enkephalin pathway and NO-cyclic GMP pathway. Br J Pharmacol. 1993;109:73–9.
60. Semos ML, Headley PM. The role of nitric oxide in spinal nociceptive reflexes in rats with neurogenic and non-neurogenic peripheral inflammation. Neuropharmacology. 1994;33:1487–97.
61. Shibuta S, Mashimoto T, Ohara A, Zhang P, Yoshiya I. Intracerebroventricular administration of a nitric oxide-releasing compound, NOC-18, produces thermal hyperalgesia in rats. Neurosci Lett. 1995;187:103–6.
62. Zhang ZG, Chopp M, Gautam S et al. Upregulation of neuronal nitric oxide synthase and mRNA, and selective sparing of nitric oxide synthase-containing neurons after focal cerebral ischemia in rat. Brain Res. 1994;654:85–95.
63. Saxon DW, Beitz AJ. Induction of NADPH-diaphorase/nitric oxide synthase in the brainstem trigeminal system resulting from cerebellar lesions. J Comp Neurol. 1996;371:41–71.
64. Coutinho SV, Su X, Sengupta JN, Gebhart GF. Role of sensitized pelvic nerve afferents from the inflamed rat colon in the maintenance of visceral hyperalgesia. Prog Brain Res. 2000; 129:375–87.

Section VIII
Role of acute bacterial infections in irritable bowel syndrome

25
Epidemiology and clinical impact of post-infectious irritable bowel syndrome

J. HAMMER

INTRODUCTION

Irritable bowel syndrome (IBS) is a chronic disorder of the gastrointestinal function that is common in the community and affects approximately 15–20% of the general population[1]. No specific pathophysiological mechanism is known; however, there is increasing evidence that some patients develop IBS after an episode of acute gastroenteritis. Data from animal studies have demonstrated that altered gut physiology can persist even after an infection and its associated inflammation have resolved[2]. In a subgroup of IBS patients symptoms begin after an acute gastrointestinal illness[3,4]. Chaudhary and Truelove suggested that 33% of patients recovering from enteric infection go on to develop symptoms of functional gastrointestinal disease, suffering mainly from symptoms of functional diarrhoea[4]. Others have suggested that a history of acute gastroenteritis is associated with chronic bile acid malabsorption that, in turn, causes chronic diarrhoea[5]. Clinical practice seems to confirm that a considerable number of patients with IBS describe an acute onset of symptoms which has been taken to indicate an infectious origin; however, this line of research has not been taken up by other investigators until recently, when the potential role of infection and low-grade inflammation and its treatment again received increasing attention.

EPIDEMIOLOGY OF POST-INFECTIOUS IBS

A history of acute gastroenteritis has been identified as a major risk factor for the development of IBS. The relative risk of developing IBS after an acute gastroenteritis is 6.6–11.9%, as suggested by two prospective studies using non-infected controls[6,7]. Among the patients with IBS consulting a physician, approximately 10–30% describe acute onset of their bowel disturbance following an acute infective enteritis. The rate of patients reporting acute onset of symptoms seems to depend on the country and subgroups of patients being referred. Seventeen per cent of IBS patients in two primary-care networks in the United Kingdom reported a history of symptoms beginning with an acute diarrhoeal illness[8]. In contrast, only 6% of patients who have been referred to a gastroenterologist in the United States reported acute onset of symptoms[8].

Several bacterial agents have been implicated in the pathogenesis of post-infectious IBS, and persistent bowel symptoms 3–12 months after infective gastroenteritis have been reported in 7–30% of patients[9–11]. Twelve out of 38 patients with *Salmonella* enteritis reported symptoms of bowel dysfunction 12 months after the acute infection despite documented clearance of the organism[9]. In 386 patients with confirmed bacterial gastroenteritis, 90 (23%) reported persistently altered bowel habits 6 months after clearance of the bacteria[10]. The majority of patients had an infection with *Campylobacter* (65%), followed by *Salmonella* (30%) and *Shigella* (5%). The prevalence of IBS symptoms 6 months after infection was independent of the bacterial species. The changes in bowel habit were mainly towards more frequent and looser stools and urgent defaecation (Table 1)[10].

The risk of developing IBS symptoms following a gastrointestinal infection increases with the duration of the acute disease, with female gender, the absence of vomiting and with the presence of psychosocial stressors during or after the time of infection[9–11]. Patients with diarrhoea lasting more than 22 days had a relative risk of 11.4 of developing IBS compared with those with diarrhoea for less than a week (Table 2). Patients who developed IBS 3 months after a bout of acute gastroenteritis had significantly higher anxiety, somatization and neurotic scores at the time of the initial illness compared to patients who did not develop IBS (Table 3). Patients who developed post-infectious IBS also reported a higher number of adverse life events – ranging from minor illness to a bereavement and a break-up in a relationship – in the 12 months leading up to the acute illness and in the 3 months following gastroenteritis[11].

Table 1 Mean number of days each week with symptoms 6 months before and 6 months after bacterial gastroenteritis in people who reported symptoms compatible with IBS (from ref. 10)

Symptom	*Mean days/week*		
	Before illness	*After illness*	p-*Value*
Abdominal pain	0.7	1.7	< 0.001
Loose/watery stools	0.8	2.4	< 0.001
Hard/lumpy stools	1.6	1.4	0.9
Straining	1.0	1.0	0.5
Rushing to the toilet	0.7	1.8	< 0.001
Reopening bowels	0.7	1.9	< 0.001
Slime or mucus	0.4	1.1	0.002
Bloated abdomen	1.3	2.7	< 0.001
Loosening clothing	0.8	1.8	< 0.001

Table 2 Relative risks for development of IBS in people after acute gastroenteritis (from ref. 10)

Factor	Adjusted relative risk (95% CI)
Gender	
Male	1.0
Female	3.39 (1.2–9.8)
Duration of diarrhoea	
< 1 week	1.0
1–2 weeks	2.94 (0.6–15)
2–3 weeks	6.46 (1.3–34)
> 3 weeks	11.37 (2.2–58)

Table 3 Psychometric scores of patients with acute gastroenteritis at the time of acute illness depending on whether they develop IBS 3 months later or not (from ref. 11) (mean ± SD)

	Three months after initial disease		
	Developed IBS	No IBS	p-Value
Anxiety score[*]	8.3 ± 4.6	5.7 ± 3.4	0.01
Somatization score	3.1 ± 2.5	1.5 ± 1.6	0.003
Neuroticism score[†]	11.7 ± 4.7	8.4 ± 4.9	0.008
Life event score[‡]			
(1 year before illness)	4.6 ± 3.3	2.4 ± 1.9	0.001
Life event score[‡]			
(3 months after illness)	2.0 ± 2.2	0.7 ± 0.9	0.001
Hypochondriasis score[§]	3.1 ± 2.5	1.7 + 1.8	0.02

* Hospital Anxiety and Depression Scale (HAD).
† Eysenck Personality Inventory.
‡ Life Event Inventory.
§ Whiteley Index of Hypochondriasis (WIH).

CLINICAL FEATURES OF POST-INFECTIOUS IBS

Patients with post-infectious IBS differ from those with non-infective disease by having more diarrhoeal features[10,12]. Six months after the acute illness, as well as 6 years thereafter, the majority of patients with post-infectious IBS have either diarrhoea-predominant or alternating IBS according to Rome II criteria[13] (Table 4).

PROGNOSIS OF POST-INFECTIOUS IBS

IBS is a chronic, yet often remitting, condition; episodes of active symptoms are followed by periods of relative inactivity. Earlier studies using less precise criteria for IBS suggested that the prognosis of post-infectious functional gastrointestinal disease might be better compared to non-post-infectious functional

Table 4 Clinical presentation of IBS 6 years after bacterial gastroenteritis*

	Post-infectious IBS	New-onset IBS
IBS subtype		
Diarrhoea-predominant IBS	36%	15%
Alternating IBS	57%	60%
Constipation-predominant IBS	7%	25%
Days with abdominal pain (mean ± SEM)	3.2 ± 0.4	2.8 ± 0.3
Loose stools (days/week)	3.4 ± 0.7	2.0 ± 0.2
Urgency (days/week)	2.6 ± 0.6	2.6 ± 0.3

* Patients with IBS who developed symptoms within 6 months after bacterial gastroenteritis (post-infectious IBS) are compared to patients with IBS who developed symptoms during the 6-year follow up (new-onset IBS)[12].

disease[4]. In a prospective follow-up study 6 years after an acute gastroenteritis, however, Neal *et al.* found that 43% of patients who had post-infectious IBS 6 months after the acute illness recovered over a 6-year period; this prognosis was statistically not different compared with the prognosis of patients who already had IBS before they experienced their infection (31%)[12]. Both female sex and past history of psychological treatment were identified as risk factors associated with a worse prognosis[12].

TREATMENT OF POST-INFECTIOUS IBS

The high prevalence of symptoms compatible with IBS following acute gastroenteritis suggests that inflammation plays a role in the pathogenesis of some patients with IBS. In view of the increasing evidence of histological abnormalities in IBS[14], interventions that might reduce the inflammation might have utility, and several agents have been tested very recently.

Corticosteroids

In a randomized, double-blind, placebo-controlled trial of prednisolone in post-infectious IBS 3 or more months after their initial infection, 31 patients received either oral prednisolone at a dose of 30 mg per day or placebo for a period of 3 weeks[15]. CD3 lymphocyte counts in the lamina propria correlated with the IBS symptom score at initial presentation. Although the CD3 counts fell similarly following both treatment with placebo and prednisolone, no reduction in symptom scores was seen with prednisolone as was seen with placebo.

Antibiotics

The use of antibiotics in IBS is controversial; antibiotics may predispose to IBS in some patients as well as protecting in other patients[16,17]. Patients receiving antibiotic therapy for *Helicobacter pylori* were significantly less likely to develop IBS in the following 2 years than those who received placebo[18]. IBS patients receiving 500 mg neomycin twice daily for 10 days showed a 39% improvement in symptoms, compared to 12% with placebo[19]. Bowel habits improved in 40% of patients receiving neomycin but in only 15% receiving placebo. However, which groups of IBS patients might benefit from antibiotic treatment, the length of therapy and safety issues remain to be determined.

Probiotics

Lactobacillus plantarum 299V has been shown to improve abdominal pain and bowel habit in constipated patients compared to placebo[20]. IBS patients who received *Bifidobacterium* sp. once daily for 8 weeks showed a significant improvement in pain, bloating, and difficulty in bowel movement[21]. Thus, although results on the effect of probiotics are encouraging, their use in IBS remains investigational for the time being.

References

1. Talley NJ, Zinsmeister AR, van Dyke C, Melton LJ. Epidemiology of colonic symptoms and the irritable bowel syndrome. Gastroenterology. 1991;1001:927–34.
2. Barbara G, De Giorgio R, Deng Y *et al*. Role of immunologic factors and cyclooxygenase 2 in persistent postinfective enteric muscle dysfunction in mice. Gastroenterology. 2001;120:1729–36.
3. Stewart GT. Post-dysenteric colitis. Br Med J. 1950;3:405–9.
4. Chaudhary NA, Truelove SC. The irritable bowel syndrome. Q J Med. 1962;123:307–22.
5. Niaz SK, Sandrasegaran K, Renny FH, Jones BJ. Postinfective diarrhoea and bile acid malabsorption. J R Coll Phys Lond. 1997;31:53–6.
6. Ilnyckyj A, Choudhri SH, Duerksen D. Association of travel-related diarrhea (TD) with irritable bowel syndrome (IBS): is post-infectious IBS a true entitiy? Gastroenterology. 1999;116:A1011.
7. Rodriguez LA, Ruigomez A. Increased risk of irritable bowel syndrome after bacterial gastroenteritis: cohort study. Br Med J. 1999;318:565–6.
8. Longstreth GF, Hawkey CJ, Mayer EA *et al*. Characteristics of patients with irritable bowel syndrome recruited from three sources: implication for clinical trials. Aliment Pharmacol Ther. 2001;15:959–64.
9. McKendrick MW, Read NW. Irritable bowel syndrome – post *Salmonella* infection. J Infect. 1994;29:1–3.
10. Neal KR, Hebden J, Spiller R. Prevalence of gastrointestinal symptoms six months after bacterial gastroenteritis and risk factors for development of the irritable bowel syndrome: postal survey of patients. Br Med J. 1997;314:779–82.
11. Gwee KA, Leong YL, Graham C *et al*. The role of psychological and biological factors in postinfective gut dysfunction. Gut. 1999;44:400–6.
12. Neal KR, Barker L, Spiller RC. Prognosis in post-infective irritable bowel syndrome: a six year follow up study. Gut. 2002;51:410–13.
13. Thompson WG, Longstreth GF, Drossman DA *et al*. Functional bowel disorders and functional abdominal pain. Gut. 1999;45(Suppl. 2):II43–7.
14. Spiller RC, Jenkins D, Thornley JP *et al*. Increased rectal mucosal enteroendocrine cells, T lymphocytes and increased gut permeability following acute *Campylobacter* enteritis and in post-dysenteric irritable bowel syndrome. Gut. 2000;47:804–11.
15. Dunlop S, Jenkins D, Naesdal J *et al*. Randomised double-blind placebo-controlled trial of prednisolone in post-infectious irritable bowel syndrome (PI-IBS). Gastroenterology. 2002;122:A60.
16. Mendall MA, Kumar D. Antibiotic use, childhood affluence and irritable bowel syndrome (IBS). Eur J Gastroenterol Hepatol. 1998;10:59–62.
17. Pimentel M, Chow EJ, Lin HC. Eradication of small intestinal bacterial overgrowth reduces symptoms of irritable bowel syndrome. Am J Gastroenterol. 2000;95:3503–6.
18. Moayyedi P, Duffett S, Mason S *et al*. The influence of antibiotics on irritable bowel syndrome: a randomised controlled trial. Gastroenterology. 2002;122:A465.
19. Pimentel M, Chow E, Lin H. Neomycin leads to a dramatic improvement in IBS symptoms that depend on lactulose breath test findings: a double blind randomized placebo controlled study. Gastroenterology. 2002;122:A60.

20. Niedzielin K, Kordecki H, Birkenfeld B. A controlled, double-blind, randomized study on the efficacy of *Lactobacillus plantarum 299V* in patients with irritable bowel syndrome. Eur J Gastroenterol Hepatol. 2001;13:1143–7.
21. Quigley E, O'Mahony L, McCarthy J *et al*. Probiotics for the irritable bowel syndrome (IBS): a randomized, double-blind, placebo-controlled comparison of *Lactobacillus* and *Bifidobacterium* strains. Gastroenterology. 2002;122:A59.

26
Potential mechanisms and therapeutic implications of bacterial infection in irritable bowel syndrome

R. C. SPILLER

NORMAL RESPONSE TO ENTERIC INFECTION

Bacterial infection is a non-random event, which is more likely in younger males, those who eat out frequently, and those who travel to tropical countries. The end result is usually diarrhoea, often associated with vomiting. This is part of a protective mechanism designed to minimize bacterial load and expel pathogens as rapidly as possible. This occurs before any antibody response and depends on 'innate' rather than 'acquired' immunity. These defensive mechanisms include gastric acid, bile salts and mucus secretion, together with a range of complex antibacterial compounds, defensins and cryptins derived from Paneth cells. Serotonin, via its interaction with mucosal nerves, also plays an important part in orchestrating the secretion of fluid and the induction of specific motor patterns such as vomiting and diarrhoea.

POST-INFECTIVE IRRITABLE BOWEL SYNDROME (PI-IBS)

These beneficial effects are usually short-lived, but when prolonged can be regarded as a disease, PI-IBS. The outcome of such an event depends on prior bowel habit; some patients who are constipated are actually improved by this illness, while for the majority of those with a normal bowel habit, increased frequency and urgency is regarded as a disorder. The outcome also depends on prior exposure, and in countries where infants or young children are exposed to multiple infections, infections are often asymptomatic and much milder[1]. This is associated with acquired immunity via the secretion of mucosal antibodies[2,3] and alterations in mucosal function and structure, which are inadequately character-ized. Following enteric infection between 7% and 17% of individuals with a normal previous bowel habit develop persistent bowel symptoms compatible with IBS[4,5]. A substantial further number (8–18%) have similar disturbed bowel function which does not meet the threshold criteria for IBS. These symptoms, which consist largely of increased bowel frequency and loose stools, may persist for many years[6]. Most studies of PI-IBS have excluded those with pre-existing IBS, but those which have examined such patients, find that they are more likely to submit a stool sample and be included in a survey[7]. They are also, by virtue of their focus on bowel symptoms, more likely to return questionnaires. In the Nottingham experience the illnesses were similar in severity to those experienced by those with previously normal bowel habit, though such people were more likely to consult their general practitioners.

INITIAL ILLNESS

The symptoms of the original illness are shown in Table 1. As shown, severity of the initial illness was greater in those with a persistent change in bowel habit. Those developing IBS, and those with a change in bowel habit not amounting to IBS, experienced a similar severity of initial symptoms but both were significantly more affected than those who recovered completely. Those with pre-existing IBS had a similar illness to the others but consulted their GP more often. Six months later, persistent symptoms showed a similar graded response, with those developing PI-IBS being most affected. Those with a change in bowel habit not amounting to IBS showed intermediate symptoms, while those who recovered completely showed the least symptoms (Table 2). As shown, symptoms at 6 months show that PI-IBS is characterized by frequent abdominal pain, urgency and loose stools with increased bowel frequency. The only difference from pre-existing IBS is a greater tendency to diarrhoea, this feature persisting for many years[8].

Bowel habit before the illness has a persisting influence on bowel habit afterwards, as can be seen by the correlation between these two parameters seen in a study of *Campylobacter* infection (Fig. 1)[6]. Infection may increase bowel frequency, but since this is influenced by many other factors, including genetics, diet, social habits, and personality, the outcome is still dependent on the initial habit.

Table 1

	Pre-existing IBS	Post-infectious IBS	Changed bowel habit but not IBS	Normal bowel habit
n	21	24	98	299
Maximum bowel frequency	27 ± 7	21 ± 5	21 ± 3	13 ± 0.1
Duration of initial illness	23 ± 7	21 ± 5	21 ± 3	13 ± 0.01
Time off work	38 ± 10	21 ± 5	14 ± 3	14 ± 0.2
Percentage consulting GP	38	29	28	7

Table 2 Symptoms at 6 months (mean ± SEM)

Symptom	Pre-existing IBS	Post-infectious IBS	Changed bowel habit but not IBS	Normal bowel habit
Days of abdominal pain	2.4 ± 0.3	3.7 ± 0.4	1.9 ± 0.3	0.6 ± 0.01
Days/week with urgency	2.5 ± 0.5	2.8 ± 0.5	1.6 ± 0.2	0.6 ± 0.01
Days/week with loose stool	1.9 ± 0.3	3.0 ± 0.3	2.2 ± 0.2	1.1 ± 0.01

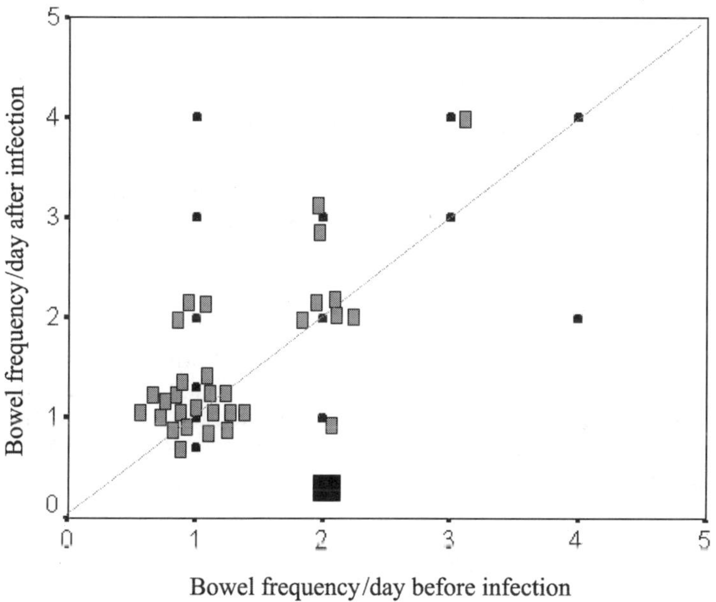

Fig. 1

PHYSIOLOGICAL CHANGES FOLLOWING INFECTION

As anyone who has ever experienced gastroenteritis knows, there is clearly a shortening in whole-gut transit time during the acute illness, and increased rectal irritability. Three months later this is still obvious, as was shown by Gwee and colleagues who demonstrated a 50% reduction in transit time[9]. All those experiencing infection showed response in the same direction, but those who developed IBS were more affected than those who did not. Gwee also studied rectal sensitivity, and showed a similar pattern with increased sensitivity. The mechanism of this is unclear, since others have shown that merely inducing diarrhoea can increase rectal sensitivity. Frequent defaecation may introduce minor trauma in the rectum which, with the release of inflammatory mediators such as prostaglandins, may contribute to rectal hypersensitivity. Other mucosal changes will be described below.

ROLE OF BACTERIAL TOXINS AND SEVERITY OF ILLNESS IN PREDICTING LONG-TERM OUTCOME

Several studies have shown that the severity of the initial illness is a predictor of subsequent outcome[4,10]. Those with an illness lasting more than 3 weeks were 11 times more likely to develop PI-IBS, the risk rising with each additional week the initial illness lasted (Table 3). The severity of the initial illness does, of course, depend on the nature of the bacterial infection. Those infected with either *Campylobacter jejuni* or *Shigella* have a 10% chance of developing PI-IBS, but there was only a 1% incidence after *Salmonella* infection[4]. Shigellosis and *Campylobacter* infection both cause severe mucosal damage characterized by painful bloody diarrhoea. Most of the *Salmonella* in our survey were *Salmonella enteritidis*, which generally gives a much milder illness. When focusing on a single bacterium such as *C. jejuni*, the presence of different toxins can be explored by the use of cell lines. When this is done the more toxigenic bacteria are shown to be more likely to induce prolonged post-infective symptoms[11].

MUCOSAL CHANGES

A number of changes have been documented following bacterial infection. Following *Campylobacter* infection there is an increase in T lymphocytes of both CD4 and CD8 varieties, an increase in activated macrophages (calprotectin positive) and an increase in entero-endocrine cells. Each of these cell types will be considered individually.

LYMPHOCYTE RESPONSE

Campylobacter infection is not the only infection to show a persistent lymphocytosis since Gwee *et al.*[9] studied a range of organisms and showed that those patients who go on to suffer PI-IBS have an increased lymphocytic infiltration in the mucosa. More recently it has been demonstrated that, in diarrhoea-predominant IBS (D-IBS), of which many patients had an acute onset, there was evidence of increased numbers of activated regulatory T lymphocytes expressing the IL-2

Table 3 Effect of duration of initial illness on relative risk of developing new PI-IBS

Duration of illness	Relative risk	95% confidence intervals
0–7 days	1.0	
8–14 days	2.9	0.6–15
15–21 days	6.5	1.3–34
>21 days	11.4	2.2–58

receptor (CD25)[12]. The increase in lymphocytes is not sufficient to meet criteria for microscopic colitis, but when quantified shows clear distinction from the normal range. Whether all D-IBS are post-infective it is not clear, but certainly not all give a history of acute onset, though when onset is many months or years prior to interview memory is an unreliable guide. However, in our own study, when we defined PI-IBS as an acute onset of symptoms, on a single day combined with two or more of the following symptoms: fever, vomiting, diarrhoea or positive stool culture, we found that both PI-IBS and non-post-infective D-IBS showed increased lymphocyte counts in the mucosa[13].

MACROPHAGES

Following *C. jejuni* infection there is a decline in resident macrophages staining with CD68 but an increase in calprotectin-positive cells, which represent incoming monocytes recruited from the circulation[14]. Chadwick *et al.*'s study[12] also showed an increase in macrophages. These may well be important mediators of altered motility, being potent sources of a range of mediators including prostaglandins, nitric oxide and interleukin-1β. Other authors have suggested that, in some patients, iNOS is increased in the mucosa of IBS patients[15]. In laboratory animals iNOS inhibitors can prevent the dysmotility resulting from iNOS activation[16]. Whether selective iNOS inhibitors could be used in humans without significant side-effects remains to be seen.

ENTERO-ENDOCRINE CELL ACTIVATION

The entero-endocrine cell is coming to be seen as a key transducer of luminal stimuli enabling nutrients, toxins and pressure to be transduced to 5-HT and neuropeptide release, which can then act as modulators of intestinal reflexes. Entero-endocrine cells originate from stem cells in the base of crypts and migrate up the crypt wall where cytoplasm projections enable them to sample the lumen. Activation of these cells, both by mechanical deformation and absorption of nutrients, activates a cascade, which involves increased cyclic AMP followed by a rise in intracellular calcium, which mediates fusion of secretory granules and exocytosis into the lamina propria. The commonest component of these granules is serotonin, but in the upper gut, CCK, secretin and motilin are common, in the midgut neurotensin, glicentin-like peptide-1 and peptide-YY (PYY) predominate while PYY and somatostatin abound in the rectum. Infection produces a striking increase in rectal entero-endocrine cells, particularly those containing serotonin. The ratio of serotonin to PYY is reversed with a much greater increase in the serotonin than the PYY cells[14]. The balance between PYY and serotonin may be important since they have opposing actions, PYY slowing transit and inhibiting secretions while stimulating absorption[17] whereas serotonin has the opposite effect with accelerated transit and increased secretions[18]. Following *C. jejuni* infection there is a striking increase in entero-endocrine cells which then declines over the next 3 months but remains elevated in some individuals for up to 1 year (Fig. 2).

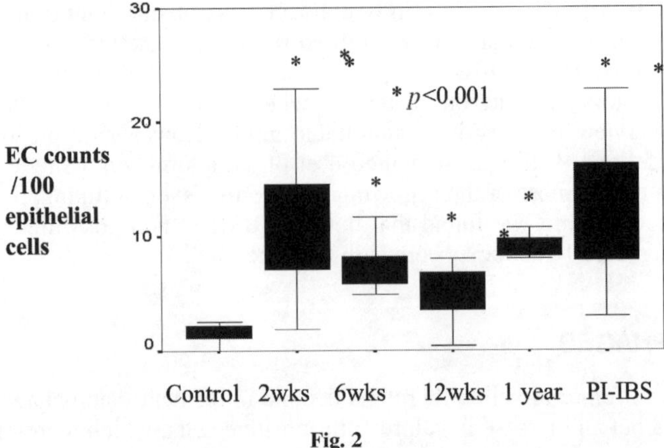

Fig. 2

SIGNIFICANCE OF INCREASED ENTERO-ENDOCRINE CELLS

Patients with persistent symptoms after infection show an increase in entero-endocrine cell numbers[13]. The importance of this may relate to serotonin release. There are two preliminary studies which indicate increased serotonin release after a test meal in D-IBS[19,20]. In the larger more recent study Houghton et al.[20] showed that IBS patients with symptoms had higher levels than those without. There is certainly a plausible explanation for this since serotonin infusions are known to stimulate motility, increase secretions and be associated with flushing and diarrhoea. The increased appearance of free serotonin in plasma after a meal must reflect an excess mucosal release of serotonin and an escape from the normal uptake mechanisms. Most serotonin which is released in the gut mucosa is rapidly taken up by enterocytes and destroyed. The serotonin transporter (SERT) which mediates this is variably expressed with genetic polymorphisms in the gene coding for this transporter which produce long and short varieties. The short ones are less effective and have been related to clinical diseases such as depression. They have also recently, in a preliminary study, been shown to relate to the response to serotonin antagonists[21]; however, the numbers so far studied are very small and the results need confirming in much larger studies. Other factors influencing the expression of the serotonin transporter include interferon-γ and TNF-α which increases its expression, and IL-4 which depresses it. It is therefore possible that the increased release seen in D-IBS may reflect either increased release of serotonin or depressed SERT, or a combination of the two.

The therapeutic implications, however, in both cases are similar, namely that 5-HT$_3$ receptor antagonists are likely to inhibit secretions and delay transit. These effects have been shown in normal controls with ondansetron and granisetron[22]. 5-HT$_3$ receptor antagonists have also been shown to be effective in D-IBS[23]. These drugs of course are effective only while being taken. The first attempt at a disease-modifying treatment was the use of prednisolone in an attempt to suppress the increase in entero-endocrine (EC) cells. A short course of

30 mg of prednisolone for 3 weeks did not, however, alter symptoms or EC cell counts, though it did reduce lymphocyte counts in biopsies taken 4 weeks after the start of treatments[24]. Side-effects are likely to limit the use of prednisolone, but whether other safer agents, which could be taken for longer, would have a chance of being effective is uncertain. Certainly, in animals there are two populations of EC, one with a half-life of 16 days and the other with a half-life of 160. Whether these very long-lived EC would require a prolonged course of treatment is not clear, though on an anecdotal basis some patients have responded.

MAST CELLS

These storehouses of neuromediators, which include substance P, histamine, NGF, mast cell proteases and PGE2, have been reported to be elevated in some patients with IBS. Weston *et al.*[25] found increased mast cells in the terminal ileum of 20 IBS patients, the highest values being found in those with diarrhoea predominance. Other reports have been conflicting, but one which looked at all segments of the colon found the changes only in the right colon[15]. Our own studies using just rectal biopsies found no increase in PI-IBS but a slight increase in D-IBS due to other causes[13]. Although there has been one clinical trial suggesting mast cell stabilizers might help in IBS with positive skinprick tests for food allergy[26] this has not been repeated. Substance P activates mast cells and in animal models of *C. difficile* infection NK2 antagonists inhibit this process[27] and have a marked anti-inflammatory effect.

BILE SALT MALABSORPTION

Salmonella and *Campylobacter* infection often produces an acute ileitis which has been associated with bile salt malabsorption[28]. This induces a profound decrease ($<5\%$) in retention of labelled bile salt (ScHCAT) and responds well to cholestyramine. This is not to be confused with the lesser degree of bile salt malabsorption (10–15% retention) which is common in all forms of diarrhoea associated with fast whole-gut transit. These patients tend not to respond to cholestyramine[29].

ALTERED GUT FLORA

The profound catharsis which occurs eliminates the normal commensal flora and there is usually some delay before the flora is fully restored. Thus all forms of diarrhoea reduce anaerobic bacterial numbers and hence short-chain fatty acid concentrations in stool causing the stool pH to rise, allowing abnormal flora to develop[30].

This has prompted attempts to reconstruct the beneficial flora using probiotics. Thus *Lactobacillus GG* has been shown to speed up recovery from Rotavirus infection in children[31,32]. Several trials of probiotics have been reported[33,34] but only one high-quality trial showed benefit[33].

There are many anecdotal reports of success in treating D-IBS with antibiotics and bismuth, but these have yet to be confirmed in randomized double-blind placebo-controlled trials.

CHANGES IN MUCOSAL NERVES

Mucosal ulceration leads to mucosal nerve damage. Studies using the DNBS colitis model[35] have documented acute loss of ganglion cells and mucosal nerves stained using antibodies to PGP9.5. Muscular innervation actually increased in the longer term, implying a degree of remodelling associated with muscular hypertrophy. Our own studies also showed a loss of PGP9.5 staining lasting up to 3 months after infection (Fig. 3)[11], suggesting neural injury, which has been shown to cause PGP9.5 to concentrate in the neuronal cell bodies which are not usually seen in superficial biopsies. More recently we have examined another example of mucosal injury: that seen after acute diverticulitis. This shows acute loss of mucosal nerves associated with an increase in small-diameter nerves in the muscular layers which show increased branching. Recurrent inflammation is commonly seen in ulcerative colitis, in which increased density of nerves staining for substance P has been reported[36]. Inflammation up-regulates the substance P receptor while substance P released by axonal reflex is proinflammatory, activating mast cells. This is well demonstrated in *C. difficile* pseudomembranous colitis in which substance P antagonists, as well as mast cell stabilizers, both substantially inhibit the inflammatory response. Neurokinin receptor$_2$ antagonists inhibit a number of neurokinin A effects on smooth muscle and also inhibit the increased sensitivity to colorectal distension seen in inflammation. Their effects are mediated both via reducing afferent nerve discharges[37] and via central anxiolytic effects[38].

These neural changes seen with inflammation may be mediated via nerve growth factors released by tissue injury. Increased expression of nerve growth factor receptor trkA is seen in acute inflammatory bowel disease[39] and nerve

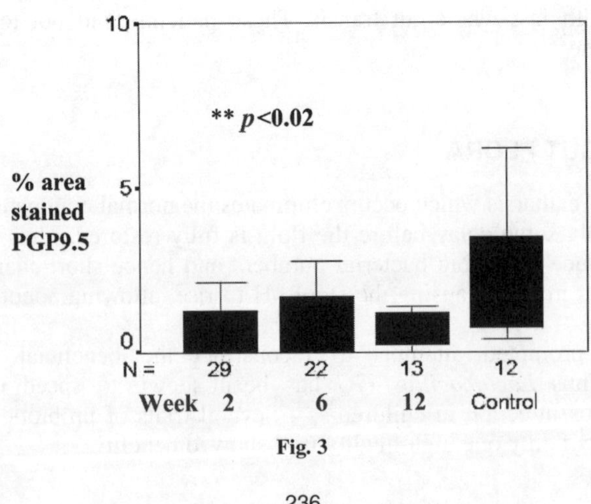

Fig. 3

growth factor is known to promote the survival and differentiation of sensory neurons acting via trkA. It may well be important in up-regulation of various ion channels such as VR1 (vanilloid receptor 1) and ASIC (acid-sensitive ion channel) which might mediate visceral hypersensitivity.

CONCLUSIONS

Several lines of study suggest that there may be an inflammatory component to IBS. This may originate from an initial infectious insult but other possibilities include chemical and allergic phenomena. The pattern of inflammatory mediators may differ, but include serotonin, substance P and mast cell products. These suggest that therapeutic interventions with anti-inflammatory agents such as steroids or serotonin, tachykinin and nerve growth factor antagonists might be worth exploring.

References

1. Young DM, Biao J, Zheng Z *et al*. Isolation of *Campylobacter jejuni* in Hunan, the People's Republic of China: epidemiology and comparison of Chinese and American methodology. Diagnost Microbiol Infect Dis. 1986;5:143–9.
2. Blaser MJ, Taylor DN, Echeverria P. Immune response to *Campylobacter jejuni* in a rural community in Thailand. J Infect Dis. 1986;153:249–54.
3. Taylor DN, Perlman DM, Echeverria PD, Lexomboon U, Blaser MJ. *Campylobacter* immunity and quantitative excretion rates in Thai children. J Infect Dis. 1993;168:754–8.
4. Neal KR, Hebden J, Spiller R. Prevalence of gastrointestinal symptoms six months after bacterial gastroenteritis and risk factors for development of the irritable bowel syndrome: postal survey of patients. Br Med J. 1997;314:779–82.
5. Parry SD, Barton R, Welfare MR. Prevalence of pre-existing functional gastrointestinal disorders (FGID) in infectious diarrhoea (ID) subjects compared to a matched community control group. Gastroenterology. 2001;120(Suppl. 1):A633.
6. Neal K, Barker L, Spiller RC. Prognosis in post infective irritable bowel syndrome: a 6 year follow up study. Gut. 2002;51:410–13.
7. Parry S, Stansfield R, Jelley D, Phillips F, Barton JR, Welfare MR. Is irritable bowel syndrome (IBS) more common in patients presenting with bactreial gastro-enteritis? A community-based case–control study. Am J Gastroenterol. 2003;98:327–31.
8. Neal KR, Barker L, Spiller RC. Prognosis in post-infective irritable bowel syndrome: a six year follow up study. Gut. 2002;51:410–13.
9. Gwee KA, Leong YL, Graham C *et al*. The role of psychological and biological factors in postinfective gut dysfunction. Gut. 1999;44:400–6.
10. Gwee KA, Graham JC, McKendrick MW *et al*. Psychometric scores and persistence of irritable bowel after infectious diarrhoea. Lancet. 1996;347:150–3.
11. Jenkins D, Thornley JP, Wright T *et al*. Enterchromaffin and mast cell hyperplasia parallels mucosal nerve damage following *Campylobacter* enteritis. Neurogastroenterol Motil. 1998;10:464.
12. Chadwick VS, Chen W, Shu D *et al*. Activation of the mucosal immune system in irritable bowel syndrome. Gastroenterology. 2002;122:1778–83.
13. Dunlop SP, Jenkins D, Spiller RC. Distinctive histological patterns of chronic inflammatory cells in rectal biopsies of patients with different clinical subtypes of IBS. Gastroenterology. 2002;122:A.
14. Spiller RC, Jenkins D, Thornley JP *et al*. Increased rectal mucosal enteroendocrine cells, T lymphocytes and increased gut permeability following acute *Campylobacter* enteritis and in post-dysenteric irritable bowel syndrome. Gut. 2000;47:804–11.
15. O'Sullivan M, Clayton N, Breslin NP *et al*. Increased mast cells in the irritable bowel syndrome. Neurogastroenterol Motil. 2000;12:449–57.

16. Turler A, Moore BA, Pezzone MA, Overhaus M, Kalff JC, Bauer AJ. Colonic postoperative inflammatory ileus in the rat. Ann Surg. 2002;236:56–66.
17. Playford RJ, Domin J, Beacham J *et al.* Preliminary report: role of peptide YY in defence against diarrhoea. Lancet. 1990;335:1555–7.
18. Spiller RC. Effects of serotonin on intestinal secretion and motility. Curr Opin Gastroenterol. 2001;17:99–103.
19. Bearcroft CP, Perrett D, Farthing MJ. 5-Hydroxytryptamine release into human jejunum by cholera toxin. Gut. 1996;39:528–31.
20. Houghton LA, Atkinson W, Whitaker P *et al.* A role for 5-hydroxytryptamine (5-HT) in the post-prandial exacerbation of symptoms in female patients with diarrhoea predominant irritable bowel syndrome (IBS). Gastroenterology. 2001;120:A636 (abstract).
21. Camilleri M, Atanasova E, Carlson PJ *et al.* Serotonin-transporter polymorphism pharmacogenetics in diarrhea-predominant irritable bowel syndrome. Gastroenterology. 2002;123:425–32.
22. Gore S, Gilmore IT, Haigh CG, Brownless SM, Stockdale H, Morris AI. Colonic transit in man is slowed by ondansetron (GR38032F), a selective 5-hydroxytryptamine receptor (type 3) antagonist. Aliment Pharmacol Ther. 1990;4:139–44.
23. Camilleri M, Mayer EA, Drossman DA *et al.* Improvement in pain and bowel function in female irritable bowel patients with alosetron, a 5-HT3 receptor antagonist. Aliment Pharmacol Ther. 1999;13:1149–59.
24. Dunlop SP, Kenkins D, Neal KR *et al.* Randomised double-blind, placebo-controlled trial of prednisolone in post-infectious irritable bowel syndrome. Aliment Pharmacol Ther. 2003 (in press).
25. Weston AP, Biddle WL, Bhatia PS, Miner PB Jr. Terminal ileal mucosal mast cells in irritable bowel syndrome. Dig Dis Sci. 1993;38:1590–5.
26. Stefanini GF, Bazzocchi G, Prati E. Efficacy of oral disodium cromoglycate in patients with irritable bowel syndrome and positive skin prick tests to foods. Lancet. 1986;1:207–8.
27. Pothoulakis C, Castagliuolo I, Lamont JT *et al.* CP-96,345, a substance P antagonist, inhibits rat intestinal responses to *Clostridium difficile* toxin A but not cholera toxin. Proc Natl Acad Sci USA. 1994;91:947–51.
28. Niaz SK, Sandrasegaran K, Renny FH, Jones BJ. Postinfective diarrhoea and bile acid malabsorption. J R Coll Phys Lond. 1997;31:53–6.
29. Williams AJK, Merrick MV, Eastwood MA. Idiopathic bile acid malabsorption – a review of clinical presentation, diagnosis, and response to treatment. Gut. 1991;32:1004–6.
30. Tazume S, Ozawa A, Yamamoto T *et al.* Ecological study on the intestinal bacterial flora of patients with diarrhea. Clin Infect Dis. 1993;16:S77–82.
31. Isolauri E, Kaila M, Mykkanen H, Ling WH, Salminen S. Oral bacteriotherapy for viral gastroenteritis. Dig Dis Sci. 1994;39:2595–600.
32. Majamaa H, Isolauri E, Saxelin M, Vesikari T. Lactic acid bacteria in the treatment of acute rotavirus gastroenteritis. J Pediatr Gastroenterol Nutr. 1995;20:333–8.
33. Nobaek S, Johansson ML, Molin G, Ahrne S, Jeppsson B. Alteration of intestinal microflora is associated with reduction in abdominal bloating and pain in patients with irritable bowel syndrome. Am J Gastroenterol. 2000;95:1231–8.
34. O'Sullivan MA, O'Morain CA. Bacterial supplementation in the irritable bowel syndrome. A randomised double-blind placebo-controlled crossover study. Dig Liver Dis. 2000;32:294–301.
35. Sanovic S, Lamb DP, Blennerhassett MG. Damage to the enteric nervous system in experimental colitis. Am J Pathol. 1999;155:1051–7.
36. Watanabe T, Kubota Y, Muto T. Substance P containing nerve fibers in rectal mucosa of ulcerative colitis. Dis Colon Rectum. 1997;40:718–25.
37. Laird JM, Olivar T, Lopez-Garcia JA, Maggi CA, Cervero F. Responses of rat spinal neurons to distension of inflamed colon: role of tachykinin NK2 receptors. Neuropharmacology. 2001;40:696–701.
38. Steinberg R, Alonso R, Griebel G *et al.* Selective blockade of neurokinin-2 receptors produces antidepressant-like effects associated with reduced corticotropin-releasing factor function. PG. J Pharmacol Exp Ther. 2001;299:449–58.
39. Di Mola FF, Friess H, Zhu ZW *et al.* Nerve growth factor and Trk high affinity receptor (TrkA) gene expression in inflammatory bowel disease. Gut. 2000;46:670–9.

27
Role of epithelium–environment interactions in down-regulation of mucosal inflammation

J. BIENENSTOCK and D. MA

The epithelium represents a natural barrier, but also an evident interface with the external environment. The present view of the epithelium as an active participant in the maintenance of homeostasis has evolved over the past few decades[1,2]. Currently, the view that it contributes significantly and is involved actively in reactions to toxins and potential and actual pathogens is widely held[3]. Evidence is clear that it synthesizes biologically active molecules, such as IL-8, a major chemoattractor, which is significant in recruitment of polymorphonuclear leucocytes, and IL-6, which promotes the synthesis of acute-phase reactants in response to various interactions[4]. Equally clear is the fact that mucosal tissues and the skin are generally in a down-regulated state with regard to inflammation. This is most evident in the intestine, which is faced with large numbers of organisms, molecules, nutrients, etc., on a constant basis and yet, in the normal healthy state, is only, if anything, mildly inflamed. This natural physiological condition is essential if the tissue is to maintain its normal physiological functions of digestion, secretion and absorption.

This chapter describes some of our recent work[5] and suggests some mechanisms whereby molecules, such as nerve growth factor (NGF) secreted in copious amounts by the normal salivary gland and found in all external excretions, may be involved in some of these processes[6]. It further ascribes some possible mechanisms whereby commensal organisms in the intestinal tract may, under normal physiological circumstances, promote down-regulation of local immune and inflammatory processes.

These studies began with the assumption that the epithelium was involved in immune regulation. For example, oral tolerance, a well-known phenomenon, may involve local interactions between the external environment and the intestinal epithelium[7]. The best-known way of inducing oral tolerance follows the observations of Czerkinsky *et al.*[8], who have shown that antigen chemically conjugated to the B subunit of cholera toxin is an extremely potent method of induction. Consequently, our earliest experiments in this area examined the effect of the holotoxin and recombinant cholera toxin B subunit (kindly provided by Professor Tim Hirst, Bristol University) and human intestinal epithelial cells (T-84). While we will in this chapter use as examples the observations obtained with T-84 they have since been repeated and confirmed with experiments using other human intestinal epithelial cell lines such as CaCo2, HT29 and, most recently, a mouse epithelial line/mode K.

In brief, holotoxin induced IL-6 and IL-8 synthesis but had no effect on other immunoregulatory cytokines, such as TGF-β or IL-10. The methods used were mostly RT-PCR, but in certain circumstances evidence for protein synthesis and secretion was also obtained using intracellular FACS, and protein quantitation by ELISA. In contrast to these findings, cholera toxin B (CTB) dose-dependently and significantly increased the mRNA for IL-10 in a relatively selective manner, since it had no effect on TGF-β, IL-6 or IL-8. The time-course for induction was optimal at 6h of incubation. Evidence for protein synthesis was obtained and intracellular increase of the protein was observed using FACS and immunohistology. Evidence for increased synthesis was observed in the culture medium within 48 h.

Because our laboratory has an interest in NGF, and because there is one report in the literature suggesting that IL-10 and NGF may have reciprocal regulatory influences in astrocytes, we examined whether IL-10 and NGF may have such reciprocal interactions on intestinal epithelial cells. Indeed this was the case. IL-10 dose-dependency increased both the mRNA for, and protein synthesis of, NGF quite selectively, having no effect on IL-6 and IL-8, TGF-β or IL-10 itself. Furthermore, murine recombinant NGF, as well as naturally occurring NGF obtained from male mouse submandibular glands, had selective effects on IL-10 synthesis. This was dose-dependent, and followed a similar time-course (within 1–2h for the effect on mRNA) and protein synthesis (within 48h). In an analogous fashion to the actions of NGF, it was relatively selective, having no effect on IL-6, IL-8, TGF-β or NGF.

Thus there appears to be an autocoid activity involving IL-10 and NGF. This is interesting since IL-10 is not generally thought to be constitutively synthesized by the epithelium[9], and has not been identified as being up-regulated in studies of effects on epithelial cytokines.

IL-10 is an extremely immunoregulatory molecule, having been shown to be widely effective in down-regulation of immune and inflammatory processes[10]. On the other hand, NGF has been shown to have both pro- and anti-inflammatory effects, depending on the circumstances[6]. NGF has mast cell degranulatory capability and has been observed experimentally to display a wide variety of pleiotropic activities[11]. These include promotion of mast cell growth and maturation, both *in vivo* and *in vitro*; promotion of the synthesis of certain IgG subtypes in *in-vitro* studies of immunoglobulin synthesis, in addition to its profound effects on growth and maturation of nervous tissue, both centrally and peripherally. Most importantly, from the point of view of our own observations, NGF appears to have potent anti-inflammatory effects. For example, it seems to reduce the inflammation consequent to the injection of carrageenan[12], and profoundly inhibits deterioration and promotes epithelialization in cases of recalcitrant corneal ulceration[13]. The injection of anti-NGF into mice, in which hapten-induced colitis was generated, significantly increased the inflammation in the tissue[14]. Matsuda *et al.*[15] have shown that NGF significantly promotes the growth and repair of skin wounds in both normal and diabetic animals. NGF markedly reduced the inflammation seen in the central nervous system in a marmoset model of acute allergic encephalomyelitis (EAE)[16]. Perhaps the most cogent example of the anti-inflammatory effects of NGF is contained in the experiments of Flugel *et al.*[17] These workers recently observed that myelin-specific T cells transduced to synthesize and express NGF could suppress the inflammation of EAE when injected even after the initiation of EAE in a rat model. This suppression was not obtained when T cells specific for ovalbumin and similarly transduced were injected, even though the same levels of NGF were found in the serum. These observations perfectly confirm the suggestion that NGF locally delivered to an inflammatory environment has general anti-inflammatory effects.

It is interesting at the same time to observe that NGF appears to be synthesized by a large variety of inflammatory cells, which include mast cells, eosinophils and T cells, especially those of the TH2 variety[6].

Because our laboratory is also interested in the effects and mechanisms of effects of probiotic organisms, we have begun to look at these from the point of view of cytokine synthesis in the various model systems described above. We have focused our interest on *Lactobacillus reuteri*, since this has been shown to have a potent anti-inflammatory effect in at least one model of colitis: the IL-10 knockout[18]. In our hands *L. reuteri* has no effect on cytokine synthesis by human epithelial cells.

Since Neish *et al.*[19] have shown that a non-pathogenic organism, *S. pullorum*, can inhibit the production of IL-8 in epithelial cells induced by TNF-α or by a pathogenic organism, *S. typhi*, we re-examined this model with *L. reuteri*. This organism dose-dependently inhibits IL-8 production induced by TNF-α, both in terms of message and protein secretion. This appears to require live organisms, adherence and attachment of these organisms to the epithelium, a necessary prerequisite to colonization. There has been no effect demonstrated on epithelium with the supernatant obtained from cultures in which the *L. reuteri* was grown. Currently, we are examining the possibility that this effect is mediated by NGF.

CONCLUSIONS

All in all, our observations support the thought that NGF may have important local anti-inflammatory effects in mucosal tissue. These may involve other molecules through a reciprocal autocoid pathway in the epithelium. However, since *L. reuteri* has an inhibitory effect on the induction of colitis in the IL-10 knockout model, it is possible and even likely that NGF, as shown in other models, has potent anti-inflammatory capacity even in the absence of IL-10. We are pursuing these observations and extending them to explore the possibility that NGF is locally involved in the production of oral tolerance, and that it may be involved in the potential protective and beneficial effects of probiotic organisms.

References

1. Kagnoff MF, Eckmann L. Epithelial cells as sensors for microbial infection. J Clin Invest. 1997;100:6–10.
2. Berin MC, McKay DM, Perdue MH. Immune–epithelial interactions in host defense. Am J Trop Med Hyg. 1999;60:16–25.
3. Gordon JI, Hooper LV, McNevin MS, Wong M, Bry L. Epithelial cell growth and differentiation. III. Promoting diversity in the intestine: conversations between the microflora, epithelium, and diffuse GALT. Am J Physiol. 1997;273:G565–70.
4. Svanborg C, Godaly G, Hedlund M. Cytokine responses during mucosal infections: role in disease pathogenesis and host defence. Curr Opin Microbiol. 1999;2:99–105.
5. Ma D, Wolvers D, Stanisz A, Bienenstock J. Interleukin-10 and nerve growth factor have reciprocal upregulatory effects on intestinal epithelial cells. Am J Physiol Regul Integr Comp Physiol. 2003;284:R1323–9.
6. Bienenstock J. Mast cell–nerve interactions: possible significance of nerve growth factor. In: Marone G, Lichtenstein LM, Galli SJ, editors. Mast Cells and Basophils. New York: Academic Press, 2000:313–23.
7. Faria AM, Weiner HL. Oral tolerance: mechanisms and therapeutic applications. Adv Immunol. 1999;73:153–264.
8. Czerkinsky C, Anjuere F, McGhee JR et al. Mucosal immunity and tolerance: relevance to vaccine development. Immunol Rev. 1999;170:197–222.
9. Eckmann L, Jung HC, Schurer-Maly C, Panja A, Morzycka-Wroblewska E, Kagnoff MF. Differential cytokine expression by human intestinal epithelial cell lines: regulated expression of interleukin 8. Gastroenterology. 1993;105:1689–97.
10. Stordeur P, Goldman M. Interleukin-10 as a regulatory cytokine induced by cellular stress: molecular aspects. Int Rev Immunol. 1998;16:501–22.
11. Levi-Montalcini R, Skaper SD, Dal Toso R, Petrelli L, Leon A. Nerve growth factor: from neurotrophin to neurokine. Trends Neurosci. 1996;19:514–20.
12. Banks BE, Vernon CA, Warner JA. Nerve growth factor has anti-inflammatory activity in the rat hindpaw oedema test. Neurosci Lett. 1984;47:41–5.
13. Lambiase A, Rama P, Bonini S, Caprioglio G, Aloe L. Topical treatment with nerve growth factor for corneal neurotrophic ulcers. N Engl J Med. 1998;338:1174–80.
14. Reinshagen M, Rohm H, Steinkamp M et al. Protective role of neurotrophins in experimental inflammation of the rat gut. Gastroenterology. 2000;119:368–76.
15. Matsuda H, Koyama H, Sato H et al. Role of nerve growth factor in cutaneous wound healing: accelerating effects in normal and healing-impaired diabetic mice. J Exp Med. 1998;187:297–306.
16. Ransohoff RM, Trebst C. Surprising pleiotropy of nerve growth factor in the treatment of experimental autoimmune encephalomyelitis. J Exp Med. 2000;191:1625–30.
17. Flugel A, Matsumuro K, Neumann H et al. Anti-inflammatory activity of nerve growth factor in experimental autoimmune encephalomyelitis: inhibition of monocyte transendothelial migration. Eur J Immunol. 2001;31:11–22.
18. Madsen KL, Doyle JS, Jewell LD, Tavernini MM, Fedorak RN. *Lactobacillus* species prevents colitis in interleukin-10 gene-deficient mice. Gastroenterology. 1999;116:1107–14.
19. Neish AS, Gewirtz AT, Zeng H et al. Prokaryotic regulation of epithelial responses by inhibition of IkappaB-alpha ubiquitination. Science. 2000;289:1560–3.

Section IX
Genetics and molecular mechanisms

28
Is irritable bowel syndrome
a genetic disorder?

N. J. TALLEY

INTRODUCTION

The functional gastrointestinal disorders are common and clinically important but the underlying pathophysiology is only beginning to emerge. One aspect of potential importance has been the recognition that functional gastrointestinal disorders can cluster in families, leading to the suspicion that genetic factors may play a key role in combination with common environmental factors[1]. There is increasing interest in studying potential genetic influences of complex disorders including the functional gastrointestinal disorders because this may shed new light on the pathogenesis, may improve the ability to identify other relevant risk factors including gene–environment interactions, and finally successful therapy may in part depend on an individual's underlying genotype; indeed recent evidence supports this hypothesis in irritable bowel syndrome (IBS).

In this chapter the epidemiological evidence that gastrointestinal disorders of function are inherited will be reviewed. Further evidence that genetic factors may be important in these disorders is discussed in relationship to those conditions that clearly overlap with, and may share a similar pathogenesis with, the functional gastrointestinal disorders. Finally, potential genetic markers will be reviewed and the difficulties in searching for a gene discussed.

FAMILIAL ASSOCIATION OF THE FUNCTIONAL GASTROINTESTINAL DISORDERS

Studies of familial aggregation of the functional gastrointestinal disorders are very limited. Locke *et al.* sent a modified version of a validated bowel disease questionnaire to 892 eligible subjects and obtained a response rate of 72%[1]. Overall, 12% had IBS and 14% dyspepsia based on the Rome I definitions. Furthermore, 24% and 22%, respectively, reported having a first-degree relative or a spouse with abdominal pain or bowel dysfunction. In a model that adjusted for age, sex, and multiple somatic symptoms, it was found that those subjects reporting a family member with a history of abdominal pain or bowel dysfunction showed a greater than two-fold increased odds of reporting IBS and a nearly two-fold increased odds of reporting dyspepsia. In contrast, the subjects who reported that their spouse had a history of abdominal pain or bowel dysfunction were not significantly more likely to report either IBS or dyspepsia[1]. One strength of this study is that somatic symptoms were controlled for, suggesting that the familial aggregation was not explained because of the familial aggregation of a somatization disorder. Other potential explanations for the findings, however, need to be considered. It remains uncertain whether people with gastrointestinal symptoms may be more aware of the symptom status of their family members or may more openly discuss symptoms with family members, leading to a reporting bias. Familial aggregation could also be due to learned illness behaviour in families or other common environmental factors such as abuse, which has been associated with IBS[1].

Few other data on familial aggregation in IBS exist. Oster (1972) reported that 50% of the mothers of children with recurrent abdominal pain had functional gastrointestinal symptoms[2]. Kalantar *et al.*[3] assessed patients attending an IBS education programme and Olmsted County residents; they were mailed a questionnaire, and a survey of first-degree relatives was also obtained, with an overall response rate of 70%. There was an over two-fold increased risk of IBS amongst patient relatives compared with spouse relatives.

TWIN STUDIES IN IBS

Twin studies are particularly suited for complex diseases including neuropsychiatric disorders and the functional gastrointestinal disorders because of the difficulty in disentangling environment from genetic factors. Monozygotic twins are genetically identical in comparison to dizygotic twins which share, on average, about half of their genes. If both twins appear affected this is referred to as being concordant. In a disorder in which genetic factors are important in the aetiology, but are not the only factor, the concordance rate for monozygotic twins will be greater than for dizygotic twins. There are four studies that have evaluated twins in order to ascertain whether IBS may be inherited.

Morris-Yates *et al.* in Australia studied 462 families with 924 twins[4]. A broad definition of functional bowel disease was applied and the presence of one or more symptoms was considered to be suitable to identify a case. There were 33 twin pairs identified with functional bowel disease, with a concordance in monozygotic twins of 33.3% and in dizygotic twins 13.3%. Based on structured linear modelling it was concluded that genetics accounted for approximately 57% of the variance in reporting of functional bowel disease symptoms.

A study from the United States by Levy *et al.* evaluated 10 699 twin respondents representing 6060 twin pairs[5]. A questionnaire obtained information on more than 80 health problems including self-reported IBS, in this US study. Here the concordance for monozygotic twins with IBS was 17.2% versus a concordance in dizygotic twins of 8.4%. This study also concluded that heredity contributed to the development of IBS, and confirmed that the concordance for IBS was about twice as great in monozygotic compared with dizygotic twins. The different concordance rates in the Australian and US studies are most likely explained based on differences in case definition. Levy *et al*. also evaluated the prevalence of IBS among mothers and fathers of the twins evaluated[5]. It can be assumed that the probability that a mother of a monozygotic twin with IBS will have the same probability as a dizygotic co-twin of a twin with IBS, because the number of shared genes should be approximately the same. They observed that having a mother with IBS accounted for as much variance as having a monozygotic co-twin. This suggests that common environmental factors in families, including perhaps social learning, are as important as genetic factors[5].

A further twin study from the United Kingdom has failed to identify any hereditary component in IBS[6], but a second US twins study confirmed previous results in IBS[7]. There are many reasons that discordant results can occur between studies. For example, concordant twin pairs are more likely, because they are rare, to come to attention and be published, and hence may not be representative of the general population in a particular study. Furthermore, twin pairs may become concordant only over time, unless the age of onset is strictly controlled. Indeed, the estimates derived from twin studies, because they are small, lead to necessarily large confidence limits. At this point, adoption studies have not been undertaken to try to further disentangle environmental factors in IBS. Studies of twins separated at birth have not been undertaken in functional gastrointestinal disorders because of a general lack of availability of such twin pairs.

It is known that a number of extra-intestinal manifestations of IBS exist, including bladder dysfunction, fibromyalgia and psychiatric disease[8]. Svedberg *et al*. undertook a study in twins to evaluate co-morbidity in IBS[9]. Both a classical case–control design (which evaluated 72 subjects with IBS and 216 age- and gender-matched controls from the cohort) and a co-twin analysis (which incorporated 58 diseased twins with IBS and their healthy co-twins) were undertaken[9]. IBS was broadly defined as one or more of the Rome II symptoms or lower abdominal pain or diarrhoea or constipation. A strength of this study is that a random subsample of twin pairs from the Swedish twin registry was utilized, and the overall response rate was 67%. In the case–control study IBS was significantly associated with obesity, eating disorders, rheumatoid arthritis, gluten intolerance and renal disease. In the co-twin control analysis for the 58 discordant twin pairs with irritable bowel, the associations mostly disappeared except for the presence of renal and urinary tract disease. These results suggest that genetic or alternatively intra-familial environmental effects are important for the association of IBS with obesity, eating disorder, gluten intolerance and rheumatoid arthritis. The diagnosis of these extra-intestinal manifestations was based on self-report; hence misclassification error is possible. Indeed, the association with gluten intolerance may reflect undiagnosed coeliac disease, while reports of rheumatoid arthritis may reflect misclassification of fibromyalgia with arthritic conditions. Further work is needed to confirm whether genetic mediators explain in part the association between IBS and other extra-intestinal manifestations.

IBS AND GASTRO-OESOPHAGEAL REFLUX DISEASE

Gastro-oesophageal reflux disease (GORD) is common and often overlaps with IBS, but an explanation for this association remains obscure. It is therefore of interest to note that Cameron *et al.* compared the concordance for GORD in monozygotic and dizygotic twins based on data from the Swedish Twin Registry[10]. The concordance for GORD was higher in monozygotic than dizygotic twins in men and women, and in twins aged 55–64 and 65 and over. It was calculated that the heritability for GORD in both sexes was 31%. It was also shown that obesity, alcohol intake and smoking had no major influence on the genetic impact for reflux disease in this study. Zaman *et al.* have also shown, in a preliminary report in younger subjects, that the pairwise concordance for GORD was 19% in monozygotic and 4.3% in dizygotic twins, confirming a modest heritability for GORD[11].

Other evidence supports a genetic predisposition in GORD. Familial aggregation of Barrett's oesophagus and oesophageal adenocarcinoma has been reported[12,13]. Seri *et al.* have shown, in a very rare syndrome comprising bilateral cataracts, gastro-oesophageal reflux and spastic paraplesis with amyotrophy, that this disorder mapped to chromosome 10[14]. Hu *et al.* mapped a gene for severe paediatric reflux disease to chromosome 13 in families with an autosomal dominant pattern of inheritance[15]. However, adult GORD is more likely a polygenic syndrome, and whether a genetic link explains the co-association of reflux disease with IBS is unclear.

IBS AND PSYCHIATRIC DISEASE

The co-association of IBS with psychiatric disease in tertiary referral centres is well established[16,17]. However, the nature of this association remains unclear. It is conceivable that a subset of IBS is a feature of a psychiatric disease rather than a separate syndrome. Referral bias has also been suggested to explain the association, as some studies have identified psychiatric disorders to be less common in IBS subjects from the community compared with patients who have sought care, although not all studies agree[16]. A further possibility is that psychiatric disease is secondary to the chronic gastrointestinal illness itself, although lower rates of psychiatric disease in patients with inflammatory bowel disease suggest this explanation is less likely[17].

Woodman *et al.* evaluated 20 patients with IBS and 20 patients as controls who had undergone laparoscopic cholecystectomy; their first-degree relatives were interviewed to obtain information on lifetime diagnoses of both functional gastrointestinal disorders and psychiatric disease[18]. Woodman *et al.* found that the probands with IBS had an increased lifetime prevalence of psychiatric disease compared with controls. More interestingly, the relatives of probands with IBS had an increased frequency of lifetime psychiatric disease compared with the relatives of control probands, and this was significant for major depression and generalized anxiety disorder. This suggests that psychiatric disorders associated with IBS may be familial. However, it was a relatively small study, and selection bias in the probands cannot be excluded. However, it is conceivable, based on these results, that both psychiatric disease and IBS are transmitted together, although whether this is due to heredity or environment, or both, is unclear. Svedberg *et al.* did not detect any association of anxiety or depression in their case–control twin study; hence further insights into a genetic component could not be determined by this investigation[9].

GENE POLYMORPHISMS

The physical site or location of a gene is referred to as its locus. At any gene site there can exist different forms of a gene. Single basepair substitutions represent the most common difference. These types of changes first occur by chance, but if passed on to future generations they persist. Any locus that has two or more alleles each with a frequency of at least 1% in the general population is referred to as being polymorphic[19]. Single nuclear type polymorphisms occur roughly at a rate of 1 in every 1000 basepairs. A gene is functionally polymorphic when its allelic variance exists stably in the population and this alters the activity of the encoded protein. Single nuclear type polymorphisms are important in explaining human physical diversity and are considered likely to explain chronic disease vulnerability. However, a complex disease is likely to be caused by multiple single nucleotide polymorphisms, making characterization very challenging. Gene polymorphisms have been identified in complex diseases such as obesity, asthma and hypertension, but it is likely there are multiple polymorphisms (perhaps 30–50) in complex disease that can increase or decrease disease expression. There has been much interest in evaluating polymorphisms in neuropsychiatric disease which, as discussed above, overlaps with IBS.

Both in IBS and psychiatric disease there has been increasing interest focused on serotonin release, serotonin receptors and serotonin transporters[20,21]. There is evidence that serotonin is released from enterochromaffin cells on stimulation by pressure or chemical stimulation that in turn initiates peristalsis, secretory reflexes and sensory nerve stimulation[22]. The serotonin transporter (SERT) is found in the epithelium and in enteric neurons. Work from Chen *et al.* showed in the guinea pig that SERT resulted in the epithelial re-uptake of serotonin, terminating its actions[20]. Furthermore, in the knockout mouse, targeted deletion of the gene encoding SERT led to diarrhoea occasionally alternating irregularly with constipation, suggesting that 5-HT receptor desensitization occurred in this model[21]. This animal work implies that polymorphisms of the SERT could be relevant in human diseases such as IBS. Camilleri *et al.* evaluated SERT polymorphisms in 30 patients with diarrhoea-predominant IBS[22]. They observed that the long homozygous SERT polymorphism (increasing re-uptake, hence resulting in less serotonin availability) was associated with slowing of colonic transit in response to alosetron, a $5-HT_3$ receptor antagonist, compared with heterozygous patients. However, it is unclear whether SERT polymorphisms could be related to disease pathogenesis, as the genotype distribution of the long polymorphism in this small and selected population of patients appeared to be similar to what would be expected in the general population[22]. On the other hand, the relationship between SERT polymorphisms and neuropsychiatric disease remains controversial[23–25].

There are many other potential targets for study in IBS in terms of polymorphisms. One area of recent interest has been in G-protein polymorphisms which have been linked to depression as well as altered alpha-2 adrenoreceptor function[26]. A recent report has identified an association between a beta subunit polymorphism of the G protein and functional dyspepsia, but further work is required to confirm and characterize this association[26].

Circadian abnormalities have been identified in patients with depression[27]. Subgroups of depressed patients can have documented circadian abnormalities in terms of mood, sleep, temperature and uroendocrine secretions. There are mutations in the clock genes that may accelerate or delay circadian cycles[27]. It is tempting to hypothesize that altered clock genes may be important in circadian changes. This may in turn be relevant in the serotonin system, as there is a modulatory role for serotonin in terms of changes in sensitivity of circadian rhythm to light. Furthermore, serotonin transporter promoter repeat length polymorphisms have been identified in this condition, perhaps tying this field together[27].

SEARCHING FOR THE IBS GENES

This is a very complex task, as it is no longer the case that researchers are looking for one or few rare mutations in a single gene[19]. The current focus is looking for a number of genes that are acting in concert to either increase or decrease the risk of developing a condition such as IBS. These alterations may often be not rare mutations, but common polymorphisms acting together[19].

One of the key issues in searching for a genetic component in IBS is accurately identifying the phenotype[19]. This remains the major challenge in IBS and other functional gastrointestinal disorders. As there are a wide variation of symptoms and severity, and almost certainly a heterogeneous collection of different diseases, narrowing the phenotype is crucial. The Rome criteria here are insufficient and subsetting, preferably with reliable disease markers, remains an absolute must; otherwise it is likely that the data sets would need to be so large as to be impractical, even with the most recent advances in gene chip technology, because even a few mis-assigned phenotypes can seriously undermine the analysis[19]. It is also essential that consensus diagnostic schemata are applied in any multicentre studies, confirming the need to continue to refine current criteria.

The next step is to confirm that IBS and the related functional disorders have a genetic component. While there is evidence from studies in twins, additional family studies and adoption studies, as well as studies of the population-based risk to relatives of probands, remain needed[19]. A very labour-intensive next step to follow is family ascertainment, at which time DNA samples can be collected and extracted. There are a number of different specific approaches for genotyping samples and analysing the data, such as applying genome-wide microarrays.

The next challenge is to identify the region of interest because of the commonness of false-positives[19]. This requires re-testing of genomic regions of interest using additional markers, or application of the results to a second independent data set. Once regions of interest harbouring susceptibility genes have been confirmed, the next step is fine mapping, which may require examining the region for genes known to have biological functions of interest, or performing saturation genotyping and analysing the data for linkage and allelic association. Subsequently identifying physical maps and looking at gene identification based on the strength of allelic association and tests in biological systems are required. The complexity of the situation is enhanced because it is likely that there are gene–environment interactions, which will need to be defined based on epidemiological studies of the identified genes and likely environmental factors[19].

CONCLUSIONS

It is clear that there is indirect evidence of heritability in IBS. It is hoped that further studies will lead to better identification of the different phenotypes of IBS, and in turn the contribution of genetic and common environmental factors. Adequate biological markers will need to be identified in order for IBS genes to be eventually identified with confidence. However, this is theoretically feasible, and it seems likely that, like other complex diseases, IBS will become amenable to better diagnosis and hopefully therapy with an understanding of its genetics.

References

1. Locke GR III, Zinsmeister AR, Talley NJ, Fett SL, Melton LJ III. Familial association in alpha functional gastrointestinal disorders. Mayo Clin Proc. 2000;75:907–12.
2. Oster J. Recurrent abdominal pain, headache and limb pains in children and adolescents. Pediatrics. 1972;50:429–36.
3. Kalantar JS, Locke GR III, Zinmeister AR, Beighley M, Talley NJ. Familial aggregation of irritable bowel syndrome: A prospective study. Gut. 2003 (in press).
4. Morris-Yates A, Talley NJ, Boyce P, Nandurkar S, Andrews G. Evidence of a genetic contribution to functional bowel disorder. Am J Gastroenterol. 1998;93:1311–17.
5. Levy RL, Jones KR, Whitehead WE, Feld SI, Talley NJ, Corey LA. Irritable bowel syndrome in twins: heredity and social learning both contribute to etiology. Gastroenterology. 2001;121: 799–804.
6. Mohammed J, Cherkas L, Riley SA, Spector TD, Trudgill N. Genetic influence in irritable bowel syndrome: a twin study. Gut. 2002;50:A1.
7. Lembo T, Zaman MS, Chavez NF, Crueger R, Jones MP, Talley NJ. Concordance of IBS among monozygotic and dizygotic twins. Gastroenterology. 2001;120(Suppl. 1):A66.
8. Zaman MS, Chavez NF, Krueger R, Talley NJ, Lembo T. Extra-intestinal symptoms in patients with irritable bowel syndrome (IBS). Gastroenterology. 2001;120(Suppl. 1):A636.
9. Svedberg P, Johansson S, Wallander MA, Hamelin B, Pedersen NL. Extra intestinal manifestations associated with irritable bowel syndrome: a twin study. Aliment Pharmacol Ther. 2002; 16:975–83.
10. Cameron AJ, Lagergren J, Henriksson C, Nyren O, Locke GR 3rd, Pedersen NL. Gastroesophageal reflux disease in monozygotic and dizygotic twins. Gastroenterology. 2002; 122:55–9
11. Zaman MS, Hur C, Jones MP, Krueger RF, Chavez NF, Talley NJ. Concordance of reflux among monoxygotic and dizygotic twins. Gastroenterology. 2002;120:A418.
12. Romero Y, Cameron AJ, Locke GR 3rd *et al*. Familial aggregation of gastroesophageal reflux in patients with Barrett's esophagus and esophageal adenocarcinoma. Gastroenterology. 1997;113: 1449–56.
13. Fahmy N, King JF. Barrett's esophagus: an acquired condition with genetic predisposition. Am J Gastroenterol. 1993;88:1262–5.
14. Seri M, Cusano R, Forabosco P *et al*. Genetic mapping to 10q23.3-q24.2, in a large Italian pedigree, of a new syndrome showing bilateral cataracts, gastroesophageal reflux, and spastic paraparesis with amyotrophy. Am J Hum Genet. 1999;64:586–93.
15. Hu FZ, Preston RA, Post JC *et al*. Mapping of a gene for severe pediatric gastroesophageal reflux to chromosome 13q14. J Am Med Assoc. 2000;19;325–34.
16. Talley NJ, Spiller R. Irritable bowel syndrome: a little understood organic bowel disease? Lancet. 2002;360:555–64.
17. Walker EA, Roy-Byrne PP, Katon WJ, Li L, Amos D, Jiranek G. Psychiatric illness and irritable bowel syndrome: a comparison with inflammatory bowel disease. Am J Psychiatry. 1990;147: 1656–61.
18. Woodman CL, Breen K, Noyes R Jr *et al*. The relationship between irritable bowel syndrome and psychiatric illness. A family study. Psychosomatics. 1998;39:45–54.
19. Haines JL, Pericak-Vance MA. Approaches to Gene Mapping in Complex Human Diseases. New York: John Wiley, 1998.

20. Chen JX, Pan H, Rothman TP, Wade PR, Gershon MD. Guinea pig 5-HT transporter: cloning, expression, distribution, and function in intestinal sensory reception. Am J Physiol. 1998; 275:G433–48.
21. Chen JJ, Li Z, Pan H *et al.* Maintenance of serotonin in the intestinal mucosa and ganglia of mice that lack the high-affinity serotonin transporter: Abnormal intestinal motility and the expression of cation transporters. J Neurosci. 2001;21:6348–61.
22. Camilleri M, Atanasova E, Carlson PJ *et al.* Serotonin-transporter polymorphism pharmacogenetics in diarrhea-predominant irritable bowel syndrome. Gastroenterology. 2002;123:425–32.
23. Stoltenberg SF, Burmeister M. Recent progress in psychiatric genetics – some hope but no hype. Hum Mol Genet. 2000;9:927–35.
24. Lotrich FE, Pollock BG, Ferrell RE. Polymorphism of the serotonin transporter: implications for the use of selective serotonin reuptake inhibitors. Am J Pharmacogenomics. 2001;1:153–64.
25. Lesch KP, Bengel D, Heils A *et al.* Association of anxiety-related traits with a polymorphism in the serotonin transporter gene regulatory region. Science. 1996;274:1527–31.
26. Holtmann G, Siffert W, Grote E *et al.* G-protein mediated receptor cell coupling as a predicator for the long-term response to treatment in patients with functional dyspepsia. Gastroenterology. 2003;124:A80.
27. Bunney WE, Bunney BG. Molecular clock genes in man and lower animals: possible implications for circadian abnormalities in depression. Neuropsychopharmacology. 2000;22:335–45.

29
Localization and functions of neurokinin and *N*-methyl-D-aspartate receptors

B. ADAM, T. LIEBREGTS, G. GERKEN and G. HOLTMANN

INTRODUCTION

Irritable bowel syndrome (IBS) is the most common disorder seen in gastroenterological practice[1]. The pathophysiology of IBS is a multifactorial feature. Altered bowel motility, visceral hypersensitivity, psychological factors, an imbalance in neurotransmitters and infection have been proposed as being involved in the development of IBS[2]. A subgroup of IBS patients reports abdominal pain associated with altered sensory thresholds which are lower compared to those of healthy people. Many studies have already shown that the threshold of visceral sensitivity in IBS patients is much lower than in healthy controls. Munakata *et al.* found that repetitive stimulation of sigmoid splanchnic afferents results in the development of central sensitization manifested as hyperalgesia and increased viscerosomatic referral during rectal distension in the absence of applied stimuli[3]. Whitehead *et al.* also confirmed that there is a reduced tolerance for balloon distension which is specific to the colon in IBS patients[4]. Many studies suggest an involvement of neurokinin and NMDA receptors in the modulation of visceral hypersensitivity.

NEUROKININ RECEPTORS

The group of neurokinin receptors (NK) is composed of three subtypes which are involved in the modulation of pain. Three tachykinin receptors, named NK-1, NK-2 and NK-3, have been characterized by molecular biology techniques[5,6]. Each of these binds with different affinities to tachykinin family polypeptides substance P (SP), neurokinin A (NKA) and neurokinin B (NKB)[7,8]. In the gut the most highly represented tachykinins are SP and NKA, and those act as excitatory transmitters directly or indirectly, through the activation of enteric neurons[9].

As neurotransmitters these peptides exert their biological activity via the activation of NK receptors that have been pharmacologically characterized and cloned[10]. SP binds preferentially to the NK-1 receptor, NKA to the NK-2 receptor, and NKB to the NK-3 receptor. However, each of the tachykinins is able, at higher concentrations, to activate all three receptors and therefore shows poor selectivity[11]. NK-1 receptors are highly expressed in both the central nervous system (CNS) and peripheral tissues, NK-2 receptors are characterized by a predominant expression in the periphery and NK-3 receptors are found primarily in the CNS. So these peptides and receptors are present in both the CNS and peripheral tissues and mediate a variety of biological functions, including the transmission of nociceptive information[12].

NK-1 receptor

Substance P is the primary ligand of the NK-1 receptor. In normal human colonic tissue NK-1 receptors are expressed in large quantities in vessels (arteries and veins) and in the outer layer of the circular smooth muscle. Moreover, a strong and topical expression of NK-1 receptors is seen in the mucosa-directed margin of the circular muscle. The longitudinal smooth muscle is mainly reported not to express NK-1 receptors, except in one study[13]. NK-1 receptors were detected in submucous (SMP) and myenteric neurons. At the deep muscular plexus NK-1 receptor was observed in mice and rats[14]. Mann *et al.* and Grady *et al.* reported the expression of NK-1 receptors in rat myenteric plexus neurons. These neurons had co-localization with NK-3-positive neurons[15,16]. Holzer suggests that an unbalanced function of the tachykinin system may profoundly influence the pathophysiology of acute and chronic intestinal inflammation, contributing to motor, secretory and immunological disturbances which characterize human inflammatory bowel disease[9,17].

To evaluate the influence of NK-1 receptors and substance P release many studies have shown the prevention of visceral hyperalgesia after application of selective antagonists. Both selective NK-1 receptor- and *N*-methyl-D-aspartate receptor antagonists attenuate or abolish the hypersensitivity of spinal neurons evoked by noxious stimulation. The combined administration of NK and NMDA receptors antagonists produces a significant enhanced inhibitory effect, suggesting a synergism between these two types of antagonists[18]. Rusin *et al.* described that protein kinase C (PKC) mediates the release of excitatory amino acids in the spinal horn by activation of NK-1 receptors. They reported that the PKC inhibitor stauroporine blocked the NK-induced synergism with NMDA receptors and suggested that PKC activation occurs after NK receptors were activated[19].

NK-2 receptor

NKA is released into the dorsal horn following noxious thermal, mechanical, electrical and chemical stimuli applied to skin[20,21] and intrathecal administration of NKA facilitates nociceptive reflexes[22,23]. Conversely, NK-2 receptors bind NKA with the highest affinity, and antagonists of this receptor attenuate the prolonged responses of dorsal horn neurons that occur acutely following cutaneous application of noxious chemical stimuli[24,25]. Furthermore, NKA may contribute to the increased excitability of spinal neurons that accompanies peripheral inflammation. There is both direct[20] and indirect[26] evidence that release of NKA is increased during the development of peripheral inflammation, and an antagonist of NK-2 receptors attenuates the hyperexcitability of spinal neurons that accompanies acute inflammation[27]. Since peripheral inflammation results in long-term changes in the expression of tachykinin in primary afferent neurons[28,29] as well as neurokinin receptors in the spinal cord[30], it is important to determine whether endogenous tachykinin contributes to the increase in excitability of spinal neurons that occurs several days after the induction of peripheral inflammation.

Jia *et al.* have shown that the activity of the electrically evoked nociceptive flexor reflex is increased in rats at 2–3 days after induction of peripheral inflammation with complete Freund's adjuvant (CFA)[31]. The ability of an NK-2 receptor antagonist to attenuate the activity of the visceromotor response in CFA-treated rats 2–3 days after the induction of inflammation implies that there is an increased activation of NK-2 receptors which is maintained during peripheral inflammation[31]. Blockade of NK-2 receptors also attenuates increased activity of spinal neurons that occurs acutely following stimulation of unmyelinated primary afferent neurons either chemically[24,25], electrically[32] or several hours after the induction[27].

The cellular location of the NK-2 receptor mediating the effects described in this study remains to be resolved. Although NK-2 receptor-mRNA is not detectable in adult rat spinal cord[6], NK-2 receptor binding sites have been localized in the dorsal horn of the spinal cord, and NKA modulates the firing of dorsal horn neurons evoked by peripheral stimuli[33]. Together these data suggest that NK-2 receptors may occur on terminals of neurons that are extrinsic to the spinal cord. Presynaptic NK-2 receptors have been localized immunohistochemically on neurons in the enteric nervous system[16]. However, NKA modulation of post-synaptic responses to excitatory amino acids[19,33] suggests that NK-2 receptors may also occur on spinal neurons. NK-2 receptors at synapses onto interneurons in the dorsal horn may contribute to hyperalgesia observed in animals with inflamed hind paws, as well as to increased motor reflexes.

There is evidence for the differential activation of NK-1 and NK-2 receptors which appears dependent upon the pattern and duration of nociceptor activation reported by Thompson and co-workers. Hence NK-2 receptor activation is involved in acute high thresholds afferent signalling, while the activation of the NK-1 receptor appears to require a sustained nociceptive afferent drive and appears to interact in a complex manner with activated NMDA receptors[34].

NK-3 receptor

The NK-3 receptor is predominantly expressed in the CNS. Immunohistological results showed that NK-3 receptors exist in neurons of the enteric plexus (submucous plexus and myenteric plexus) in the duodenum, jejunum, ileum and colon but not in the oesophagus or stomach of mice[35]. NK-3 receptor antagonists given intrathecally significantly reduced the responses to colorectal distensions in both normal (saline-treated) and hyperalgesic (zymosan-treated) rats, suggesting that the NK-3 receptor mediates normal responses to acute visceral pain at the level of the spinal cord[36].

Previous studies *in vitro* have shown that NK-3 receptors exist on primary afferent terminals in rat spinal cord and mediate potentiation of the depolarization-evoked substance P (SP) release. Zaratin *et al.* have investigated the role of the NK-3 receptor-mediated SP release system in a model of inflammatory pain. The data suggest that neurokinin B acting at NK-3 receptors mediates SP release within the spinal cord to play a role in inflammation. The NK-3 receptors may therefore represent appropriate targets in the therapy of inflammatory pain[37]. Using immunohistochemistry, Carpentier and Baude demonstrated that neurons of the rat dorsal vagal complex (DVC) express NK-3 receptors. The density of NK-3-immunoreactive neurons depends on the different subnuclei of the nucleus tractus solitarii. The efferent vagal neurons of the dorsal vagal nucleus highly express NK-3. No NK-3 immunoreactivity has been detected in the area postrema. Ultrastructural examination shows that NK-3 immunoreactivity is principally present at non-synaptic membranes of somatic and dendritic profiles. Therefore, neurokinin B and/or other ligands may act through a process of volume transmission on non-synaptic NK-3 receptors in the DVC[38].

In the presence of atropine (1 μM), guanethidine (3 μM) and of the tachykinin NK-1 (SR 140,333 0.1 μM) and NK-2 (GR 94,800 3 μM) receptor antagonists, the application of the tachykinin NK-3 receptor selective agonist senktide, or of neurokinin B, produced concentration-dependent sustained non-adrenergic non-cholinergic (NANC) relaxation of mucosa-free circular muscle strips from the proximal guinea-pig colon. These findings indicate that a neuronal NK-3 receptor mediates NANC hyperpolarization and relaxation of the circular muscle of the proximal guinea-pig colon, principally through the release of nitric oxide (NO). NO generation/release in response to NK-3 receptor stimulation does not require calcium influx through N-type calcium channels[39].

NK-4 receptor

Donaldson *et al.* have shown that a cloned receptor, highly homologous to the NK-3–tachykinin peptide receptor, encodes a novel functional tachykinin receptor NK-4. They also reported the expression by Northern blot analysis of a tachykinin NK-4 receptor in human skeletal muscle, lung and liver, but not in the brain[40]. Sarau *et al.* were not able to detect the NK-4 receptor sequence in the human genome by using different molecular biological techniques, although this receptor was almost identical to the known human tachykinin NK-3 receptor[41]. Page *et al.* failed to show that there are four different NK receptors[42].

N-METHYL-D-ASPARTE RECEPTORS

Gulutamate receptors play an important role in synaptic plasticity[43]. NMDA receptors belong to the ionotropic receptor group. These complexes contain integral cation-specific ion channels and do not correspond by intracellular signalling through G proteins such as metabotropic receptors and NK receptors[44].

Both NMDA receptors and NK-1 receptors are located in the rat spinal cord[5]. There is evidence that both transmitters, SP and glutamate, coexist in the dorsal root ganglion cell bodies and primary afferent neurons[45]. NMDA receptors may play a role in processing nociceptive input to the spinal dorsal horn. NMDA receptors are also present in presynaptic terminals of primary afferents in the dorsal horn where they stimulate the release of SP[46,47].

The intrathecal administration of SP and glutamate induces hyperalgesia in rats[48]. Both spinal SP and NMDA receptors are involved in the central processing of nociception[49]. Rusin *et al.* earlier suggested that there is a synergism in the interaction of SP and NMDA[19]. The implications of the findings by Ren *et al.* are a co-activation of the NMDA and NK-1 receptor systems in response to peripheral inflammation, but an independent contribution to the development of hyperalgesia[50]. There is no supra-additive effect after administration of both transmitters[48,51].

CONCLUSION

Functional bowel disorders are linked to alterations in sensory function. Many receptor systems are involved in the processing of nociceptive input. The administration of NK-1 receptor antagonists or NMDA receptor antagonists, and the co-administration, attenuate the hyperalgesia caused by local instillation of complete Freund's adjuvant. This implies that such antagonists are possible drugs for treatment of acute and chronic pain. To characterize the interaction of these two systems further studies are necessary.

References

1. Longstreth GF, Wolde-Tsadik G. Irritable bowel-type symptoms in HMO examinees: prevalence, demographics and clinical correlates. Dig Dis Sci. 1993;38:1581–9.
2. Horwitz BJ, Fisher RS. The irritable bowel syndrome. N Engl J Med. 2001;344:1846–50.
3. Munakata J, Naliboff B, Harraf F *et al.* Repetitive sigmoid stimulation induces rectal hyperalgesia in patients with irritable bowel syndrome. Gastroenterology. 1997;112:55–63.
4. Whitehead WE, Holtkotter B, Enck P *et al.* Tolerance for rectosigmoid distension in irritable bowel syndrome. Gastroenterology. 1990;98.1187–92.
5. Hershey AD, Krause JE. Molecular characterization of a functional cDNA encoding the rat substance P receptor. Science. 1990;247:958–62.
6. Shigemoto R, Yokota Y, Tsuchida K, Nakanishi S. Cloning and expression of a rat neuromedin K receptor cDNA. J Biol Chem. 1990;265:623–8.
7. Maggi CA, Patacchini R, Rovero P, Giachetti A. Tachykinin receptors and tachykinin receptor antagonists. J Auton Pharmacol. 1993;13:193–9.
8. Regoli D, Boudon A, Fauchere JL. Receptors antagonists for substance P and related peptides. Pharmacol Rev. 1994;46:551–99.
9. Holzer P, Holzer-Petsche U. Tachykinins in the gut. Part I. Expression, release and motor function. Pharmacol Ther. 1997;73:173–217.
10. Maggi CA. The mammalian tachykinin receptors. Gen Pharmacol. 1995;26:911–44.
11. Maggi CA, Schwartz TW. The dual nature of the tachykinin NK1 receptor. Trends Pharmacol Sci. 1997;18:351–5.
12. Nakanishi S. Mammalian tachykinin receptors. Annu Rev Neurosci. 1991;14:123–36.
13. Rettenbacher M, Reubi JC. Localization and characterization of neuropeptide receptors in human colon. Naunyn-Schmiedeberg's Arch Pharmacol. 2002;364:291–304.
14. Vannucchi MG, Faussone-Pellegrini MS. NK1, NK2 and NK3 tachykinin receptor localization and tachykinin distribution in the ileum of the mouse. Anat Embryol. 2000;202:247–55.
15. Mann PT, Southwell BR, Ding YQ, Shigemoto R, Mizuno N, Furness JB. Localization of neurokinin 3 (NK3) receptor immunoreactivity in the rat gastrointestinal tract. Cell Tissue Res. 1997;289:1–9.

16. Grady EF, Baluk P, Baihm S *et al*. Characterization of antisera specific to NK1-NK2, NK3 neurokinin receptors and their utilization to localize receptors in the rat gastrointestinal tract. J Neurosci. 1996;16:6975–86.
17. Holzer P. Implications of tachykinins and calcitonin gene-related peptide in inflammatory bowel disease. Digestion. 1998;59:269–83.
18. Urban L, Naeem S, Patel IA, Dray A. Tachykinin induced regulation of excitatory amino acid responses in the rat spinal cord *in vitro*. Neurosci Lett. 1994;168:185–8.
19. Rusin KI, Ryu PD, Randic M. Modulation of excitatory amino acid responses in rat dorsal horn neurons by tachykinins. J Neurophysiol. 1992;68:265–8.
20. Hope PJ, Jarrott B, Schaible HG, Clarke RW, Duggan AW. Release and spread of immunoreactive neurokinin A in the cat spinal cord in a model of acute arthritis. Brain Res. 1990;533:292–9.
21. Hua XY, Saria A, Gamse R, Theodorsson-Norheim E, Brodin E, Lundberg JM. Capsaicin induced release of multiple tachykinins (substance P, neurokinin A, and eledoisin-like material) from guinea-pig spinal cord and ureter. Neuroscience. 1986;19:313–19.
22. Cridland RA, Henry JL. Comparison of the effects of substance P, neurokinin A, physalamin, and eledoisin in facilitating a nociceptive reflex in the rat. Brain Res. 1986;381:93–9.
23. Fleetwood-Walker SM, Mitchell R, Hope PJ, El Yassir N, Molony V, Bladon CM. The involvement of neurokinin receptor subtypes in somatosensory processing in the superficial dorsal horn of the cat. Brain Res. 1990;519:169–82.
24. Dougherty PM, Palecek J, Paleckova V, Willis WD. Neurokinin 1 and 2 antagonists attenuate the responses and NK1 antagonists prevent the sensitization of primate spinothalamic tract neurons after intradermal capsaicin. J Neurophysiol. 1994;72:1464–75.
25. Munro FE, Fleetwood-Walker SM, Parker RM, Mitchell R. The effects of neurokinin receptor antagonists on mustard oil-evoked activation of rat dorsal horn neurons. Neuropeptides. 1993;25:299–305.
26. Parker RM, Fleetwood-Walker SM, Rosie R, Munro FE, Mitchell R. Inhibition by NK2 but not NK1 antagonists of carrageenan-induced preprodynorphin mRNA expression in rat dorsal horn lamina I neurons. Neuropeptides. 1993;25:213–22.
27. Neugebauer V, Rumenapp P, Schaible HG. The role of spinal neurokinin-2 receptors in the processing of nociceptive information from the joint and the generation and maintenance of inflammation-evoked hyperexcitability of dorsal horn neurons in the rat. Eur J Neurosci. 1996;8:249–60.
28. Donaldson LF, Harmar AJ, McQueen DS, Seckl JR. Increased expression of preprotachykinin, calcitonin gene-related peptide, but not vasoactive intestinal peptide messenger RNA in dorsal root ganglia during the development of adjuvant monoarthritis in the rat. Brain Res Mol Brain Res. 1992;16:143–9.
29. Minami M, Kuraishi Y, Kawamura M *et al*. Enhancement of preprotachykinin A gene expression by adjuvant-induced inflammation in the rat spinal cord: possible involvement of substance P-containing spinal neurons in nociception. Neurosci Lett. 1989;98:105–10.
30. McCarson KE, Krause JE. NK-1 and NK-3 type tachykinin receptor mRNA expression in the rat spinal cord dorsal horn is increased during adjuvant or formalin-induced nociception. J Neurosci. 1994;14:712–20.
31. Jia YP, Seybold VS. Spinal NK2 receptors contribute to the increased excitability of the nociceptive flexor reflex during persistent peripheral inflammation. Brain Res. 1997;751:169–74.
32. Xu XJ, Maggi CA, Wiesenfeld-Hallin Z. On the role of NK-2 tachykinin receptors in the mediation of spinal reflex excitability in the rat. Neuroscience. 1991;44:483–90.
33. Cumberbatch MJ, Chizh BA, Headley PM. Modulation of excitatory amino acid responses by tachykinins and selective tachykinin receptor agonists in the rat spinal cord. Br J Pharmacol. 1995;115:1005–12.
34. Thompson SW, Urban L, Dray A. Contribution of NK1 and NK2 receptor activation to high threshold afferent fibre evoked ventral root responses in the rat spinal cord *in vitro*. Brain Res. 1993;625:100–8.
35. Wang H, Zhang YQ, Ding YQ, Zhang JS. Localization of neurokinin B receptor in mouse gastrointestinal tract. World J Gastroenterol. 2002;8:172–5.
36. Kamp EH, Beck DR, Gebhart GF. Combinations of neurokinin receptor antagonists reduce visceral hyperalgesia. J Pharmacol Exp Ther. 2001;299:105–13.
37. Zaratin P, Angelici O, Clarke GD *et al*. NK3 receptor blockade prevents hyperalgesia and the associated spinal cord substance P release in monoarthritic rats. Neuropharmacology. 2000;39:141–9.

38. Carpentier C, Baude A. Immunocytochemical localisation of NK 3 receptors in the dorsal vagal complex of rat. Brain Res. 1996;734:327–31.
39. Maggi CA, Zagorodnyuk V, Giulani S. Tachykinin NK3 receptor mediates NANC hyperpolarization and relaxation via nitric oxide release in the circular muscle of the guinea-pig colon. Regul Pept. 1994;53:259–74.
40. Donaldson LF, Haskell CA, Hanley MR. Functional characterization by heterologous expression of novel cloned tachykinin peptide receptor. Biochem J. 1996;320:1–5.
41. Sarau HM, Mooney JL, Schmidt DB et al. Evidence that the proposed novel human 'neurokinin-4' receptor is pharmacologically similar to the human neurokinin-3 receptor but is not of human origin. Mol Pharmacol. 2000;58:552–9.
42. Page NM, Bell NJ. The human tachykinin NK-1 (short form) and tachykinin NK-4 receptor: a reappraisal. Eur J Pharm. 2002;437:27–30.
43. Choi DW, Rothman SM. The role of glutamate neurotoxicity in hypoxic–ischemic neuronal death. Annu Rev Neurosci. 1990;13:171–82.
44. Nakanishi S, Masu M. Molecular diversity and functions of glutamate receptors. Annu Rev Biophys Biomol Struct. 1994;23:319–48.
45. Battaglia G, Rustioni A. Coexistence of glutamate and substance P in dorsal root ganglion neurons of the rat and monkey. J Comp Neurol. 1988;277:302–12.
46. Liu H, Mantyh PW, Basbaum AI. NMDA-receptor regulation of substance P release from primary afferent nociceptors. Nature. 1997;386:721–4.
47. McRoberts JA, Coutinho SV, Marvizon JC *et al.* Role of peripheral N-methyl-D-aspartate (NMDA) receptors in visceral nociception in rats. Gastroenterology. 2001;120:1737–48.
48. Aanonsen LM, Lei S, Wilcox GL. Excitatory amino acid receptors and nociceptive neurotransmission in rat spinal cord. Pain. 1990;41:309–21.
49. Xu XJ, Dalsgaard CJ, Wiesenfeld-Hallin Z. Spinal substance P and N-methyl-D-aspartate receptors are coactivated in the induction of central sensitization of the nociceptive flexor reflex. Neuroscience. 1992;51:641–8.
50. Ren K, Iadarola MJ, Dubner R. An isobolographic analysis of the effects of N-methyl-D-aspartate and NK1 tachykinin receptor antagonists on inflammatory hyperalgesia in the rat. Br J Pharmacol. 1996;117:196–202.
51. Aanonsen LM, Wilcox GL. Nociceptive action of excitatory amino acids in the mouse: effects of spinally administered opioids, phencyclidine and sigma agonists. J Pharmacol Exp Ther. 1987;243:9–19.

30
Replacing physiological variability by genetic variability – from gene to function

W. SIFFERT

INTRODUCTION

Physiological variability is a common experience for all those actively involved in research on biological human and non-human materials, as well as in animals or human subjects. This variability is evident in experiments on freshly isolated or cultured cells but also in whole organs. Moreover, patients with seemingly identical disorders show a huge variation regarding responses to common drugs, a field covered by pharmacogenetics[1]. Finally, patients with apparently identical diseases may represent totally different disease outcomes or altered progression to defined endpoints. All these variations have earlier been referred to as 'physiological variability'. Now, as the human genome project begins to prosper, we will have to ask the question: how much of what we refer to as physiological variability is in fact genetic variability. The human genome, with its estimated 30 000–60 000 genes, harbours a huge number of nucleotide exchanges commonly referred to as single nucleotide polymorphisms (SNPs). Many of these SNPs can be found in public databases; however, their function remains to be elucidated. Some SNPs will have clearly predictable functional consequences, e.g. if they change an encoded amino acid or promoter responsiveness. SNPs in introns, on the other hand, have long been regarded as 'gene junk', although such variations can have an impact on proper mRNA processing, e.g. splicing.

In contrast to mutations, which are rare and sometimes lead to monogenic diseases, many SNPs are frequent, and if their frequencies exceed 1% in a given population they are termed 'genetic polymorphisms'. Most of these polymorphisms are not by themselves harmful. However, they can alter the function of their encoded gene product and can thereby contribute to disease susceptibility, altered drug responses or disease outcomes. SNP analysis provides us with the unique opportunity to learn, by DNA genotyping, about altered functions of biological components which by conventional biochemical methods cannot (or cannot conveniently) be analysed using routine laboratory techniques.

WHICH SNPs – WHICH TARGETS?

At first glance it appears most attractive to investigate SNPs in genes which alter the expression of proteins or SNPs in genes which alter receptor function. A good example of this latter approach are SNPs in the gene encoding the β_2-adrenoceptor[2–4]. These SNPs affect down-regulation and desensitization of the β_2-adrenoceptor and are associated with altered cardiovascular responses to drugs and with an increased risk for obesity and hypertension[5–7]. We, on the other hand, focus on SNPs in bottleneck components of intracellular signal transduction as represented by human G proteins.

FUNCTION OF G PROTEINS

G proteins are heterotrimeric proteins composed of α, β and γ subunits[8,9]. They are predominantly localized at the plasma membrane and mediate intracellular signal transduction by heptahelical receptors but also by receptors with intrinsic tyrosine kinase activity, e.g. receptors for insulin, insulin-like growth factor and platelet-derived growth factors, to name but a few. The $\beta\gamma$ dimers form a functional monomer and the composition of various $\beta\gamma$ subunit isoforms determines receptor-G-protein coupling specificity[10]. On receptor activation the α-subunit releases bound GDP in exchange for GTP with a subsequent dissociation of α and $\beta\gamma$ subunits. The α as well as the $\beta\gamma$ subunits can inhibit or activate a variety of intracellular effectors including ion channels, phospholipases, adenylyl cyclase isoforms, the PI3 kinase, the MAP kinase pathway, etc. Due to the intrinsic GTPase activity the α subunit hydrolyses bound GTP to GDP, α and $\beta\gamma$ subunits reassociate, and the complex is ready for the next activation cycle. Thus, G protein activation is the bottleneck for intracellular signal transduction. Therefore, it is sensible to assume that mutations or genetic polymorphisms which affect G protein function or expression have a strong impact on intracellular signal transduction, thereby modulating cell function, disease susceptibility, the natural course of given disorders, and drug responses. There are few examples for somatic and germ-line mutations in G protein genes in rare disorders[8].

The human G protein family consists of at least 16 different α subunits, five different β subunits, and 12 γ subunits encoded by different genes; splice variants are being mentioned here[11].

THE GNB3 C825T POLYMORPHISM – PART OF
A COMPLEX HAPLOTYPE

Following systematic sequencing of genes encoding for G protein subunits expressed in lymphoblasts and fibroblasts from patients with essential hypertension we detected a silent C825T polymorphism in exon 10 of the gene *GNB3* which encodes the β3 subunit of heterotrimeric G proteins[12]. The 825T allele was strictly associated with a truncated albeit functionally active splice variant of the Gβ3 protein generated through alternative splicing of exon 9 and was referred to as Gβ3s. Thus, in cells from homozygous 825C allele carriers only the wild-type protein or mRNA is expressed. In contrast, both homozygous and heterozygous 825T allele carriers show both the wild-type protein and the shortened splice variant. Moreover, the 825T allele was strictly associated with enhanced G protein activation. In these experiments it remained unresolved how a remote nucleotide exchange in exon 10 could affect splicing of exon 9, especially as these exons are separated by an intron of >1000 base pairs[13]. Meanwhile additional polymorphisms have been detected in the promoter[14] and in intron 9 which, surprisingly, are in almost complete linkage disequilibrium[15]. These nucleotide exchanges define a complex 'C haplotype' and 'T haplotype'. For practical reasons C825T polymorphism can be used for genotyping due to its one-to-one coupling with the other polymorphisms in *GNB3*. Alternative splicing of *GNB3* in 825T allele carriers thus seems to result from a complex, coordinate interaction of multiple polymorphisms located in intron 9 and exon 10, and modelling studies show that the respective pre-mRNA of the 'T-haplotype' differs significantly from that associated with the 'C haplotype'[15].

BIOLOGICAL FUNCTIONS OF Gβ3s

Using reverse transcription-PCR the mRNA encoding Gβ3s has been detected in all tissues examined so far. In human adipocytes, however, Gβ3s escaped detection by Western blot analysis[16]. However, in cells from 825T allele carriers the amount of wild-type Gβ3 protein was reduced, which may indicate a reduced production of this protein due to formation of Gβ3s from one or two 825T alleles. Reconstitution studies have shown that Gβ3s is operative in G protein heterotrimers consisting of Gαi2 and Gγ5-Gβ3s[12]. On overexpression of Gβ3s in COS-7 cells an enhanced chemotaxis was observed[17]. It should be noted, however, that results on the biological function of Gβ3s have so far been exclusively obtained in overexpressing systems. Although this has partially reconstituted the original phenotype originally observed in hypertensive cell lines, these experiments do not unequivocally prove that the same mechanism is operative *in vivo*. It is also conceivable that the effect of alternative splicing ultimately affects the amount of wild-type Gβ3 protein with a concomitant disturbance of the delicate interaction between α, β, and γ subunits.

ETHNIC DISTRIBUTIONS OF 825T ALLELE FREQUENCIES

After the detection of the 825T allele we studied its worldwide prevalence in various races[18]. Interestingly, 'old' ethnicities, e.g. bushmen, pygmies, Australian aborigines, black Africans, and African Americans, showed highest frequencies of the 825T allele in the range of 70–80%. East Asians, e.g. Chinese, Koreans, and Japanese, display intermediate frequencies of approximately 50–60%, whereas the lowest frequencies were found in Caucasians with ranges from 20% to 40%. In non-human primates, e.g. gorilla and orangutan, the 825T allele appears to be absent. This observation is interesting from different aspects. First, these findings show that the 825T allele represents the 'wild-type' allele in humans. Second, its distribution tracks exactly the origin and migration of modern humans out of Africa. Third, its frequency is highest in populations who are at highest risk for obesity and cardiovascular disorders such as hypertension and stroke if they give up their natural lifestyle and adopt the typical sedentary lifestyle of industrialized societies.

THE PARADIGM: GNB3 825T ALLELE AS A GENETIC MARKER FOR THE EFFICACY OF INTRACELLULAR SIGNAL TRANSDUCTION EXPLAINING PHYSIOLOGICAL VARIABILITY

Present knowledge regarding the promise of genotyping the GNB3 C825T polymorphism can be summarized as follows: genotyping predicts alternative splicing of *GNB3* in 825T allele carriers with – potentially – an allele–dose effect, i.e. alternative splicing is strongest in homozygous 825T allele carriers (TT genotype) and intermediate in heterozygous 825T allele carriers (TC genotype). A minor amount of the splice variant is seen in mRNA from cells originating from individuals with CC genotype. In most cases 825T allele carrier status is associated with enhanced signal transduction via G protein-coupled receptors. As the TT genotype is relatively rare (approximately 10%) in the Caucasian population, it is sometimes difficult to discriminate between TC and TT genotypes, and for ease of statistical analysis TC and TT genotypes are frequently combined and compared versus CC genotype.

GNB3 C825T POLYMORPHISM AND *IN-VITRO* CELL FUNCTION

Huge variability exists if cell functions from different individuals are determined *in vitro*. One typical example is cell migration or chemotaxis which is frequently determined in a classical Boyden chamber assay. It has been shown that cell migration is mainly initiated by G protein $\beta\gamma$ subunits released from the α subunit on stimulation of appropriate G protein-coupled receptors[19]. This made genetic changes in a G protein β subunit a good candidate to influence cell migration. We have determined the migration of human neutrophils on stimulation with two agonists, IL-8 and the peptide fMLP. It could be shown that neutrophils from 825T allele carriers responded more sensitively (by a factor of two) to stimulation by IL-8 and fMLP[17,20]. Thus, neutrophils from 825T allele carriers started to migrate at very low agonist concentrations (10^{-10} M fMLP) while cells from individuals with CC genotype hardly migrated at such low concentrations[20]. These findings were confirmed in human T lymphocytes. Resting as well as PHA/IL-2 preactivated CD4$^+$ T cells from 825T allele carriers displayed a two-fold enhanced migration compared to CC cells on stimulation of the CXCR4 receptor by stromal cell-derived factor 1α[21]. Moreover, peripheral blood mononuclear cells (PBMC) from 825T allele carriers proliferate more vigorously in response to recall antigens (tetanus, *Candida albicans*, HSV type 1) and to IL-2 in a classical cellular *in-vitro* proliferation assay[21]. The same findings were obtained on PBMCs from individuals who received a booster vaccination against HBV or their first basic immunization[22]. Again, T cell responses from 825T allele carriers were significantly enhanced. These findings not only underscore the fact that physiological variability as frequently seen in cell-based assays is largely determined by genetic host factors. They may also point to differential immune cell responses in 825T allele carriers versus individuals with CC genotype. How this potentially relates to the susceptibility for allergies or the pathogenesis or outcome of inflammatory bowel diseases such as Crohn's disease or ulcerative colitis, remains to be determined.

GNB3 C825T POLYMORPHISM AND *IN-VIVO* ORGAN RESPONSIVENESS

Baumgart *et al.* determined coronary vasoconstriction on bolus injection of an α_1-adrenoceptor agonist and an α_2-adrenoceptor agonist into the left coronary arteries of patients undergoing coronary angiography[23]. Both agonists induce a reduction of coronary blood flow with a huge variation ranging from 10% to almost 80%. While α_1-adrenoceptor agonist-mediated vasoconstriction was independent of *GNB3* genotypes, α_2-adrenoceptor-mediated reduction in blood flow was strictly dependent on *GNB3* genotypes. In summary, coronary vasoconstriction in 825T allele carriers was more pronounced (by a factor of two) than that in individuals with CC genotype. In accordance with these findings, 825T allele carriers showed signs of clinical myocardial ischaemia. Using different compounds these findings were confirmed by others[24].

Wenzel and co-workers determined vasoconstriction in the skin microcirculation on injection of noradrenaline, angiotensin II, and endothelin 1[25]. Again, they observed a huge variability regarding vasoconstriction in young healthy individuals. However, on genotyping for the *GNB3* polymorphism this variation disappeared to an impressive extent, and it was shown that 825T allele carriers displayed a more pronounced vasoconstriction on application of these agonists. Finally, a similar result was seen on intravenous infusion of the β-adrenoceptor blocker propanolol[26]. Carriers of an 825T allele displayed most marked reductions in cardiac stroke volume. These findings nicely underscore the notion that physiological variability in terms of variable responses to endogenous hormones is largely determined by genetic host factors.

GNB3 C825T POLYMORPHISM AND DRUG RESPONSES

Many currently available drugs block or activate G protein-coupled receptors. A general alteration in signal transduction, as associated with the *GNB3* C825T polymorphism, is therefore also expected to be associated with genotype-dependent drug responses. Patients with major depression carrying an 825T allele were shown to respond better to various antidepressants compared to patients with CC genotype[27]. In a large study on black patients and white patients with essential hypertension, individuals with an 825T allele displayed the strongest blood pressure decrease on therapy with a thiazide diuretic[28]. It is expected that *GNB3* genotypes will determine the responses to many other drugs, and related studies are in progress.

SUMMARY AND PERSPECTIVES

Available evidence supports the notion that common SNPs in G proteins contribute a major part to what we previously referred to as 'physiological variability'. It is expected that *GNB3* genotypes will make their way into clinical applications as soon as more indications have been unravelled. It is tempting to speculate that SNPs in other genes encoding G protein subunits will show similar effects.

References

1. Roden DM, George AL Jr. The genetic basis of variability in drug responses. Nat Rev Drug Discov. 2002;1:37–44.
2. Hoit BD, Suresh DP, Craft L, Walsh RA, Liggett SB. Beta$_2$-adrenergic receptor polymorphisms at amino acid 16 differentially influence agonist-stimulated blood pressure and peripheral blood flow in normal individuals. Am Heart J. 2000;139:537–42.
3. McGraw DW, Liggett SB. Coding block and 5 leader cistron polymorphisms of the beta$_2$-adrenergic receptor. Clin Exp Allergy. 1999;29(Suppl. 4)43–5.
4. Weir TD, Mallek N, Sandford AJ *et al*. Beta$_2$-adrenergic receptor haplotypes in mild, moderate and fatal/near fatal asthma. Am J Respir Crit Care Med. 1998;158:787–91.
5. Gratze G, Fortin J, Labugger R *et al*. Beta-2 adrenergic receptor variants affect resting blood pressure and agonist-induced vasodilation in young adult Caucasians. Hypertension. 1999;33:1425–30.
6. Timmermann B, Mo R, Luft FC *et al*. Beta-2 adrenoceptor genetic variation is associated with genetic predisposition to essential hypertension: the Bergen Blood Pressure Study. Kidney Int. 1998;53:1455–60.
7. Meirhaeghe A, Helbecque N, Cottel D, Amouyel P. β$_2$-Adrenoceptor gene polymorphism, body weight, and physical activity. Lancet. 1999;353:896.
8. Farfel Z, Bourne HR, Iiri T. The expanding spectrum of G protein diseases. N Engl J Med. 1999;340:1012–20.
9. Hamm HE, Gilchrist A. Heterotrimeric G proteins. Curr Opin Cell Biol. 1996;8:189–96.
10. Gautam N, Downes GB, Yan K, Kisselev O. The G-protein beta–gamma complex. Cell Signal. 1998;10:447–55.
11. Downes GB, Gautam N. The G protein subunit gene families. Genomics. 1999;62:544–52.
12. Siffert W, Rosskopf D, Siffert G *et al*. Association of a human G-protein beta$_3$ subunit variant with hypertension. Nat Genet. 1998;18:45–8.
13. Iiri T, Bourne HR. G proteins propel surprise. Nat Genet. 1998;8–10.
14. Rosskopf D, Busch S, Manthey I, Siffert W. G protein beta 3 gene: structure, promoter, and additional polymorphisms. Hypertension. 2000;36:33–41.
15. Rosskopf D, Manthey I, Siffert W. Identification and ethnic distribution of major haplotypes in the gene GNB3 encoding the G-protein beta3 subunit. Pharmacogenetics. 2002;12:209–20.
16. Ryden M, Faulds G, Hoffstedt J, Wennlund A, Arner P. Effect of the (C825T) Gbeta(3) polymorphism on adrenoceptor-mediated lipolysis in human fat cells. Diabetes. 2002;51:1601–8.
17. Virchow S, Ansorge N, Rosskopf D, Rübben H, Siffert W. The G protein beta$_3$ subunit splice variant Gbeta$_3$-s causes enhanced chemotaxis of human neutrophils in response to interleukin-8. Naunyn Schmiedeberg Arch Pharmacol. 1999;360:27–32.
18. Siffert W, Forster P, Jöckel KH *et al*. Worldwide ethnic distribution of the G protein beta3 subunit 825T allele and its association with obesity in Caucasian, Chinese, and Black African individuals. J Am Soc Nephrol. 1999;10:1921–30.

19. Neptune ER, Bourne HR. Receptors induce chemotaxis by releasing the beta-gamma subunit of Gi, not by activating Gq or Gs. Proc Natl Acad Sci USA. 1997;94:14489–94.
20. Virchow S, Ansorge N, Rübben H, Siffert G, Siffert W. Enhanced fMLP-stimulated chemotaxis in human neutrophils from individuals carrying the G protein beta3 subunit 825 T-allele. FEBS Lett. 1998;436:155–8.
21. Lindemann M, Virchow S, Ramann F *et al.* The G protein beta$_3$ subunit 825T allele is a genetic marker for enhanced T cell response. FEBS Lett. 2001;495:82–6.
22. Lindemann M, Barsegian V, Siffert W, Ferencik S, Roggendorf M, Grosse-Wilde H. Role of G protein beta$_3$ subunit C825T and HLA class II polymorphisms in the immune response after HBV vaccination. Virology. 2002;297:245–52.
23. Baumgart D, Naber C, Haude M *et al.* G protein beta$_3$ subunit 825T allele and enhanced coronary vasoconstriction on alpha(2)-adrenoceptor activation. Circ Res. 1999;85:965–9.
24. Meirhaeghe A, Bauters C, Helbecque N *et al.* The human G-protein beta3 subunit C825T polymorphism is associated with coronary artery vasoconstriction. Eur Heart J. 2001;22:845–8.
25. Wenzel RR, Siffert W, Bruck H, Philipp T, Schäfers RF. Enhanced vasoconstriction to endothelin-1, angiotensin II and noradrenaline in carriers of the GNB3 825T allele in the skin microcirculation. Pharmacogenetics. 2002;12:489–95.
26. Schäfers RF, Nürnberger J, Rutz A *et al.* Haemodynamic characterization of young normotensive men carrying the 825T-allele of the G-protein beta3 subunit. Pharmacogenetics. 2001;11:461–70.
27. Zill P, Baghai TC, Zwanzger P *et al.* Evidence for an association between a G-protein beta$_3$-gene variant with depression and response to antidepressant treatment. Neuroreport. 2000;11:1893–7.
28. Turner ST, Schwartz GL, Chapman AB, Boerwinkle E. C825T Polymorphism of the G protein beta(3)-subunit and antihypertensive response to a thiazide diuretic. Hypertension. 2001;37:739–43.

Section X
The brain, the gut and the genes

31
Gut function and dysfunction in functional gastrointestinal disorders: a personal view

E. M. M. QUIGLEY

INTRODUCTION

In recent years we have witnessed a quantum leap in our understanding of such functional gastrointestinal disorders as non-cardiac chest pain (NCCP), functional dyspepsia (FD) and irritable bowel syndrome (IBS). Contemporary advances in pathophysiology, facilitated by technological innovation, and comprehensive epidemiological approaches have taken us from an era which focused on the presence, or absence, of various motor patterns in the gut to an integrated approach to the gut–brain axis, in all of its complexity. Along the way progress has, at times, been frustrated by attempts to emphasize, depending on one's background and expertise, events at the periphery of this axis (i.e. in the gut) at the expense of central (i.e. corticospinal) phenomena, and vice-versa (Fig. 1). For some, and for those of us whose background is primarily gastrointestinal, in particular, the ever-increasing complexity of central neural circuitry has, at times, proven daunting (Fig. 2) and has, perhaps understandably, led us to retreat to the more familiar confines of the gut that we have come to know and love. The goal of this review will be to evaluate, from the perspective of a 'peripheralist', the current status of dysfunction, at the level of the enteric neuromuscular apparatus, in the pathophysiology and presentation of those functional disorders which continue to represent a formidable challenge in clinical practice.

MOTILITY AND FUNCTIONAL GASTROINTESTINAL DISORDERS (FGID); MOVING TO NEW PARADIGMS

For many years studies in FGID focused on motor events as recorded in the constituent organs of the gut[1,2]. Thus, diffuse spasm and the 'nutcracker' oesophagus were described among patients with NCCP, gastroparesis in those with FD and a variety of small intestinal and colonic motor events documented in IBS.

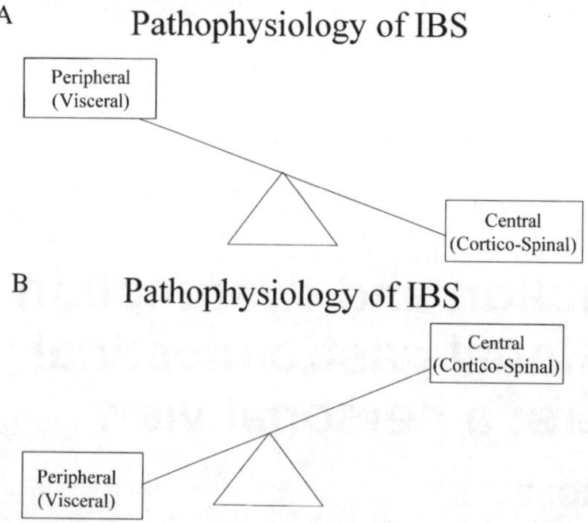

Fig. 1 Approaches to the pathophysiology of IBS; competing research strategies have alternately emphasized the central importance of peripheral, or visceral (**A**), and central, or corticospinal (**B**), events

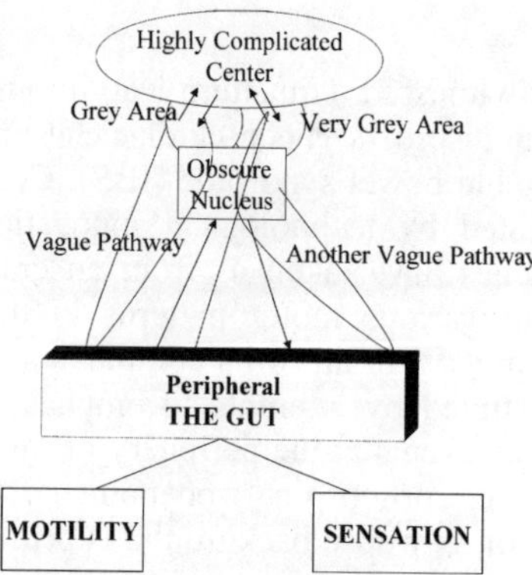

Fig. 2 The brain–gut axis in FGID; perceptions of a befuddled gastroenterologist!

These studies employed either techniques to measure whole-organ transit or intraluminal manometry. Over time some of these findings, such as myolectrical abnormalities in the sigmoid colon, have not been consistently reproduced and others, such as delayed gastric emptying or abnormal intestinal or colonic transit, have proven to be non-specific. Several of these observed abnormalities, such as gastroparesis or 'clustered' contractions, do not correlate well with symptoms and have therefore proven to be an unreliable target for therapeutic intervention. This is not to dismiss motility in FGID; rather, more recent studies, facilitated by technological advances, have identified more subtle abnormalities in motor function which appear to bear a close relationship with selected symptoms.

In the oesophagus, for example, intraluminal ultrasound probes have led to the identification of contractions of the longitudinal muscle which appear to relate to unexplained chest pain[3]. Transabdominal ultrasound, magnetic resonance imaging, impedance systems and the barostat have revolutionized our understanding of gastric motor physiology and have provided valuable clues to pathophysiology[4]. The stomach is now viewed as a complex organ comprising functionally distinct segments which collaborate to ensure the efficient and appropriate delivery of the meal to the intestine. Accommodation of the incoming meal is a primary role of the fundus; this function is impaired in approximately 40% of patients with FD and is associated with the symptoms of early satiety, postprandial fullness and weight loss[5]. This phenomenon has attracted considerable interest; initial studies have shown that this abnormality may be reversed, in patients with chronic dyspepsia, by serotonin $5\text{-}HT_1$ agonists, such as sumatriptan and buspirone[6]. Interestingly, impaired accommodation is even more prevalent among those with FD whose symptoms were of acute onset, a situation in which an infectious aetiology is often suspected, though rarely proven[7]. Based on a re-evaluation, with current technology, of the role of various factors in FD a new approach to subgrouping has been proposed and is summarized in Table 1[8]. Whether this approach, more firmly rooted in a 'peripheral' approach to pathophysiology, will prove more helpful in guiding evaluation and therapy than former efforts is unknown at this time and awaits prospective trials.

Innovative approaches have also led to progress in IBS. Especially intriguing has been the work on intestinal gas transit by the Barcelona group. 'Gas-related' symptoms are common in IBS, result in appreciable distress and are notoriously resistant to therapy[9]. While the balance of evidence suggests that gas production is not actually increased in IBS, in general, there is now a sufficient body of data to suggest that gas transit through the intestine is impaired in IBS. Normal individuals rapidly transit gas through the small intestine; delayed transit, whether spontaneous or iatrogenic, results in bloating and distension[10]. In IBS gas transit is delayed, and this delay correlates with usual symptoms and with measurable abdominal distension[11]. Furthermore, acceleration of this retarded transit, by a prokinetic agent such as neostigmine, will alleviate symptoms and reduce distension[12]. These findings have led these researchers to hypothesize that impaired gas transit may reflect a selective motor dysfunction and IBS. This work also illustrates the importance of focusing on 'real' motor events, such as transit of a component of normal intestinal contents, rather than on contractile events whose relationship with function is unclear.

Table 1   A new subgrouping of dyspepsia

Subgroup	Symptom(s)	Prevalence (%)
Acid-related	Heartburn, acid regurgitation	38
Delayed gastric emptying	Nausea, vomiting	13
Impaired fundic accommodation	Early satiety, postprandial fullness	40
Visceral hypersensitivity	Pain, discomfort	7

Based on data from ref. 8.

These, and other recent studies, by their attention to motor phenomena that have direct functional consequences and that bear directly on symptom development, have reinvigorated the motility approach to FGID. While motor dysfunction may not be, in truth, the fundamental issue in IBS, the observations on regional gastric function and intestinal gas transit illustrate the continuing potential for motor events to serve as a valid therapeutic target.

VISCERAL HYPERSENSITIVITY; SENSATION, PERCEPTION AND IBS

The development and validation of techniques for the assessment of visceral sensation and its central perception, in humans, have opened up a completely new area of research in FGID. Visceral hypersensitivity and hyperalgesia are ubiquitous in FGID, balloon distension and other intraluminal stimuli leading to symptoms and pain at lower levels on stimulation of the oesophagus, stomach, small intestine, colon and rectum in NCCP, FD and IBS, respectively[13]. This has led some to propose rectal hypersensitivity as a diagnostic test for IBS; the development of pain on distension at balloon pressures below 40 mmHg being 95.5% sensitive and 71.8% specific for IBS, in one study[14]. This hypersensitivity also appears to differentiate IBS from functional abdominal pain[15]. Using highly sophisticated methodologies such as functional magnetic resonance imaging (fMRI) and positron emission tomography (PET), pioneering studies have advanced our understanding of the central appreciation of visceral events in humans, and have indicated deviations between how the brain perceives 'normal' and 'abnormal' visceral events in FGID[16]. Whether this reflects abnormal transmission to, or processing within, the brain remains to be established. Such findings also raise the possibility, supported by evidence of dysfunction in the hypothalamic–pituitary axis (HPA)[17], of a primary central nervous system (CNS) abnormality in FGID which, in turn, drives the motor and sensory dysfunctions recorded at the periphery. Where do the influences of stress and psychopathology fit in? Could the aforementioned perceptual abnormalities thus reflect an aberrant response to environmental stimuli? These intriguing questions await answers.

INFECTION, INFLAMMATION AND FGID; THE MISSING LINK?

Evidence accumulates to suggest a role for inflammation in IBS and other functional gastrointestinal disorders. The role of inflammation in the pathogenesis of motor dysfunction has been amply defined in a variety of animal models, and is exemplified in humans by the myriad of motor syndromes associated with infection with *Trypanosoma cruzei*, Chagas' disease[18]. Inflammation has also been shown, in experimental models, to promote visceral hypersensitivity and hyperalgesia and to modify the transmission of peripheral sensory events to and through the CNS[19]. Furthermore, a variety of inflammatory gastrointestinal disorders have been associated with motor dysfunction and some, including coeliac disease[20] and inflammatory bowel disease[21], have been directly linked with IBS.

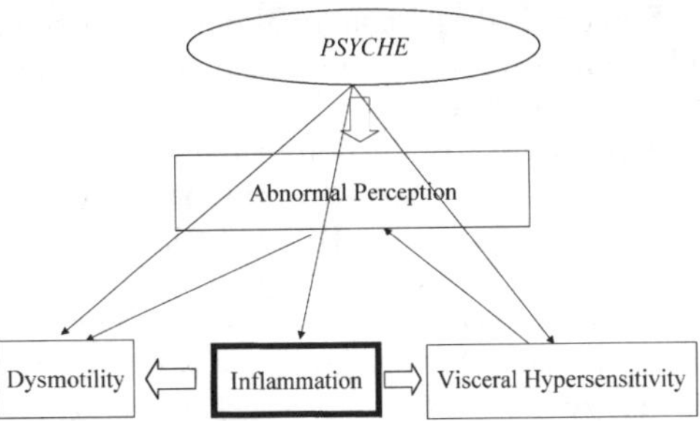

Fig. 3 The central role of inflammation in IBS. This schema hypothesizes a central role for mucosal inflammation in IBS. Note the potential for inflammation to disrupt motility, potentiate visceral sensation and modulate the transmission of peripheral sensory events to the central nervous system. Note also the ability of the psyche, representing the interaction between the individual and the environment, to modify these events at all levels; thus establishing a direct interaction between the periphery, the centre and the external environment

Clinicians have for some time recognized a subgroup of patients with FGID whose disorder is of acute onset, and apparently triggered by an infectious illness. This association has already been referred to in relation to some patients with dyspepsia; others have documented the development of gastroparesis following a presumed acute viral illness[22]. However, it is the link between IBS and prior gastroenteritis that has generated the greatest interest. Several prospective and retrospective studies have now confirmed what clinicians have recognized for decades; some individuals go on to develop chronic gastrointestinal symptoms which satisfy criteria for IBS following a single episode of bacteriologically confirmed gastroenteritis[23–26]. In one such study, Gwee and colleagues described the new onset of IBS in 23% of 94 individuals who had an episode of bacterial gastroenteritis[26]. Factors predictive of post-infectious IBS included being female, possessing certain pre-morbid psychological traits and revealing persistence of a chronic inflammatory infiltrate in the rectal mucosa 3 months following the initial infectious insult. The latter finding established a direct link between inflammation, generated in response to the infection, and bowel dysfunction and symptoms. This link has been further supported by others who have documented mucosal inflammation in IBS, regardless of the mode of onset of their illness or of its linkage to an acute infection. Most recent and striking was the report of Chadwick and colleagues, who found evidence of inflammatory cell activation, of some degree, in all the patients with IBS that they studied[27]. Clearly such dramatic findings deserve replication, but have placed inflammation at the centre of the FGID debate, and it seems not unreasonable to propose, pending further studies, a unifying hypothesis for the pathogenesis of IBS, and perhaps all FGID, centred on inflammation (Fig. 3).

CONCLUSIONS

All the FGIDs are associated with reproducible abnormalities in both motility and sensation which have been identified by recent and more detailed studies of these parameters. Some of these abnormalities are associated with certain symptoms and could well prove targets for new therapeutic interventions. Of late, the focus in research has moved from descriptive studies detailing peripheral events to a more comprehensive evaluation of the interplay between the periphery, the gut, and the centre, the CNS – the gut–brain axis. Abnormalities have been described at all levels of this axis in IBS and other FGIDs; which are primary and which are secondary remains to be clarified. While the search for primary triggers continues, recent evidence has presented a strong case for inflammation as a basic common factor in some instances. What is important is that we continue to sustain and emphasize this holistic approach to these common symptoms; recent history tells us that an isolationist approach will prove fruitless.

References

1. McKee DP, Quigley EMM. Intestinal motility and the irritable bowel syndrome – is IBS a motility disorder? Part 1. Definition of IBS and colonic motility. Dig Dis Sci. 1993;38:1761–72.
2. McKee DP, Quigley EMM. Intestinal motility and the irritable bowel syndrome – is IBS a motility disorder? Part 2. Motility of the small bowel, esophagus, stomach and gall bladder. Dig Dis Sci. 1993;38:1773–82.
3. Balaban DH, Yamamoto Y, Liu J et al. Sustained esophageal contraction: a marker of esophageal chest pain identified by intraluminal ultrasonography. Gastroenterology. 1999;116:29–37.
4. Quigley EMM. Gastric motor and sensory function and motor disorders of the stomach. In: Feldman F, Friedman LS, Sleisenger MH, editors. Gastrointestinal and Liver Disease. Pathophysiology/Diagnosis/Management, 7th edn. Philadelphia: WB Saunders, 2002:691–714.
5. Tack J, Piessevuax H, Coulie B, Caenepeel P, Janssens J. Role of impaired gastric accommodation to a meal in functional dyspepsia. Gastroenterology. 1998;115:1346–52.
6. Tack J, Demedts I, Dehondt G et al. Clinical and pathophysiological characteristics of acute-onset functional dyspepsia. Gastroenterology. 2002;122:1738–47.
7. Tack J, Coulie B, Wilmer A, Andrioli A, Janssens J. Influence of sumatriptan on gastric fundus tone and on the perception of gastric distension in man. Gut. 2000;46:468–73.
8. Coulie B, Camilleri M, Revecki D, Dubois D. Symptoms suggestive of pathophysiological disturbances provide a basis for novel classification of functional upper gastrointestinal disorders. Gastroenterology. 2002;122:A571.
9. Quigley EMM. Aerophagia and intestinal gas. Curr Treat Options Gastroenterol. 2002;5:259–65.
10. Serra J, Azpiroz F, Malagelada J-R. Intestinal gas dynamics and tolerance in humans. Gastroenterology. 1998;115:542–50.
11. Serra J, Azpiroz F, Malagelada J-R. Impaired transit and tolerance of intestinal gas in the irritable bowel syndrome. Gut. 2001;48:14–19.
12. Caldarella MP, Serra J, Azpiroz F, Malagelada JR. Prokinetic effects in patients with intestinal gas retention. Gastroenterology. 2002;122:1748–55.
13. Camilleri M. Testing the sensitivity hypothesis in practice: tools and methods, assumptions and pitfalls. Gut. 2002;51(Suppl. 1):i34–40.
14. Bouin M, Plourde V, Boivin M et al. Rectal distention testing in patients with irritable bowel syndrome: sensitivity, specificity, and predictive values of pain sensory thresholds. Gastroenterology. 2002;122:1771–7.
15. Van Ginkel R, Voskuijl WP, Benninga MA, Taminiau JAJM, Boeckxstaens GE. Alterations in rectal sensitivity and motility in childhood irritable bowel syndrome. Gastroenterology. 2001;120:31–8.
16. Aziz Q, Thompson DG. Clinical relevance of the gut–brain axis. Gastroenterology. 1997;114:559–78.
17. Dinan TG, Scott LV, Brady D, McNamara D, Keeling PW. Altered hypothalamic cholinergic responses in patients with nonulcer dyspepsia: a study of pyridostigmine-stimulated growth hormone release. Am J Gastroenterol. 2002;97:1937–40.
18. de Oliveira RB, Troncon LE, Dantas RO, Menghelli UG. Gastrointestinal manifestations of Chagas' disease. Am J Gastroenterol. 1998;93:884–9.

19. Mayer EA, Collins SM. Evolving pathophysiologic models of functional gastrointestinal disorders. Gastroenterology. 2002;122:2032–48.
20. O'Leary C, Wieneke P, Buckley S *et al.* Celiac disease and irritable bowel-type symptoms. Am J Gastroenterol. 2002;97:1463–7.
21. Simrén M, Axelsson J, Gillberg R *et al.* Quality of life in inflammatory bowel disease in remission: the impact of IBS-like symptoms and associated psychological factors. Am J Gastroenterol. 2002;97:389–96.
22. Oh JJ, Kim CH. Gastroparesis after a presumed viral illness: clinical and laboratory features and natural history. Mayo Clin Proc. 1990;65:636–42.
23. McKendrick MW, Read MW. Irritable bowel syndrome – post-*Salmonella* infection. J Infect. 1994;29:1–3.
24. Neal KR, Hebdon J, Spiller R. Prevalence of gastrointestinal symptoms six months after bacterial gastroenteritis and risk factors for development of the irritable bowel syndrome. Br Med J. 1997;314:779–82.
25. Garcia Rodriguez LA, Ruigomez A. Increased risk of irritable bowel syndrome after bacterial gastroenteritis: cohort study. Br Med J. 1999;318:565–6.
26. Gwee K-A, Leong Y-L, Graham C *et al.* The role of psychological and biological factors in post-infective gut dysfunction. Gut. 1999;44:400–6.
27. Chadwick VS, Chen W, Shu D *et al.* Activation of the mucosal immune system in irritable bowel syndrome. Gastroenterology. 2002;122:1778–83.

Index

bismuth   67
bladder
  afferent innervation   26
  dysfunction   247
  irritation   26
bladder–bowel–sphincteric interaction   26
bladder-to-colon cross-sensitization
      19, 21–3
BOND study   200
bowel habits, alterations   110(table),
      111(fig.), 112
bradykinin   121, 124, 157
bradykinin-induced mechanical hyperalgesic
      behaviour   80, 84–90
brain stem   79, 81(fig.)
breath test   177
buspirone   271

C3H-HeJBir mice   38
C-fibre afferent innervation   27
C-reactive protein   54
Campylobacter   224
Campylobacter jejuni   235
  enteritis   57
  post-infective-IBS   232–3
capsaicin   85, 112, 124, 207–8
capscizepine   160
CD4CD25+ T cells   35
central nervous system   111–12
central stress response system   14
  see also stress
Chagas' disease   272
chemoreceptors   151
cholecystokinin   83, 233
cholera toxin   240
cholestyramine   235
chromosome-10   248
chromosome-13   248
chronic fatigue syndrome   12(table), 14
chronic gut inflammation   113–14
chronic idiopathic intestinal
      pseudo-obstruction   177
cinchophen   129
cingulate cortex   59(fig.), 60
cisapride   67
clarithromycin   199
  resistance   199
Clostridium difficile pseudomembranous
      colitis   236
co-morbid conditions   12–13
"co-sensitization"   18
coeliac disease   116(fig.)
coeliac sprue   117

coeliac vagal branches   93
collagenous colitis   117
colon, afferent innervation   26
colon-to-bladder cross-sensitization   19, 21–3
colonic motility, postprandial   105
colonic sensory pathways   120
colonic spinal primary afferents (study)   120–5
  chemosensitivity   123–4
  mechanosensitivity   123
colorectal balloon distention   124
colorectal cancer   7
colorectal motility disorders   136–45
constipation   111(fig.)
  chronic   112–13
  "sensory form"   117
  slow-transit   136
      patients with   136–7, 140, 143–4
corticopontine circuitry   115–16
corticosteroids   107, 164, 226
Crohn's disease   117
  gender distribution   5
  genetic components   7
  incidence   5
  prevalence   6
cromolyn sodium   164
cryptins   229
cytokines
  proinflammatory, vagal afferent pathway,
      effect on   131
  secretion profile   40–1
  vagal afferent sensitivity   127(fig.)

defensins   229
depression   6, 13–14
  circadian abnormalities   250
derealization   29
diarrhoea   111(fig.)
  chronic   117
  irritable bowel syndrome vs. inflammatory
      bowel disease   7
discrete clustered contractions   181(table)
dissociation   29–32
  abuse history   31(fig.)
  health care behaviour   32(fig.)
  health care utilization, excessive   32
  lower abdominal pain   31(fig.)
  sexual trauma   32
Dissociative Experiences Scale/subscales
      (DES)   30
dissociative mental disturbances, visceral
      hyperalgesia   29–32
distal colonic overdistention   26
DNQX   215

Falk Symposium Series

82B. Paumgartner G, Beuers U, eds.: *Bile Acids in Liver Diseases.* International Falk Workshop. 1995 ISBN 0-7923-8891-7

83. Dobrilla G, Felder M, de Pretis G, eds.: *Advances in Hepatobiliary and Pancreatic Diseases: Special Clinical Topics.* Falk Symposium 83. 1995. ISBN 0-7923-8892-5

84. Fromm H, Leuschner U, eds.: *Bile Acids – Cholestasis – Gallstones: Advances in Basic and Clinical Bile Acid Research.* Falk Symposium 84. 1995 ISBN 0-7923-8893-3

85. Tytgat GNJ, Bartelsman JFWM, van Deventer SJH, eds.: *Inflammatory Bowel Diseases.* Falk Symposium 85. 1995 ISBN 0-7923-8894-1

86. Berg PA, Leuschner U, eds.: *Bile Acids and Immunology.* Falk Symposium 86. 1996 ISBN 0-7923-8700-7

87. Schmid R, Bianchi L, Blum HE, Gerok W, Maier KP, Stalder GA, eds.: *Acute and Chronic Liver Diseases: Molecular Biology and Clinics.* Falk Symposium 87. 1996 ISBN 0-7923-8701-5

88. Blum HE, Wu GY, Wu CH, eds.: *Molecular Diagnosis and Gene Therapy.* Falk Symposium 88. 1996 ISBN 0-7923-8702-3

88B. Poupon RE, Reichen J, eds.: *Surrogate Markers to Assess Efficacy of TReatment in Chronic Liver Diseases.* International Falk Workshop. 1996 ISBN 0-7923-8705-8

89. Reyes HB, Leuschner U, Arias IM, eds.: *Pregnancy, Sex Hormones and the Liver.* Falk Symposium 89. 1996 ISBN 0-7923-8704-X

89B. Broelsch CE, Burdelski M, Rogiers X, eds.: *Cholestatic Liver Diseases in Children and Adults.* International Falk Workshop. 1996 ISBN 0-7923-8710-4

90. Lam S-K, Paumgartner P, Wang B, eds.: *Update on Hepatobiliary Diseases 1996.* Falk Symposium 90. 1996 ISBN 0-7923-8715-5

91. Hadziselimovic F, Herzog B, eds.: *Inflammatory Bowel Diseases and Chronic Recurrent Abdominal Pain.* Falk Symposium 91. 1996 ISBN 0-7923-8722-8

91B. Alvaro D, Benedetti A, Strazzabosco M, eds.: *Vanishing Bile Duct Syndrome – Pathophysiology and Treatment.* International Falk Workshop. 1996 ISBN 0-7923-8721-X

92. Gerok W, Loginov AS, Pokrowskij VI, eds.: *New Trends in Hepatology 1996.* Falk Symposium 92. 1997 ISBN 0-7923-8723-6

93. Paumgartner G, Stiehl A, Gerok W, eds.: *Bile Acids in Hepatobiliary Diseases – Basic Research and Clinical Application.* Falk Symposium 93. 1997 ISBN 0-7923-8725-2

94. Halter F, Winton D, Wright NA, eds.: *The Gut as a Model in Cell and Molecular Biology.* Falk Symposium 94. 1997 ISBN 0-7923-8726-0

94B. Kruse-Jarres JD, Schölmerich J, eds.: *Zinc and Diseases of the Digestive Tract.* International Falk Workshop. 1997 ISBN 0-7923-8724-4

95. Ewe K, Eckardt VF, Enck P, eds.: *Constipation and Anorectal Insufficiency.* Falk Symposium 95. 1997 ISBN 0-7923-8727-9

96. Andus T, Goebell H, Layer P, Schölmerich J, eds.: *Inflammatory Bowel Disease – from Bench to Bedside.* Falk Symposium 96. 1997 ISBN 0-7923-8728-7

97. Campieri M, Bianchi-Porro G, Fiocchi C, Schölmerich J, eds. *Clinical Challenges in Inflammatory Bowel Diseases: Diagnosis, Prognosis and Treatment.* Falk Symposium 97. 1998 ISBN 0-7923-8733-3

98. Lembcke B, Kruis W, Sartor RB, eds. *Systemic Manifestations of IBD: The Pending Challenge for Subtle Diagnosis and Treatment.* Falk Symposium 98. 1998 ISBN 0-7923-8734-1

Falk Symposium Series

99. Goebell H, Holtmann G, Talley NJ, eds. *Functional Dyspepsia and Irritable Bowel Syndrome: Concepts and Controversies.* Falk Symposium 99. 1998
ISBN 0-7923-8735-X

100. Blum HE, Bode Ch, Bode JCh, Sartor RB, eds. *Gut and the Liver.* Falk Symposium 100. 1998
ISBN 0-7923-8736-8

101. Rachmilewitz D, ed. *V International Symposium on Inflammatory Bowel Diseases.* Falk Symposium 101. 1998
ISBN 0-7923-8743-0

102. Manns MP, Boyer JL, Jansen PLM, Reichen J, eds. *Cholestatic Liver Diseases.* Falk Symposium 102. 1998
ISBN 0-7923-8746-5

102B. Manns MP, Chapman RW, Stiehl A, Wiesner R, eds. *Primary Sclerosing Cholangitis.* International Falk Workshop. 1998.
ISBN 0-7923-8745-7

103. Häussinger D, Jungermann K, eds. *Liver and Nervous System.* Falk Symposium 102. 1998
ISBN 0-7924-8742-2

103B. Häussinger D, Heinrich PC, eds. *Signalling in the Liver.* International Falk Workshop. 1998
ISBN 0-7923-8744-9

103C. Fleig W, ed. *Normal and Malignant Liver Cell Growth.* International Falk Workshop. 1998
ISBN 0-7923-8748-1

104. Stallmach A, Zeitz M, Strober W, MacDonald TT, Lochs H, eds. *Induction and Modulation of Gastrointestinal Inflammation.* Falk Symposium 104. 1998
ISBN 0-7923-8747-3

105. Emmrich J, Liebe S, Stange EF, eds. *Innovative Concepts in Inflammatory Bowel Diseases.* Falk Symposium 105. 1999
ISBN 0-7923-8749-X

106. Rutgeerts P, Colombel J-F, Hanauer SB, Schölmerich J, Tytgat GNJ, van Gossum A, eds. *Advances in Inflammatory Bowel Diseases.* Falk Symposium 106. 1999
ISBN 0-7923-8750-3

107. Špičák J, Boyer J, Gilat T, Kotrlik K, Mareček Z, Paumgartner G, eds. *Diseases of the Liver and the Bile Ducts – New Aspects and Clinical Implications.* Falk Symposium 107. 1999
ISBN 0-7923-8751-1

108. Paumgartner G, Stiehl A, Gerok W, Keppler D, Leuschner U, eds. *Bile Acids and Cholestasis.* Falk Symposium 108. 1999
ISBN 0-7923-8752-X

109. Schmiegel W, Schölmerich J, eds. *Colorectal Cancer – Molecular Mechanisms, Premalignant State and its Prevention.* Falk Symposium 109. 1999
ISBN 0-7923-8753-8

110. Domschke W, Stoll R, Brasitus TA, Kagnoff MF, eds. *Intestinal Mucosa and its Diseases – Pathophysiology and Clinics.* Falk Symposium 110. 1999
ISBN 0-7923-8754-6

110B. Northfield TC, Ahmed HA, Jazwari RP, Zentler-Munro PL, eds. *Bile Acids in Hepatobiliary Disease.* Falk Workshop. 2000
ISBN 0-7923-8755-4

111. Rogler G, Kullmann F, Rutgeerts P, Sartor RB, Schölmerich J, eds. *IBD at the End of its First Century.* Falk Symposium 111. 2000
ISBN 0-7923-8756-2

112. Krammer HJ, Singer MV, eds. *Neurogastroenterology: From the Basics to the Clinics.* Falk Symposium 112. 2000
ISBN 0-7923-8757-0

113. Andus T, Rogler G, Schlottmann K, Frick E, Adler G, Schmiegel W, Zeitz M, Schölmerich J, eds. *Cytokines and Cell Homeostasis in the Gastrointestinal Tract.* Falk Symposium 113. 2000
ISBN 0-7923-8758-9

114. Manns MP, Paumgartner G, Leuschner U, eds. *Immunology and Liver.* Falk Symposium 114. 2000
ISBN 0-7923-8759-7

115. Boyer JL, Blum HE, Maier K-P, Sauerbruch T, Stalder GA, eds. *Liver Cirrhosis and its Development*. Falk Symposium 115. 2000   ISBN 0-7923-8760-0

116. Riemann JF, Neuhaus H, eds. *Interventional Endoscopy in Hepatology*. Falk Symposium 116. 2000   ISBN 0-7923-8761-9

116A. Dienes HP, Schirmacher P, Brechot C, Okuda K, eds. *Chronic Hepatitis: New Concepts of Pathogenesis, Diagnosis and Treatment*. Falk Workshop. 2000
ISBN 0-7923-8763-5

117. Gerbes AL, Beuers U, Jüngst D, Pape GR, Sackmann M, Sauerbruch T, eds. *Hepatology 2000 – Symposium in Honour of Gustav Paumgartner*. Falk Symposium 117. 2000
ISBN 0-7923-8765-1

117A. Acalovschi M, Paumgartner G, eds. *Hepatobiliary Diseases: Cholestasis and Gallstones*. Falk Workshop. 2000   ISBN 0-7923-8770-8

118. Frühmorgen P, Bruch H-P, eds. *Non-Neoplastic Diseases of the Anorectum*. Falk Symposium 118. 2001   ISBN 0-7923-8766-X

119. Fellermann K, Jewell DP, Sandborn WJ, Schölmerich J, Stange EF, eds. *Immuno-suppression in Inflammatory Bowel Diseases – Standards, New Developments, Future Trends*. Falk Symposium 119. 2001   ISBN 0-7923-8767-8

120. van Berge Henegouwen GP, Keppler D, Leuschner U, Paumgartner G, Stiehl A, eds. *Biology of Bile Acids in Health and Disease*. Falk Symposium 120. 2001
ISBN 0-7923-8768-6

121. Leuschner U, James OFW, Dancygier H, eds. *Steatohepatitis (NASH and ASH)*. Falk Symposium 121. 2001   ISBN 0-7923-8769-4

121A. Matern S, Boyer JL, Keppler D, Meier-Abt PJ, eds. *Hepatobiliary Transport: From Bench to Bedside*. Falk Workshop. 2001   ISBN 0-7923-8771-6

122. Campieri M, Fiocchi C, Hanauer SB, Jewell DP, Rachmilewitz R, Schölmerich J, eds. *Inflammatory Bowel Disease – A Clinical Case Approach to Pathophysiology, Diagnosis, and Treatment*. Falk Symposium 122. 2002   ISBN 0-7923-8772-4

123. Rachmilewitz D, Modigliani R, Podolsky DK, Sachar DB, Tozun N, eds. *VI International Symposium on Inflammatory Bowel Diseases*. Falk Symposium 123. 2002
ISBN 0-7923-8773-2

124. Hagenmüller F, Manns MP, Musmann H-G, Riemann JF, eds. *Medical Imaging in Gastroenterology and Hepatology*. Falk Symposium 124. 2002   ISBN 0-7923-8774-0

125. Gressner AM, Heinrich PC, Matern S, eds. *Cytokines in Liver Injury and Repair*. Falk Symposium 125. 2002   ISBN 0-7923-8775-9

126. Gupta S, Jansen PLM, Klempnauer J, Manns MP, eds. *Hepatocyte Transplantation*. Falk Symposium 126. 2002   ISBN 0-7923-8776-7

127. Hadziselimovic F, ed. *Autoimmune Diseases in Paediatric Gastroenterology*. Falk Symposium 127. 2002   ISBN 0-7923-8778-3

127A. Berr F, Bruix J, Hauss J, Wands J, Wittekind Ch, eds. *Malignant Liver Tumours: Basic Concepts and Clinical Management*. Falk Workshop. 2002   ISBN 0-7923-8779-1

128. Scheppach W, Scheurlen M, eds. *Exogenous Factors in Colonic Carcinogenesis*. Falk Symposium 128. 2002   ISBN 0-7923-8780-5

129. Paumgartner G, Keppler D, Leuschner U, Stiehl A, eds. *Bile Acids: From Genomics to Disease and Therapy*. Falk Symposium 129. 2002   ISBN 0-7923-8781-3

129A. Leuschner U, Berg PA, Holtmeier J, eds. *Bile Acids and Pregnancy*. Falk Workshop. 2002   ISBN 0-7923-8782-1

Falk Symposium Series

130. Holtmann G, Talley NJ, eds. *Gastrointestinal Inflammation and Disturbed Gut Function: The Challenge of New Concepts.* Falk Symposium 130. 2003
ISBN 0-7923-8783-X

131. Herfarth H, Feagan BJ, Folsch UR, Schölmerich J, Vatn MH, Zeitz M, eds. *Targets of Treatment in Chronic Inflammatory Bowel Diseases.* Falk Symposium 131. 2003
ISBN 0-7923-8784-8

132. Galle PR, Gerken G, Schmidt WE, Wiedenmann B, eds. *Disease Progression and Carcinogenesis in the Gastrointestinal Tract.* Falk Symposium 132. 2003
ISBN 0-7923-8785-6